Obstetric *and* Gynecologic Emergencies

Obstetric *and* Gynecologic Emergencies

Edited by

Guy I. Benrubi, M.D.

Professor
Division of Gynecologic Oncology
Department of Obstetrics and Gynecology
University of Florida Health Science Center
Jacksonville, Florida

with 31 contributors

J. B. Lippincott Company   *Philadelphia*

Acquisitions Editor: Lisa McAllister
Assistant Editor: Emilie Moyer
Project Editor: Bridget C. Hannon
Indexer: Sandi Schroeder
Design Coordinator: Kathy Kelley-Luedtke
Interior Designer: Holly Reid McLaughlin
Cover Designer: Tom Jackson
Production Manager: Caren Erlichman
Production Coordinator: David Murphy
Compositor: Pine Tree Composition, Inc.
Printer/Binder: Arcata Graphics/Kingsport
Pre-Press: Jay's Publishers Service
Illustrator: Jennifer S. Smith

Copyright © 1994, by J. B. Lippincott Company. All rights reserved. No part of this book may be used or reproduced in any manner whatsoever without written permission except for brief quotations embodied in critical articles and reviews. Printed in the United States of America. For information write J. B. Lippincott Company, 227 East Washington Square, Philadelphia, Pennsylvania 19106.

6 5 4 3 2

Library of Congress Cataloging-in-Publication Data

Obstetric and gynecologic emergencies / editor, Guy I. Benrubi ; with
   31 contributors
       p.   cm.
   Includes bibliographical references and index.
   ISBN 0-397-51352-6
   1. Obstetrical emergencies. 2. Gynecologic emergencies.
   I. Benrubi, Guy I.
   [DNLM: 1. Emergencies. 2. Pregnancy Complications—diagnosis.
   3. Pregnancy Complications—therapy. 4. Genital Diseases, Female—
   diagnosis. 5. Genital Diseases, Female—therapy. WQ 240 01325
   1993]
   RG571.0245 1993
   618'.0425—dc20
   DNLM/DLC
   for Library of Congress   93–25997
                                                                  CIP

The authors and publisher have exerted every effort to ensure that drug selection and dosage set forth in this text are in accord with current recommendations and practice at the time of publication. However, in view of ongoing research, changes in government regulations, and the constant flow of information relating to drug therapy and drug reactions, the reader is urged to check the package insert for each drug for any change in indications and dosage and for added warnings and precautions. This is particularly important when the recommended agent is a new or infrequently employed drug.

To Freddie, Poonch, N.B., and my parents

Things which you do not hope, happen more frequently, than things which you do hope.

Titus Maccius Plautus
254–184 B.C.

... Don't put off things till it's too late. You are the DJ of your fate.

Vikram Seth
"The Golden Gate"
1986

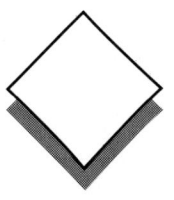

Contributors

Tracey Abner, M.D.
Attending Physician
Yale University Health Services
New Haven, Connecticut

Guy I. Benrubi, M.D.
Professor
Division of Gynecologic Oncology
Department of Obstetrics and
 Gynecology
University of Florida Health Science
 Center
Jacksonville, Florida

Richard A. Boothby, M.D.
Director Gynecologic Oncology
Assistant Director Medical Education
Orlando Regional Medical Center
Orlando, Florida

Gerardo O. Del Valle, M.D.
Assistant Professor
Division of Maternal-Fetal Medicine
Department of Obstetrics and
 Gynecology
University of Florida Health Science
 Center
Jacksonville, Florida

Isaac Delke, M.D.
Associate Professor
Division of Maternal-Fetal Medicine
Department of Obstetrics and
 Gynecology
University of Florida Health Science
 Center
Jacksonville, Florida

Lynnette Doan-Wiggins, M.D.
Assistant Professor
Department of Medicine
Loyola University of Chicago Stritch
 School of Medicine
Associate Director
Emergency Department
Loyola University Medical Center
Maywood, Illinois

Charles J. Dunton, M.D.
Assistant Professor
Department of Obstetrics and
 Gynecology
Thomas Jefferson University
Philadelphia, Pennsylvania

Daniel P. Eller, M.D.
Assistant Professor
Maternal-Fetal Medicine
Department of Obstetrics and
 Gynecology
Medical University of South Carolina
Charleston, South Carolina

Francisco L. Gaudier, M.D.
Assistant Professor
Division of Maternal-Fetal Medicine
Department of Obstetrics and
 Gynecology
University of Florida Health Science
 Center
Jacksonville, Florida

Ann Harwood-Nuss, M.D.
Professor
Department of Emergency Medicine
University of Florida Health Science
 Center
Jacksonville, Florida

Benson J. Horowitz, M.D.
Associate Clinical Professor
Department of Obstetrics and
 Gynecology
University of Connecticut College of
 Medicine
Farmington, Connecticut
Chairman
Vaginitis Section
International Society for the Study of
 Vulvar Disease
Houston, Texas
Attending Physician
Mt. Sinai and Hartford Hospital
Hartford, Connecticut

James L. Jones, M.D., Ph.D.
Assistant Professor
Department of Obstetrics and
 Gynecology
University of Florida Health Science
 Center
Jacksonville, Florida

Andrew M. Kaunitz, M.D.
Associate Professor
Director
Division of Ambulatory Care
University of Florida Health Science
 Center
Jacksonville, Florida

Kristi Morgan Mulchahey, M.D.
Attending Physician
Atlanta Gyn Associates
Atlanta, Georgia

Marcia E. Murakami, M.D.
Clinical Assistant Professor
Department of Radiology
University of Florida Health Science
 Center
Jacksonville, Florida

Roger B. Newman, M.D.
Associate Professor and Director
Maternal-Fetal Medicine
Department of Obstetrics and
 Gynecology
Medical University of South Carolina
Charleston, South Carolina

Robert C. Nuss, M.D.
Professor
Director
Division of Gynecologic Oncology
Department of Obstetrics and
 Gynecology
University of Florida Health Science
 Center
Jacksonville, Florida

Joseph G. Pastorek, II, M.D.
Professor of Obstetrics and
 Gynecology
Chief, Section of Infectious Disease
Member, Section of Maternal-Fetal
 Medicine
Department of Obstetrics and
 Gynecology
Louisiana State University Medical
 Center
New Orleans, Louisiana

Philip Samuels, M.D.
Associate Professor
Department of Obstetrics and
  Gynecology
The Ohio State University College of
  Medicine
Columbus, Ohio

Luis Sanchez-Ramos, M.D.
Associate Professor
Director
Division of Maternal-Fetal Medicine
Department of Obstetrics and
  Gynecology
University of Florida Health Science
  Center
Jacksonville, Florida

Lance A. Sang, M.D.
Assistant Professor
Department of Obstetrics and
  Gynecology
University of Florida College of
  Medicine
Jacksonville, Florida

Steven J. Sondheimer, M.D.
Professor
Division of Human Reproduction
Department of Obstetrics and
  Gynecology
University of Pennsylvania Medical
  Center
Philadelphia, Pennsylvania

Joy D. Steinfeld, M.D.
Assistant Professor
Department of Obstetrics and
  Gynecology
University of Medicine and Dentistry
  of New Jersey
Cooper Hospital
University Medical Center
Camden, New Jersey

Richard J. Stock, M.D.
Captain
MC
USN
Residency Program Director
Department of Obstetrics and
  Gynecology
Portsmouth Naval Hospital
Portsmouth, Virginia

I. Keith Stone, M.D.
Professor
Director
Women's Health Group
Chief
Division of Gynecology
University of Florida College of
  Medicine
Gainesville, Florida

Gregory P. Sutton, M.D.
Hulman Professor and Chief
Section of Gynecologic Oncology
Department of Obstetrics and
  Gynecology
Indiana University School of Medicine
Indianapolis, Indiana

Mark W. Todd, Pharm. D.
Associate Director
Department of Pharmacy
University Medical Center
Clinical Associate Professor
University of Florida College of
  Pharmacy
Jacksonville, Florida

D. Scott Wells, M.D.
Assistant Professor
Department of Obstetrics and
  Gynecology
University of Florida Health Science
  Center
Jacksonville, Florida

J.M. Whitworth, M.D.
Associate Professor
Department of Pediatrics
University of Florida Health Science
 Center
Medical Director
Children's Crisis Center
Jacksonville, Florida

Donald Willis, M.D.
South Florida Perinatal Medicine
Miami, Florida

Captain Hugh D. Wolcott, M.D.
Residency Program Director
Department of Obstetrics and
 Gynecology
Portsmouth Naval Hospital
Portsmouth, Virginia

Gregory C. Wynn, M.D.
Assistant Professor
Department of Radiology
University of Florida Health Science
 Center
Jacksonville, Florida

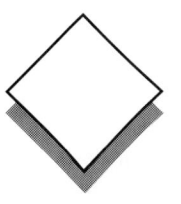

Preface

Physicians are faced, increasingly, with diagnosis and management decisions in obstetrics and gynecology emergency settings. Whether the setting is in the emergency department of a busy inner city hospital or in the office of a gynecologist or other primary care provider, understanding of the pathophysiology and management considerations of this disease is critical to good patient care. During the last decade, it has become increasingly apparent that a large proportion of young women and children, who are at greatest risk for obstetric and gynecologic emergencies, increasingly fall out of the health care system. In several areas of the country, up to 25 percent of women receive no prenatal care. In other areas, close to 50 percent of young women have no primary care providers to handle emergencies. To this must be coupled the increasing demands on the health care dollar and the increasing percentage of care delivered under managed systems which puts a premium on either no hospitalization or early discharge. Consequently, complications of delivery as well as gynecologic surgery are not recognized until after the patient has left the hospital. Therefore, management must be provided in emergent care settings whether in the hospital or the office.

This book is intended to address the need for the continuing up-to-date understanding of these obstetric and gynecologic emergencies. It seeks its audience among obstetricians, gynecologists, emergency department physicians, family practitioners, and other primary health care providers. The book is organized in two main sections: one on obstetric emergencies and the other on gynecologic emergencies. Though it is organized along the traditional major emergencies that occur in these two disciplines, several problems are addressed by different authors from different perspectives. It is the editor's belief that additional understanding of the management of these conditions can be gained through divergent points of view. Finally, it must be recognized that obstetric and gynecologic emergencies change with time. What are frequent problems today may become relatively infrequent tomorrow. New challenges face the physician. For example, approximately 80% of women in this country do not have legal abortion services available to them. It is, therefore, a probability that physicians will see emergency situations arising from illegal abortions. Additionally, violence has become a pervasive disease in our society and physicians who treat women must be conversant with problems which arise from rape and other trauma to the reproductive organs. Several chapters in this book address these and similar problems.

I would like to thank all of the contributors for their excellent work, and their diligent, careful, and astute analysis of the issues raised. Thanks is also due to Lisa McAllister of J. B. Lippincott for her encouragement in the initiation of the project and to Emilie Moyer for her efficiency, editing skills, and patience during the completion of the manuscript. A special thanks is due to Ms. Georgette Henderson for her incessant good nature, organizational skills, and ability to keep the project on track while being subjected to abominable time and deadline demands no other individual would tolerate—a special thanks is due for her ever present smile.

Guy I. Benrubi, M.D.

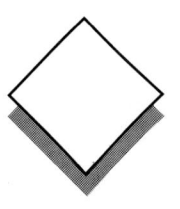

Contents

Part I OBSTETRICS 1

1. *Medical Emergencies in the Pregnant Patient* 3
   Joy D. Steinfeld ♦ Philip Samuels

2. *Acute Abdominal Pain in Pregnancy* 25
   Richard Boothby

3. *Ectopic Pregnancy* 41
   Hugh D. Wolcott ♦ Richard J. Stock ♦ Andrew M. Kaunitz

4. *Trauma in Pregnancy* 57
   Lynnette Doan-Wiggins

5. *Cardiopulmonary Resuscitation During Pregnancy* 77
   Lynnette Doan-Wiggins

6. *Perimortem Cesarean Section* 87
   Lance Sang

7. *Hypertensive Disorders of Pregnancy: Preeclampsia/Eclampsia* 93
   Luis Sanchez-Ramos

8. *Infections in Pregnancy* 103
   Joseph G. Pastorek II

9. *Bleeding in Pregnancy* 127
   Donald Willis

10. *Delivery in the Emergency Department* 139
    Isaac Delke

11. *Postpartum Emergencies* 155
    Daniel P. Eller ♦ Roger B. Newman

12. *Role of Imaging Modalities in Obstetric Emergencies* 171
Francisco L. Gaudier ♦ Gerardo O. Del Valle

13. *Drug Therapy in Pregnancy* 185
Mark W. Todd

14. *Complications of Legal and Illegal Abortion* 197
Andrew M. Kaunitz

15. *Equipment Needs in the Emergency Department* 203
D. Scott Wells

Part II GYNECOLOGY 209

16. *Sexually Transmitted Diseases* 211
I. Keith Stone

17. *Vulvar and Vaginal Disease* 233
Benson J. Horowitz

18. *Menorrhagia and Abnormal Vaginal Bleeding* 251
Steven J. Sondheimer

19. *Pelvic Mass* 263
Robert C. Nuss

20. *Torsion of the Ovary* 275
Charles J. Dunton

21. *Postoperative Emergencies* 283
Gregory Sutton

22. *Oncologic Emergencies* 305
Guy I. Benrubi ♦ Robert C. Nuss ♦ Ann Harwood-Nuss

23. *Gynecologic Emergencies in Childhood and Adolescence* 315
Kristi Morgan Mulchahey

24. *Emergency Evaluation and Treatment of the Sexual Assault Victim* 339
J.M. Jones ♦ James Whitworth

25. *Gynecologic Trauma* 355
Tracey Abner

26. *Imaging in Gynecologic Emergencies* 365
Marcia E. Murakami ♦ Gregg C. Wynn

Index 407

Obstetric *and* Gynecologic Emergencies

PART I

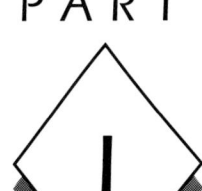

OBSTETRICS

Obstetric and Gynecologic Emergencies, edited by
Guy I. Benrubi. J.B. Lippincott Company,
Philadelphia © 1994.

CHAPTER

Medical Emergencies in the Pregnant Patient

Joy D. Steinfeld
Philip Samuels

Pulmonary Embolism

Pulmonary embolus complicates between 0.09 and 0.7 of every 1000 pregnancies.[1] Because untreated pulmonary embolus carries a 12.8% mortality rate, any patient with a suspicion of pulmonary embolization must be rapidly evaluated, diagnosed, and treated.[2] Even if these untreated patients survive the initial event, more than 30% will have recurrent emboli.[3] With treatment the mortality rate from the acute event drops to 0.7%.[2] The vast majority of these blood clots arise from the deep femoral and pelvic veins. During pregnancy the prevalence of thrombi in these veins is approximately 0.4 per 1000, a figure that is six times higher than that in nonpregnant women.[4] Often the emergency department physician is the first to see the gravida presenting with signs and symptoms of pulmonary embolism.

Patient Presentation

The gravida with acute pulmonary embolus often presents to the emergency department with chest pain and shortness of breath. She may not mention that she is pregnant. If she is not in the third trimester, the physician may not even notice that she is pregnant. It is important that the physician ask every woman in the child-bearing years who presents with any problem about the possibility of pregnancy. On examination tachypnea will be noted and a pleural friction rub may be auscultated. This is often difficult to hear because of the patient's tachypnea.

Massive pulmonary emboli are easily diagnosed, as they are most often complicated by hypotension and cardiovascular collapse. Conversely, patients with small emboli often have only subtle signs and symptoms. Because these small clots may be the harbingers of a massive embolus, it is imperative to reach a correct diagnosis rapidly. Furthermore, the sudden onset of blindness due to hypotension caused by pulmonary embolus may occur in the absence of other signs and symptoms.[5,6]

Diagnostic Tests

If the patient appears to be in severe distress an arterial blood gas should be obtained immediately. In acute pulmonary embolus the arterial blood gas usually demonstrates a decreased PO_2 and a slightly more decreased PCO_2. The pH is often normal or slightly elevated in the early stages of the process. If the patient is hypercapneic, it usually suggests a poor outcome.[7] A chest radiograph should be obtained with abdominal shielding. Many physicians will not obtain a chest radiograph because they fear a fetal risk from ionizing radiation. The fetal exposure from a single posteroanterior chest radiograph without abdominal shielding is approximately 2.5 mrad. It is even less with abdominal shielding.[8,9] Approximately 200 unshielded posteroanterior and lateral chest radiographs would be required to deliver to the conceptus an amount of radiation equal to that received during gestation from cosmic rays and naturally existing radioactive matter, such as C-14, present in organic food supplies.[10]

Radiation exposure to the fetus must be minimized. It is imperative, however, to make a correct diagnosis because there are risks both from failure to diagnose an embolus and from inappropriate treatment with prolonged anticoagulation. If the patient has a normal chest radiograph, a nuclear medicine pulmonary perfusion ventilation scan may be able to establish the diagnosis of pulmonary embolus firmly. Calculations have shown that the maximum fetal radiation exposure from this type of study is 50 mrem.[11] The fetus receives 85% of its radiation exposure from radioisotopes in the maternal bladder, as isotopes used in these tests are excreted through the maternal urinary tract. Frequent micturition and brisk diuresis should be employed to lower fetal exposure. If necessary, a Foley catheter can be used to empty the bladder and remove the radiation source from the proximity of the fetus.

If the patient's chest radiograph is abnormal or if the ventilation-perfusion nuclear medicine scan is equivocal, selected pulmonary angiography should be undertaken immediately. To minimize fetal exposure to ionizing radiation, abdominal shielding should be used. If the patient is in late gestation, the technician should be careful not to cover the base of the lungs with the shield, which would interfere with interpretation of the test. In experienced hands selected pulmonary angiography carries a morbidity of less than 1%. In pregnancy plasma volume is increased by approximately 40% and there is peripheral vasodilatation. These two factors make cannulating the veins easier, and the procedure can usually be accomplished successfully in less time than in a nonpregnant patient.

There does appear to be a small increase in the risk of childhood cancer following radiation exposures of less than 5 rad.[12] According to Wagner and colleagues, there is a 0.07% risk of any child developing a malignancy.[13] After 1 rad of fetal radiation exposure in the first trimester, this risk is raised to 0.25%. If the exposure occurs in the second or third trimesters, this risk is 0.122%.[13] It appears that deep venous thrombosis in the pelvis can be diagnosed with fetal exposure to ionizing radiation of less than 0.5 rad. Furthermore, pulmonary embolus can be diagnosed with fetal exposure of less than 0.05 rad.[12] Because of this minimal exposure these procedures should be undertaken without hesitation when clinically indicated.

Therapy

Heparin therapy is the cornerstone of treatment for pulmonary embolus. Heparin is a large, negatively charged protein with a molecular weight of 20,000, and it does not cross the placenta.[14] Therefore it will not anticoagulate the fetus in utero. If a pulmonary embolus is strongly suspected in the pregnant patient and if there is going to be a long delay before the definitive radiologic procedure can be performed, heparin therapy should be instituted empirically. As previously mentioned, there is great risk in delaying therapy for pulmonary embolus.

Once the diagnosis is established, therapy should be initiated without delay. As in a nonpregnant patient, the main complication of heparin therapy is bleeding. With meticulous attention to dosage and frequent monitoring of the activated partial thromboplastin time (APTT), this complication can be greatly reduced. Hemorrhage occurs in approximately 8 to 33% of heparin anticoagulation patients.[15] Other potential complications of heparin include osteoporosis, alopecia, bronchoconstriction secondary to histamine release, and profound thrombocytopenia.[16] Platelet counts therefore should be ascertained twice weekly during the first 2 weeks of therapy and monthly thereafter. They should also be obtained at any time if petechiae or purpura develops. In the emergency department, the initial heparin loading dose of 70 IU/kg total body weight should be administered intravenously. This should be followed by a continuous infusion of 1000 IU per hour. This dose must be adjusted to keep the APTT approximately twice normal or the heparin titer at 0.2 to 0.4 IU/mL. Often pregnant women need large doses of heparin to maintain anticoagulation. This may be due partly to the size of the clot and partly to the fact that the concentrations of most of the coagulation factors increase greatly during pregnancy. In clinically stable patients, intravenous anticoagulation should continue for approximately 10 days.

After this initial therapy the patient may be discharged on a moderate dose of subcutaneous heparin. The usual dose of 7500 to 10,000 IU every 8 to 12 hours is often sufficient to keep the APTT approximately 1.5 times normal and the heparin titer between 0.1 and 0.2 IU/mL.[17] Continuous subcutaneous heparin pumps also may be used for this purpose on an outpatient basis. It is important to realize that there is great variation in the amount of heparin absorbed and whether the patient administers it to herself subcutaneously or accidentally injects it intramuscularly. Therefore the emergency department physician must be prepared to check an APTT immediately on any pregnant woman who presents with bleeding complications while taking subcutaneous heparin. Because of the changes in clotting factors, the doses may have to be changed frequently. If the patient is bleeding and the

APTT is prolonged, then protamine may have to be administered. These therapeutic guidelines will undoubtedly be altered with the introduction of low molecular weight heparin to the United States, which is anticipated in the next few years. Low molecular weight heparin does not prolong the APTT.

Anticoagulation should be continued until the patient starts labor. Then it should be discontinued during labor and delivery but can be restarted several hours postpartum. The patient may be started on oral Coumadin in the postpartum period.

Oral anticoagulation should never be used during gestation. These vitamin K antagonists readily cross the placenta and are teratogenic when used in early pregnancy. In the first trimester these medications have been associated with facial dysmorphisms, hypoplastic digits, stippled epiphyses, and mental retardation.[18,19] Use of oral anticoagulants in the second trimester has been associated with optic nerve atrophy, faulty brain development, and developmental retardation.[18] As these drugs readily cross the placenta, the fetus is anticoagulated, which may result in severe fetal hemorrhage in the event of trauma or premature delivery.

Recently, surgical intervention has been advocated in the patient with thrombophlebitis and pulmonary embolus during pregnancy.[4,20,21] Mogensen and coworkers treated eight pregnant women suffering from acute iliofemoral venous thrombosis by thrombectomy, and all did well.[4] Belgvad and colleagues successfully treated a woman during the second trimester who developed severe right ventricular failure caused by 85% obstruction of the pulmonary arterial circulation by performing a pulmonary embolectomy.[20] Splinter and colleagues reported an open embolectomy performed immediately following cesarean section with both mother and child fully recovering.[21] The surgical approach is still investigational. It is, however, an option in the gravida with pulmonary embolus who is not responding to conventional therapy.

Asthma

Asthma is among the most common medical complications seen with pregnancy. This obstructive respiratory disorder complicates approximately 1% of all pregnancies, with status asthmaticus complicating approximately 0.2% of pregnancies.[22,23] The emergency department physician must be able to diagnose and treat the gravida with asthma rapidly. In the general population the mortality rate from asthma is 1% to 3%, which indicates that this disorder is responsible for nearly 4000 annual deaths in the United States.[24]

When a woman with a history of asthma becomes pregnant, the course of her disease over the next 9 months is unpredictable. In their review of 1054 pregnancies complicated by asthma, Turner and coworkers reported that the severity of asthma remained unchanged in 50% of patients, improved in 30%, and worsened in 20%.[25] Unfortunately, the course of a patient's asthma in one pregnancy is not a predictor of how the asthma will respond in other pregnancies.[26,27] Women who begin pregnancy with severe asthma, however, tend to experience a worsening of their disease.[28]

The effect of asthma on pregnancy is not entirely delineated. Some researchers have found an increased rate of preterm labor in women who experience asthma during pregnancy.[29] In a recent study Mabie and colleagues found the rate of preterm delivery in asthmatics to be 16%, which was not significantly different from the 17.7% rate in their control population.[30] Another study found the perinatal mortality rate in women with severe asthma to be 28%.[31] This seems excessive and probably can be explained by the fact that the study was published in 1970. Antenatal fetal assessment has improved greatly in the 22 years since that study was published. Hence the present perinatal mortality rate probably does not approach that level. In this same study four of 16 (25%) women with severe asthma died.[31] This is a small sample size and with improved therapy and intensive-care techniques, this number should be much lower. Even with improved intensive care, asthma in the gravida should never be taken lightly. In 1984 Gelber and coworkers reported the case of a pregnant woman with a previous history of mild asthma who developed life-threatening status asthmaticus that was refractory to all therapy.[32] Scoggins and colleagues, in 1977, reported a maternal mortality rate of 40% when mechanical ventilation was required for women with asthma.[33]

It is important to remember that in pregnancy, the minute ventilation increases 40% from approximately 7.5 to 10.5 L per minute. This is primarily caused by an increase in the tidal volume. The respiratory rate is only minimally increased as a result of increased respiratory drive triggered by progesterone. This leaves the patient in a mild state of compensated respiratory alkalosis.

Differential Diagnosis

To treat the gravida with asthma properly, an accurate diagnosis is mandatory. Many pregnant women experience a subjective shortness of breath, which is known as dyspnea of pregnancy.[34] This diagnosis is difficult to make over the telephone, and if a gravida complains of shortness of breath, she should be seen immediately. A rare cause of dyspnea in pregnancy is aspiration pneumonitis. Because there is an increased residual volume in the stomach in pregnancy as well as a decrease in the lower esophageal sphincter tone, the risk of aspiration during sleep increases. The risk is even greater as the uterus increases in size, placing more pressure on the stomach and its contents. Other differential diagnoses that must be excluded are pulmonary embolus, pulmonary edema, and heart failure.

Pathophysiology of Asthma

Contraction of bronchial smooth muscle, secretion of mucus, and edema of the bronchiolar mucosa are the hallmarks of asthma.[35] The primary mediators of these responses that are released include histamine, slow-reacting substance of anaphylaxis (SRS-A), eosinophil chemotactic factor (ECF), and platelet-activating factor (PAF).[35,36] These substances may be released in response to allergens, respiratory infections, or strenuous exercise. These primary mediators of asthma lead to an inflammatory response that is responsible for most of the difficulty in breathing. Secondarily, they lead to hypertrophy of bronchial smooth muscle, which until recently had been thought to be the primary mechanism for airway obstruction during pregnancy. Hence the focus of asthma therapy has changed. Where previously the emphasis was on increasing dilatation of bronchial smooth muscle, the focus now is on decreasing the inflammatory response.

Emergency Therapy

In both the pregnant and nonpregnant asthmatic presenting to the emergency department, assurance of an adequate airway is of the utmost importance. Auscultation should be used to ensure that the patient is moving air adequately. Expiratory wheezing does not always correlate with the extent of airway disease. A patient who is experiencing wheezing is moving air. One who is not wheezing may, in fact, not be moving any air. Tachycardia and pulsus paradoxus are often present. Acrocyanosis is often present in the patient with a severe asthma attack. Central cyanosis, however, is often the harbinger of a poor outcome in an asthmatic patient. Objective measurements of the patient's pulmonary function are crucial, because subjective complaints do not always mirror the true physiology of the problem.[37] A forced expiratory volume at one second (FEV_1) is an easily obtained pulmonary function test that often gives important information. A patient may feel that symptoms have resolved and still only have an FEV_1 that is 20% of the predicted value.[37] Several investigators have shown that when a patient's breathing is so inhibited that it interferes with normal speech patterns, the FEV_1 is consistently lower than 0.45 L.[36,38,39] If FEV_1 measurements cannot be obtained easily in the emergency setting, peak expiratory flow rates can be used. Corre and Rothstein concluded that rates of less than 100 L per minute correlate with severe obstruction.[39]

Because clinical signs and symptoms of asthma are often inaccurate and because the FEV_1 may not be reliable, patients with acute asthma should undergo arterial blood gas determination. Because there are increased critical closing volumes during pregnancy, normal maternal PO_2 may drop from a normal 108 mmHg to between 92 and 100 mmHg in the third trimester of pregnancy.[38] As previously mentioned, there is an increase in the minute ventilation during pregnancy. This causes the PCO_2 in pregnancy to fall to between 27 and 32 mmHg and increases the normal pH to about 7.45.[40] If the FEV_1 is less than 1 L or less than 20% of the predicted value, the patient will probably respond poorly to therapy, and outpatient management should probably be avoided.

An intravenous line should be placed immediately in the patient. Because most of these patients are tachypneic, their insensible water losses will be increased. Often they have also been unable to drink because of the tachypnea. It is therefore reasonable to administer quickly a liter of isotonic IV fluid with or without dextrose. Following this initial fluid therapy, if the patient does not appear dehydrated, a regular maintenance rate of fluid should be used. Supplemental oxygen is a mainstay in the therapy for asthma. After obtaining the initial blood gas on room air, oxygen may be administered at 3 to 5 L per minute by mask. A pulse oximeter should be placed to follow the oxygen saturation. Pharmacologic therapy must then be considered and initiated.

Pharmacologic Agents

Despite many changes in asthma therapy, epinephrine remains the first-line drug. It has a rapid onset of action and stimulates the beta receptors, promoting the conversion of ATP to cyclic AMP (cAMP). This causes bronchial smooth muscle relaxation. The alpha-adrenergic activity decreases pulmonary vascular congestion. There have been some theoretical concerns about decreasing uterine blood flow with the alpha-adrenergic activity of epinephrine. This, however, has never been shown in vivo. The usual dose is 0.3 mL of a 1:1000 solution of epinephrine given subcutaneously. The effects are usually seen in 5 minutes. If no adverse side-effects are seen, the dose may be repeated every 20 minutes for three or four doses. If the patient has good results from the epinephrine, Sus-Phrine 1:200 may be given subcutaneously in a dose of 0.15 mL before the patient is discharged. Patients also may be discharged on aerosolized beta-adrenergic agents. These meter-dosed inhalers or nebulizers result in fewer side-effects than systemic administration of adrenergic agents. These agents must be used with care in patients with a history of cardiac disease, as they induce tachycardia and cardiac dysrhythmias, since none of these drugs has pure beta-2 selectivity.

Inhaled glucocorticoids, along with inhaled beta mimetics, have become the mainstays in asthma treatment over the past few years. Previously, the theophylline derivatives had been the focus of chronic therapy. Because they are dealing with unknown fetal effects, obstetricians have always been slow to accept new pharmacologic therapeutic alternatives. They are, however, beginning to join the mainstream in treating patients with inhaled glucocorticoids.

In the acute asthmatic, intravenous glucocorticoids should be administered without delay if the patient does not respond rapidly to sympathomimetics. For parenteral use hydrocortisone and methylprednisolone are safe for use during pregnancy. Very little of these glucocorticoids actually crosses the placenta. The majority is metabolized by placental 11-beta-ol-dehydrogenase to form an inactive 11-keto-metabolite. Chapman and coworkers studied 93 nonpregnant patients with acute asthma and found that using an oral glucocorticoid decreased the relapse rate fourfold during the first 10 days after the attack.[41] Littenberg and Gluck found that the early administration of intravenous glucocorticoids decreased the need for hospitalization in patients with acute asthma.[42] It is clear that glucocorticoid use is becoming more frequent in the pregnant asthmatic. Acutely, hydrocortisone can be administered in doses of 2 mg/kg every 4 hours until the attack diminishes. Methylprednisolone, which has less mineralocorticoid activity, can be administered in a dose of 60 to 100 mg every 6 to 8 hours. After the patient's asthma clears, she may be switched to oral prednisone. The usual oral initial dose of 60 to 100 mg is tapered over several days to several weeks, depending on the severity of the disease. Chronically, the patient can be maintained on inhaled corticosteroids such as beclomethasone. These agents have almost no systemic action and do not really affect lung parenchyma. However, they do help relieve the inflammatory response that is responsible for so many of the asthma symptoms.

One must stress to the patient that glucocorticoids do not appear to have teratogenic potential.[43,44] Conversely, studies have shown that worse fetal outcomes are noted in women with poorly controlled asthma who are noncompliant with their medications.[45]

Aminophylline inhibits phosphodiesterase activity and results in an increase in cAMP, which relaxes bronchial smooth muscle. Until recently, aminophylline derivatives were recommended as the drugs of choice to treat chronic asthma. Because inflammation has been found to play a larger role in asthma, inhaled corticosteroids have largely replaced theophylline. If a patient is encountered who has previously responded very well to theophylline, continuation of the drug is advisable. If the patient has been receiving this medication chronically but has not taken it in some time, it must be initially administered parenterally. An aminophylline loading dose of 6 mg/kg is given intravenously, followed by a continuous infusion of 0.5 to 0.7 mg/kg per hour.[45] One of the advantages of aminophylline is that serum levels can be measured and the therapeutic range is between 10 and 20 mg/mL.[46] Serum levels must be followed closely in pregnancy as clearance increases early in pregnancy but decreases in late pregnancy.[47] The half-life of theophylline is shorter in smokers. Many oral theophylline preparations are available. In summary, aminophylline is recommended only for those patients who have responded well to it before. Nausea, vomiting, central nervous system irritability, and cardiac dysrhythmias are all possible side-effects.

Status Asthmaticus

If the patient's P_{CO_2} is above 40 mmHg, the P_{O_2} is less than 60 mmHg, or the O_2 saturation is less than 90 mmHg, or if the mother is exhausted, endotracheal intubation should be carried out.[48] Humidified oxygen should be used to enhance the clearance of inherent bronchial mucus. Sedation may be required. These patients often do better when continuous positive-airway pressure is used. Transfer to an intensive-care unit should be prompt. Ideally, a maternal fetal medicine as well as pulmonary medicine consultation should be available.

Thyroid Storm

Thyroid storm is most commonly seen in patients with undiagnosed or undertreated hyperthyroidism. It is also seen occasionally in patients with toxic multinodular goiter. This emergent condition is more common in women in the middle decades and is rare in pregnancy. Thyroid storm was noted in less than 1% of pregnancies complicated by thyrotoxicosis at Los Angeles County–University of Southern California Medical Center.[49] The onset is generally abrupt, and the disease is usually fatal if left untreated. Early and aggressive therapy has decreased mortality to between 10% and 20%.[49] A precipitating event can be identified in 50% to 75% of cases. The most common precipitating events are listed in Table 1-1.

Diagnostic Criteria

Fever in excess of 37.8°C (100°F) is present. The fever is invariable and may be as high as 41.1°C (106°F), with or without concurrent infection. Marked diaphoresis may occur, leading to significant insensible fluid loss. Tachycardia is often present

TABLE 1-1
Events That May Precipitate Thyroid Storm

Infection, especially pulmonary
Nonthyroidal surgery
Acute surgical emergencies
Trauma
Induction of anesthesia
Diabetic complications/DKA
Myocardial infarction
Vascular accident
Pulmonary embolus

and out of proportion to the fever. Exaggerated peripheral manifestations of thyrotoxicosis are present. Dysfunction of the cardiovascular, gastrointestinal, or central nervous system may be present.

Cardiovascular abnormalities are seen in 50% of patients. Tachycardia is usual. Atrial fibrillation and premature ventricular contractions may be seen, and complete heart block may occur rarely during storm. A widened pulse pressure is generally present, because of increased stroke volume, cardiac output, and myocardial oxygen consumption. Congestive heart failure is common and may be the presenting symptom in patients with thyroid storm. Progressive cardiac dysfunction leading to pulmonary edema and, subsequently, cardiogenic shock may occur.

Central nervous system dysfunction is seen in 90% of patients with thyroid storm. Manifestations vary from restlessness, anxiety, and agitation to the extremes of delirium, disorientation, and psychosis. Tremor and proximal muscle weakness are common. Emotional lability, obtundation, and coma may be seen.

In the weeks preceding storm the patient often experiences weight loss despite increased appetite. Diarrhea or hyperdefecation may herald the onset of storm. During storm, anorexia, nausea, vomiting, and crampy abdominal pain, which may mimic an acute abdomen, may be present. Occasionally, jaundice and/or tender hepatomegaly are noted. The combination of increased temperature and physical findings such as these has led to inappropriate and unfortunate exploratory laparatomies.

Differential Diagnosis

Thyroid storm should be suspected in any thyrotoxic patient with fever. The emergency physician should attempt to elicit a history of Graves' disease and should examine the patient for a palpable goiter or eye signs suggestive of Graves' ophthalmopathy. Thyroid storm may be confused with other hyperkinetic states.[50] The differential diagnosis is listed in Table 1-2.

Evaluation should include a history and physical examination directed toward antecedent thyrotoxicosis and Graves' disease. A careful medication history should be obtained. Table 1-3 lists the most commonly occurring physical findings in patients experiencing thyroid storm.

**TABLE 1-2
Differential Diagnosis of Thyroid Storm**

Anxiety states
Psychosis
Cocaine toxicity, other toxic ingestion
Pheochromocytoma
Heat stroke
Malignant neuroleptic syndrome
Diabetes mellitus, out of control
Chronic obstructive pulmonary disease, end stage
Acute abdomen
Congestive heart failure
Alcoholic complications
Sepsis

Laboratory Evaluation

Thyroid function tests do not distinguish storm from uncomplicated thyrotoxicosis because the values overlap. The results of these tests are usually unavailable immediately. Hyperglycemia is common, and hypercalcemia may be seen in 25% of patients. Plasma cortisol levels are noted to be inappropriately low for the level of stress.

Management

General supportive care should be initiated immediately. The goals of management are outlined in Table 1-4. Hydration with intravenous fluids and electrolytes to replace gastrointestinal and insensible losses is essential. Hypercalcemia and hyperglycemia should be corrected, if present. Supplemental oxygen should be administered, and continuous cardiac monitoring should be employed. Fever should be controlled with antipyretics and, if necessary, a cooling blanket. Congestive failure

**TABLE 1-3
Common Physical Findings in Thyroid Storm**

Fever
Tachycardia
Widened pulse pressure
CNS dysfunction
Muscle tremor
Weakness, especially proximal muscle groups
Arrhythmias, especially atrial fibrillation
Congestive heart failure
Goiter, often with a thrill or bruit
Eye signs (stare, lid lag, Graves' ophthalmopathy)

TABLE 1–4
Goals of Management in Thyroid Storm

I. General supportive care
II. Identify and treat precipitating factor
III. Inhibit thyroid hormone synthesis
IV. Inhibit thyroid hormone release
V. Block peripheral effects of hyperthyroidism

should be treated the same as in the nonpregnant individual, but patients may be refractory to digoxin and require larger doses.[51] Control of tachycardia with beta-blockade may pose problems in the face of recalcitrant congestive heart failure. Glucocorticoids should be administered intravenously in a dose equivalent to hydrocortisone, 300 mg daily. Glucocorticoids also inhibit peripheral tissue conversion of T_4 to T_3, decreasing the peripheral manifestations of thyrotoxicosis. Frequent vital signs and physical exams to monitor clinical status and response to treatment are necessary.

Broad-spectrum antibiotic coverage should be initiated early and continued until final cultures are negative, unless another precipitating cause is identified.

Thyroid hormone synthesis should be blocked with propylthiouracil (PTU), which inhibits both the organification of tyrosine residues and the peripheral conversion of T_4 to T_3.[50] A 900- to 1200-mg loading dose should be given, followed by 300 to 600 mg daily.[51] As PTU is only available in oral form, administration via nasogastric tube may be necessary. Although PTU begins to act in the first hour after administration, the full therapeutic effect is not achieved for 3 to 6 weeks.[50] In pregnancy the drug of choice for medical treatment of hyperthyroidism is PTU, rather than methimazole. It provides a more rapid clinical response and has a good safety record for the fetus. Newborns of treated mothers generally have small goiters, if one is present at all, and mild hypothyroidism, which resolves shortly after birth. Although the evidence linking methimazole to aplasia cutis in the newborn is somewhat tenuous, practitioners still hesitate to use the drug unless the patient cannot tolerate PTU.

Thyroid hormone release should be inhibited by administration of iodide (SSKI, 5 drops orally, or by nasogastric tube every 8 hours, or sodium iodide, 1 g every 24 hours by slow intravenous infusion). Iodide administration should not be initiated until an hour after PTU or methimazole therapy has begun, so that there is no further buildup of hormone stores.

Propranolol will control tachycardia, block the peripheral conversion of T_4 to T_3, and improve fever, tremor, and restlessness. One milligram per minute intravenously, up to 10 mg, or 40 to 80 mg orally every 4 hours may be administered. Plasmapheresis and peritoneal dialysis are reserved for patients who fail conservative therapy.

After initial clinical improvement, iodine and glucocorticoid therapy can be discontinued. Antithyroid medications should be continued until the patient is euthyroid. Ablative therapy with surgery or radioactive iodine is indicated in all patients after storm (although this should be postponed until after delivery). Although the half-life of ^{131}I is approximately 8 days, avoidance of pregnancy for 6 months after ablative treatment is recommended. If storm occurs early in pregnancy, a subtotal thyroidectomy can be performed in the second trimester. Utilization of the preceding management protocol has resulted in a decrease in mortality to 10% to 20%.[49] Death is usually the result of cardiac failure or intercurrent infection.[51]

Diabetic Ketoacidosis

Diabetic ketoacidosis (DKA) constitutes a medical and obstetric emergency in the pregnant patient. Despite improved supportive care, DKA is still a significant cause of mortality. Maternal mortality in DKA has been reduced to less than 1%,[52] but fetal loss rates remain as high as 50%.[53]

Pathophysiology

DKA is seen in known insulin-dependent diabetics or may be the first manifestation of previously undiagnosed diabetes mellitus. Cases have been documented in gestational diabetics[54] as well as in conjunction with beta-mimetic therapy in insulin-dependent diabetics.[55] Beta-mimetic therapy may initiate DKA by breaking down glycogen to glucose, as well as increasing cellular metabolism, resulting in lactic acidosis. DKA has also been documented in a pregnant woman with no prior history of glucose intolerance who was treated with terbutaline and betamethasone.[56]

Two basic metabolic derangements are present in DKA. A relative or absolute insulin deficiency results in decreased peripheral utilization of glucose and subsequent hyperglycemia. This causes an osmotic diuresis, which leads to volume depletion and electrolyte loss. Water is excreted in proportion to the increase in osmotic pressure. Electrolytes are lost with the free water. Concomitant increased ketogenesis causes a metabolic acidosis. The syndrome is rarely due to inadequate insulin alone. A concurrent stressor, often infection, is usually present, which can cause release of glucagon, catecholamines, growth hormone, and cortisol. These glucose counterregulatory hormones cause increased gluconeogenesis, which increases circulating glucose levels and decreases amino acid stores in the liver.

The natural progression of the osmotic diuresis results in decreased cardiac output, lowered blood pressure, and ultimately, vascular collapse and shock. Metabolic acidosis causes an increased respiratory rate, in an attempt to compensate, but this results in even further fluid loss.

Diagnosis

Patients may present with malaise, headache, dry mouth, weight loss, nausea, and vomiting. Polydipsia, polyuria, and shortness of breath are often seen. The more severe the patient's acidosis, the more obtunded she will appear. Because of increased acetone production, the patient may have characteristic "fruity" breath.

Diagnostic criteria are listed in Table 1-5. An increased anion gap (>12 mEq/L) is indicative of a decreased serum bicarbonate concentration. Large fluid shifts re-

TABLE 1-5
Diagnostic Criteria for Diabetic Ketoacidosis

Maternal pH ≤ 7.30
HCO_3 ≤ 15
Serum ketones are present
Blood glucose ≥ 300 mg/dL

*DKA may develop in pregnant patients with blood glucose < 200 mg/dL.

sult in peripheral vascular depletion. As a result, patients may suffer from dehydration and hypotension. Prerenal azotemia may also be evident.

Emergency Treatment

Prompt and aggressive treatment of the pregnant patient with DKA is essential. Fluid replacement is critical. Water is lost in excess of electrolytes. The water deficit is often 100 mL/kg body weight but may be as high as 150 mL/kg. This results in a total body water deficit of 4 to 10 L. This deficit should be replaced over the first 24 hours of treatment. A liter of normal saline should be administered over the first hour. Then 250 to 500 mL of saline per hour should be given until approximately 75% of the deficit is corrected. Solutions containing lactate should be avoided. Urine output must be monitored closely, and each void should be checked with a dipstick for glucose and ketones. If the patient has extreme malaise or is obtunded, an indwelling bladder catheter should be used. After initial blood work has been drawn and hydration begun, insulin therapy should be started. Insulin administration is most easily controlled with an intravenous drip of regular insulin. Initially, 0.1 units per kilogram body weight should be given as an intravenous push; then eight to 10 units per hour should be administered. Blood sugar should be checked every 1 to 2 hours, and if a decrease of 25% or more is not achieved within the first 2 hours, the infusion rate should be increased. Insulin resistance is common in patients with DKA. After the blood sugar is less than 250 mg/dL, the IV solution should be changed to 5% dextrose with 0.45% NaCl, and the insulin infusion rate should be decreased by one half. Blood sugars should be checked hourly. After the blood sugar is less than 150 mg/dL, a basal rate of 1 to 2 units of insulin per hour usually maintains homeostasis. After acidosis and dehydration are corrected and the blood sugar is less than 150 mg/dL, the patient can eat and return to split dosing of insulin. The insulin drip may be tapered over 4 to 6 hours and then discontinued.

Electrolyte replacement is necessary. Potassium loss due to vomiting and massive osmotic diuresis is usually in the range of 5 to 10 mEq/kg of body weight. Acidosis causes displacement of intracellular potassium to the extracellular space, giving the clinician a spurious reassurance that potassium stores are adequate. Correcting the acidosis drives potassium back into the cell, rapidly decreasing the serum potassium. Potassium chloride, up to 40 mEq/L, should be added to the IV and the serum electrolytes should be checked every 2 to 4 hours.

Bicarbonate replacement is controversial and should be considered only if the pH is less than 7.1. One ampule (44 mEq $NaHCO_3$) may be administered in a liter of half-normal saline. Administration of bicarbonate does not affect the recovery of outcome variables (rate of decrease of glucose and ketone levels, rate of increase in pH or bicarbonate) in the mother.[53] Bicarbonate is broken down to hydrogen ions and CO_2 by carbonic anhydrase. Free hydrogen ions may cross the placenta and therefore exacerbate acidosis in the fetus.

It is necessary to treat the precipitating cause of the acidosis. A thorough search for infection should be undertaken in the first 30 minutes, including examination of the skin, urine, lungs, and sputum. Chorioamnionitis should be ruled out as a possible source. Broad-spectrum antibiotics should be administered empirically pending culture results.

If the fetus is viable, fetal heart tones should be monitored. Late decelerations and decreased beat-to-beat variability (both signs of fetal distress) may be seen, but the mother should be stabilized before any consideration is given to delivery. The fetal heart rate abnormalities will usually resolve as the maternal status normalizes, and thus delivery can often be delayed until the fetus reaches maturity.[57,58]

Hospital Management

After the mother is completely stabilized, the following days in the hospital should be used to regulate the patient's insulin doses and treat any underlying infection. A return to the usual two or three divided daily doses of insulin required by pregnant diabetics is expected. Fetal surveillance should be continued as it would be for outpatient pregnant diabetics and should include daily determination of fetal activity. Weekly nonstress tests beginning at 28 weeks and increasing to twice weekly testing at 34 weeks is a commonly used protocol. This will depend upon the class of the patient's diabetes. Close follow-up of maternal and fetal status, including glycemic control and assessment of fetal growth and well-being, is requisite for the remainder of the pregnancy.

Seizure Disorders

The major causes of seizures in pregnancy are eclampsia and idiopathic seizure disorders. Approximately 7% of pregnancies are complicated by preeclampsia, a condition associated with high blood pressure, proteinuria, edema, and other laboratory and clinical manifestations. A small number of these patients progress to eclampsia, which is characterized by tonic/clonic seizures or coma. This usually occurs in the third trimester of pregnancy, although rare cases of second-trimester eclampsia can occur. Idiopathic epilepsy, conversely, affects 0.5% of the population of North America. It complicates approximately 0.15% of pregnancies. These seizures can be categorized as generalized tonic/clonic seizures, partial complex seizures that may or may not generalize, and absence seizures. Often pregnant patients stop taking their anticonvulsant medications because they are worried about fetal effects. These patients usually have more seizures. It is therefore not uncommon for a pregnant patient to be brought into the emergency department after having a tonic/clonic seizure.

Eclampsia is associated with high blood pressure, proteinuria, edema, and an unusual elevation of the serum uric acid level. Rapid weight gain in the third trimester is a result of edema. As with all seizures, the patient that has experienced eclampsia will be in a postictal state. The patient may also present with status epilepticus. Blood analysis will often show elevated uric acid level, serum creatinine >1 mg/dL, a blood urea nitrogen >10 mg/dL, an occasional elevation of the liver transaminases, or a depressed platelet count. A serum alkaline phosphatase level cannot be used to assess liver function, as the placenta produces alkaline phosphatase and this will give a misleading elevated result. It is important to note, however, that these blood tests are not always uniformly abnormal in the eclamptic and that often elevated blood pressure may be the only objective sign seen in these patients. If the patient is in the third trimester of pregnancy, if she has had an excessive weight gain in the past few weeks, and if she has been experiencing a headache that has not been responsive to acetaminophen or right-upper-quadrant pain, it is very likely the patient's tonic/clonic seizures are due to eclampsia. Conversely, the patient with an idiopathic seizure disorder presents in any trimester of pregnancy. She has often had no symptoms or prodromal signs other than her usual aura before the seizure.

Effect of Pregnancy on Epilepsy

In a review of 155 pregnancies complicated by epilepsy between 1938 and 1976, seizure frequency increased in 45% of the patients, remained unchanged in 43%, and decreased in 12%.[59,60] Another more recent study compared seizure frequency during pregnancy in 78 pregnancies in 66 patients with epilepsy. No statistical difference was noted between the seizure frequency before and during pregnancy.[61] This difference in findings may be due to our present ability to measure levels of anticonvulsant drugs in epileptic patients. Pregnancy changes the disposition of anticonvulsant medications. The increase in plasma volume, the presence of fetal and placental compartments, and the increase in extracellular fluid all increase the volume of distribution of anticonvulsant medications and can lower the total serum concentration of these medicines. However, only the free, unbound drug is pharmacologically active. Bardy and colleagues measured serum phenytoin levels during pregnancy in 111 patients and concluded that they are lowest at the time of delivery.[62] In this study the drug dosage had to be increased in 48% of patients to combat an increased seizure frequency. Furthermore, many patients experience nausea and vomiting in the first trimester of pregnancy, which reduces the absorption of anticonvulsant drugs from the gastrointestinal tract. Barbiturates and phenytoin induce hepatic microsomal enzymes, which hasten their own metabolism. In addition, pregnancy increases the liver's ability to hydroxylate these medications. This is only a brief example of the many ways in which serum anticonvulsant levels can change during a normal pregnancy and of why it is important to measure these drug levels in patients with epilepsy who are seen after a seizure.

Effect of Anticonvulsant Medications on the Fetus

Untreated epilepsy and epilepsy treated with pharmacologic agents result in an increase in major malformations.[63] The fetal hydantoin syndrome consists of microcephaly, mild to moderate mental retardation, developmental delay, growth retardation, facial clefts, facial dysmorphisms, and limb abnormalities.[64] The hands may exhibit fingerlike thumbs as well as distal phalangeal and nail hypoplasia.[65] Hanson and coworkers reported some features of this syndrome in 11% of the infants exposed to phenytoin in utero.[64] Other researchers, however, consider this figure an overestimation of the frequency of malformations associated with phenytoin.[66,67] One of the most common malformations found with this syndrome is cleft palate. In the general population the incidence of cleft palate is approximately three to five per 1000 live births. In the patient exposed in utero to phenytoin the incidence is approximately 18 per 1000.[68]

Carbamazepine has been considered a safe anticonvulsant agent to use during pregnancy. Recent studies, however, have reported cranial/facial defects and facial dysmorphisms in 11% of infants exposed to this agent in utero.[67,69] Valproate is an excellent anticonvulsant but should be avoided in women of childbearing age because of its teratogenic potential. It has been associated with neural tube defects as well as some craniofacial defects.[70-72] Therefore any woman exposed to valproate during gestation should be offered either serum or amniotic fluid alpha-fetoprotein testing as well as targeted ultrasound in an attempt to rule out these malformations. The teratogenic potentials of phenobarbital and primidone (which is metabolized to phenobarbital) are debatable. Generally, carbamazepine and phenobarbital are considered to have the least teratogenic potential. Phenytoin and valproate, in general, should be avoided during pregnancy. Nonetheless, patients should not change anticonvulsants once they are pregnant. When physicians and patients attempt to change medications at this time, seizure activity usually increases, jeopardizing both mother and fetus. More important, teratogenesis occurs in the first 2 months of pregnancy, and any negative effects of anticonvulsants have often occurred by the time the patient realizes that she is pregnant.

Management of the Patient With an Acute Seizure

In the patient experiencing a tonic/clonic convulsion, it is impossible to distinguish between idiopathic epilepsy and eclampsia without further history or laboratory investigation. If, however, the patient presents to the emergency department with seizures and she is noticeably pregnant, more than likely she has eclampsia. These patients should be treated as if they are eclamptic until further studies and history can be obtained. Generally, these tonic/clonic convulsions last from 60 to 70 seconds and can be divided into two phases. The first phase, which lasts for about 30% to 50% of the duration of the seizure, begins with facial twitching and corpus rigidity (tonus). In the second phase of the seizure the muscles of the body alternately contract and relax. This is the clonic phase of the seizure. The patient is usually in a postictal state after these seizures. Although the patient is apneic during the seizure, slow, deep respirations usually begin as soon as the seizure ends. There are several steps in managing the patient with an eclamptic seizure:

1. It is necessary to prevent maternal injury. If possible, a tongue blade should be inserted between the patient's teeth to prevent biting of the tongue. The patient should be suctioned to keep the airway clear and to prevent aspiration of

secretions or vomitus. The patient should be watched carefully to prevent bodily injury, lacerations, and fractures.[73]
2. An adequate airway must be maintained by keeping the patient on her left side and keeping the pharynx clear with suctioning. This will allow adequate oxygenation after the patient's respirations resume following the convulsion.
3. The physician should reduce the risk of maternal aspiration. The patient should be suctioned carefully and kept on her left side. In pregnancy the pressure placed upon the stomach by the enlarging uterus and the decreased lower esophageal sphincter tone (secondary to progesterone) cause the pregnant patient to be at increased risk for aspiration. If there is any question of this, the patient should undergo a chest radiograph following the seizure. If it appears that aspiration has occurred, appropriate therapy should be initiated without delay.
4. If an eclamptic seizure is the working diagnosis, the patient should be treated with intravenous magnesium sulfate, if possible. Magnesium sulfate is marketed in several different strengths. It is imperative to read the ampule label carefully before administering the drug, as overdoses can lead to respiratory depression, and inadequate doses can result in continued seizures. The usual initial dose is 6 g administered slowly intravenously over a 15- to 20-minute period. If the patient is conscious, she will feel flushed during the administration of this medication. If it is given too quickly, projectile vomiting will ensue. Approximately 15% of women will have a second convulsion after receiving a loading dose of magnesium sulfate.[74] If this occurs, another 2 g of magnesium sulfate may be given intravenously.

The usual maintenance dose of magnesium sulfate is 2 g per hour. Patients who have had a seizure should have a Foley catheter placed. If their urine output is adequate they will not become toxic on 2 g per hour of magnesium sulfate. Often, however, eclamptic patients have renal involvement of their disease, and this results in a decreased creatinine clearance and a diminished urine output. These patients must be watched carefully using serum magnesium levels to make certain that they do not become magnesium toxic. Severe magnesium toxicity may lead to apnea and cardiac arrest because of electrical-mechanical disassociation.

Although magnesium sulfate is the treatment of choice for eclampsia, it is *not* the only appropriate anticonvulsant. If magnesium sulfate is not readily available, the physician should use whatever medications are customarily used in the treatment of acute seizures. Diazepam and the other benzodiazepines can be used to treat seizures acutely until the patient can be transported to a labor floor and treated appropriately for eclampsia. Diazepam, in large doses, can lead to maternal and neonatal respiratory depression and loss of beat-to-beat variability in the fetal heart rate tracing. This may lead the physician to a false diagnosis of fetal distress.

If the patient's family gives a history of epilepsy, she should be treated with the parenteral form of the medication she has been taking. Carbamazepine, which is commonly used to treat epilepsy during gestation, is not available in a parenteral form. If this is the patient's customary anticonvulsant, however, phenobarbital can be used to control the seizures until the patient is able to take and absorb oral medications. Then she can be restarted on carbamazepine. If the etiology of the seizures is uncertain, phenytoin may be used to treat patients acutely. The usual loading dose is 10 to 15 mg/kg pregnancy weight given intravenously over an hour. The patient should be placed on a cardiac monitor while the phenytoin is being administered. Subsequently, the patient should be given 200 mg either orally or intravenously beginning 12 hours after the bolus. This dosage regimen also has been used successfully to treat eclampsia.[75]

The fetus must also be attended. Fetal heart tones must be auscultated. Often during a tonic/clonic seizure the fetus will experience an episode of bradycardia. The initial response may be to rush the mother to the operating room and perform an emergency cesarean section to save the fetus. This approach has several hazards. Needless to say, performing major surgery and administering an anesthetic to the unstable mother can be life-threatening to her. Furthermore, until the gestational age of the fetus has been documented, a previable fetus may be delivered. During the 15 minutes following a seizure, the fetus will often regain a normal fetal heart rate. This is especially true if the mother is well oxygenated and placed on her left side so that the uterus is not compressing the inferior vena cava. Patience and vigilance therefore must be used when evaluating the fetus after a maternal seizure.

Occasionally, a seizure will lead to placental abruption, which will necessitate fetal delivery to ensure both fetal and maternal well-being. In these instances the uterus will usually be very hard with a tetanic contraction. Most women in this situation experience vaginal bleeding. Usually, both mother and fetus can be stabilized so that the mother can be transferred to a labor floor where she can be further evaluated.

REFERENCES

1. Aaro LA, Jergens JL. Thrombophlebitis associated with pregnancy. Am J Obstet Gynecol 17:165, 1974
2. Villa Santa U. Thromboembolic disease in pregnancy. Am J Obstet Gynecol 93:142, 1965
3. Barritt DW, Jorden SC. Anticoagulant drugs in the treatment of pulmonary embolism: a controlled trial. Lancet 1:1309, 1960
4. Mogensen K, Skibsted L, Wadt J, Nissen F. Thrombectomy of acute iliofemoral venous thrombosis during pregnancy. Surg Gynecol Obstet 169:50, 1989
5. Stiller RJ, Leone-Tomaschoff S, Cuteri J, Beck L. Postpartum pulmonary embolus as an unusual cause of cortical blindness. Am J Obstet Gynecol 162:696, 1990
6. Stein LB, Robert RI, Marx J, Rossoff L. Transient cortical blindness following an acute hypotensive event in the postpartum period. NY State J Med 89:682, 1989
7. Girz BA, Heiselman DE. Fatal intrapartum pulmonary embolus during tocolysis. Am J Obstet Gynecol 158:145, 1988
8. Bonebarak CR, Noller KL, Loehnen CP et al. Routine chest roentgenography in pregnancy. JAMA 240:2747, 1978
9. Swartz HM, Reichling BA. Hazards of radiation exposure for pregnant women. JAMA 239:1907, 1978
10. Wagner LF, Lester RG, Saldena LR. Exposure of the pregnant patient to diagnostic radiations: a guide to medical management, p 11. Philadelphia: JB Lippincott, 1985
11. Macus CS, Mason GR, Kuperus JH, Mena I. Pulmonary imaging in pregnancy: maternal risk and fetal dosimetry. Clin Nucl Med 10:1, 1985
12. Ginsberg JS, Hirsh J, Rainbow AJ, Coates G. Risks to the fetus of radiologic procedures

used in the diagnosis of maternal venous thromboembolic disease. Thromb Haemost 61:189, 1989
13. Wagner LF, Lester RG, Saldena LR. Exposure of the pregnant patient to diagnostic radiations: a guide to medical management, p 69. Philadelphia: JB Lippincott, 1985
14. Qaso LA, Juergens JL. Thrombophlebitis associated with pregnancy. Am J Obstet Gynecol 109:1128, 1971
15. Gervin AS. Complications of heparin therapy. Surg Gynecol Obstet 140:789, 1975
16. Merrill LK, VerBurg DJ. The choice of long term anticoagulants for the pregnant patient. Obstet Gynecol 47:711, 1976
17. Baskin HF, Murray JM, Harris RE. Low dose heparin for the prevention of thromboembolic disease in pregnancy. Am J Obstet Gynecol 129:590, 1977
18. Stevenson R, Burton DM, Ferlavto GJ, Taylor HA. Hazards of oral anticoagulants during pregnancy. JAMA 243:1549, 1980
19. Harrod MJE, Sherrod PS. Warfarin embryopathy in siblings. Obstet Gynecol 57:673, 1981
20. Belgvad S, Lund O, Nielsen TT, Guldholt I. Emergency embolectomy in a patient with massive pulmonary embolism during second trimester pregnancy. Acta Obstet Gynecol Scand 68:267, 1989
21. Splinter WM, Dwane PD, Wigle RD, McGrath MJ. Anaesthetic management of emergency cesarean section followed by pulmonary embolectomy. Can J Anaesth 36:689, 1989
22. Hernandez E, Angell CS, Johnson JWG. Asthma in pregnancy: current concepts. Obstet Gynecol 55:739, 1980
23. Weinstein AM, Dubin BD, Podleski WK, Spector SL, Raff RS. Asthma and pregnancy. JAMA 241:1161, 1979
24. Corre KA, Rothstein RJ. Assessing severity of adult asthma and need for hospitalization. Ann Emerg Med 14:45, 1985
25. Turner ES, Greenberger PA, Patterson R. Management of the pregnant asthmatic. Ann Intern Med 14:588, 1988
26. Stenius-Aarniala B, Pririla P, Teramo K. Asthma and pregnancy: a prospective study of 198 pregnancies. Thorax 43:12, 1988
27. Schatz M, Harden KM, Forsythe a et al. The course of asthma during pregnancy, postpartum, and with successive pregnancies: a prospective analysis. J Allergy Clin Immunol 81:509, 1988
28. Gluck JC, Cluck PA. The effects of pregnancy on asthma: a prospective study. Ann Allergy 37:164, 1976
29. Bahna SL, Bjerkedal T. The course and outcome of pregnancy in women with bronchial asthma. Acta Allergy 27:397, 1972
30. Mabie WC, Barton JR, Wasserstrum N, Sibai BM. Clinical observations on asthma in pregnancy. J Matern Fetal Med 1:45, 1992
31. Gordon M, Niswander KR, Berendes H, Kantor AG. Fetal morbidity following potentially anoxigenic obstetric conditions: bronchial asthma. Am J Obstet Gynecol 106:421, 1970
32. Gelber M, Sidi Y, Gassner S, et al. Uncontrollable life-threatening status asthmaticus: an indicator for termination of pregnancy by cesarean section. Respiration 46:320, 1984
33. Scoggins CH, Sahn SA, Petty TL. Status asthmaticus: a nine-year experience. JAMA 238:1158, 1977
34. Weinberger SE, Weiss ST, Cohen WR, Weiss JW, Johnson TS. Pregnancy and the lung. Am Rev Respir Dis 121:559, 1980
35. Greenberger PA, Patterson R. Managing of asthma during pregnancy. N Engl J Med 313:518, 1985

36. Woolcock AJ. Asthma. In Murray JF, Nadel JA (eds): Textbook of respiratory medicine, p 1030. Philadelphia: WB Saunders, 1988
37. McFadden ER, Kiser R, de Groot WJ. Acute bronchial asthma: relations between clinical and physiologic manifestations. N Engl J Med 288:221, 1973
38. Hankins DV, Cunningham FG. Asthma complicating pregnancy. In Cunningham FG, MacDonald P, Gant N (eds): Williams Obstetrics. Appleton & Lange 1991:Supplement 15
39. Corre KA, Rothstein RJ. Assessing severity of adult asthma and need for hospitalization. Ann Emerg Med 14:45, 1985
40. Noble PW, Lavee AE, Jacobs NM. Respiratory diseases in pregnancy. Obstet Gynecol Clin North Am 15:391, 1988
41. Chapman KR, Verbeek PR, White JG, Rebuck AS. Effect of a short course of prednisone in the prevention of early relapse after the emergency room treatment of acute asthma. N Engl J Med 324:788, 1991
42. Littenberg B, Gluck EH. A controlled trial of methylprednisolone in the emergency treatment of acute asthma. N Engl J Med 314:150, 1986
43. Fanta CH, Rossing TH, McFadden ER. Emergency room treatment of asthma: relationships among therapeutic combinations, severity of obstruction and time course of response. Am J Med 72:416, 1982
44. Greenberger PA, Patterson R. The outcome of pregnancy complicated by severe asthma. Allergy Proc 9:539, 1988
45. Fitzsimons R, Greenberger PA, Patterson R. Outcome of pregnancy in women requiring corticosteroids for severe asthma. J Allergy Clin Immunol 78:349, 1986
46. Marx CM, Fraser DG. Treatment of asthma in pregnancy. Obstet Gynecol 57:766, 1981
47. Carter BL, Criscoll CE, Smith GD. Theophylline clearance during pregnancy. Obstet Gynecol 68:555, 1986
48. Hankins GDV. Acute pulmonary injury and respiratory failure during pregnancy. In Clark SL, Phelan JP, Cotton DB (eds): Critical Care Obstetrics, p 290. Oradell, NJ: Medical Economics Books, 1987
49. Mestman, J. Severe hyperthyroidism in pregnancy. In Clark SL, Phelan JP, Cotton DB (eds): Critical Care Obstetrics, p 262. Oradell, NJ: Medical Economics Books, 1987
50. Saltman RJ, Goldberg AC. Endocrine and lipid disorders. In Dunagan WC, Ridner ML (eds): Manual of Medical Therapeutics, 26th ed. Boston: Little, Brown, 1989
51. Ingbar SH, Woeber KA. Diseases of the thyroid. In Petersdorf RG, Adams RD, Braunwald E, Isselbacher KJ, Martin JB, Wilson JD (eds): Harrison's Principles of Internal Medicine, 10th ed. New York: McGraw-Hill, 1983
52. Gabbe SG, Mestman JH, Hibbard LT. Maternal mortality in diabetes mellitus: an 18-year survey. Obstet Gynecol 48:549, 1976
53. Drury MI, Greene AT, Stronge JM. Pregnancy complicated by clinical diabetes mellitus: a study of 600 pregnancies. Obstet Gynecol 49:519, 1977
54. Richards SR, Klingelberger CE. Intravenous ritodrine as a possibly provocative predictive test in gestational diabetes: a case report. J Reprod Med 32(10):798, 1987
55. Tibaldi JM, Lorber DL, Nerenberger A. Diabetic ketoacidosis and insulin resistance with subcutaneous terbutaline infusion: a case report. Am J Obstet Gynecol 163(2):509, 1990
56. Bernstein IM, Catalano PM. Ketoacidosis in pregnancy associated with the parenteral administration of terbutaline and betamethasone. A case report. J Reprod Med 35(8):818, 1990
57. Rhodes RW, Ogburn PL, Jr. Treatment of severe diabetic ketoacidosis in the early third trimester in a patient with fetal distress. A case report. J Reprod Med 29:621, 1984
58. Hughes AB. Fetal heart rate changes during diabetic ketosis. Acta Obstet Gynecol Scand 66:713, 1987

59. Ramsay RE, Strauss RG, Wilder J, Wilmore LJ. Status epilepticus in pregnancy: effect of phenytoin malabsorption on seizure control. Neurology 28:85, 1978
60. So EL, Penry JK. Epilepsy in adults. Ann Neurol 9:3, 1978
61. Gjerde IO, Strandjord RE, Ulstein M. The course of epilepsy during pregnancy: a study of 78 cases. Acta Neurol Scand 78:198, 1988
62. Bardy AH, Hiilesmaa VK, Teramo KA. Serum phenytoin during pregnancy, labor and puerperium. Acta Neurol Scand 75:374, 1987
63. Nakane Y, Okuma T, Takashishi R et al. Multi-institutional study on the teratogenicity and foetal toxicity of anti-epileptic drugs: a report of a collaborative study group in Japan. Epilepsia 21:663, 1980
64. Hanson JW, Myrianthopoulos NC, Sedgwick MA et al. Risks to the offspring of women treated with hydantoin anticonvulsants, with emphasis on the fetal hydantoin syndrome. J Pediatr 89:662, 1976
65. Nagy R. Fetal hydantoin syndrome. Arch Dermatol 117:593, 1981
66. Committee on Drugs, American Academy of Pediatrics. Anticonvulsants and pregnancy. Pediatrics 63:331, 1979
67. Shapiro S, Sloan D, Hartz SC et al. Are hydantoins (phenytoins) human teratogens? J Pediatr 90:673, 1977
68. Bartoshesky LE, Bhan I, Nagpul K, Pashyan H. Severe cardiac and ophthalmologic malformation in an infant exposed to diphenylhydantoin in utero. Pediatrics 69:202, 1982
69. Jones KL, Larco RV, Johnson KA, Adams J. Pattern of malformations in the children of women treated with carbamazepine during pregnancy. N Engl J Med 320:1661, 1989
70. Kallen B, Robert E, Mastroiacova P et al. Anticonvulsant drugs and malformations: is there a drug specificity? Eur J Epidemiol 5:31, 1989
71. Chitayat D, Farrell K, Anderson L, Hall JG. Congenital abnormalities in two sibs exposed to valproic acid in utero. Am J Med Genet 31:369, 1988
72. Tsuru N, Maeda C, Tsuruoka M. Three cases of delivery under sodium valproate-placental transfer, milk transfer and probable teratogenicity of sodium valproate. Jpn J Psychiatr Neurol 42:89, 1988
73. Gedekoh RH, Hayashi TT, McDonald HM. Eclampsia at Magee-Women's Hospital, 1970–1980. Am J Obstet Gynecol 140:860, 1981
74. Pritchard JA, Cunningham FG, Pritchard SA. The Parkland memorial protocol for the treatment of eclampsia: evaluation of 245 cases. Am J Obstet Gynecol 148:951, 1984
75. Ryan G, Lange IR, Naugler MA. Clinical experience with phenytoin prophylaxis in severe preeclampsia. Am J Obstet Gynecol 161:1297, 1989

CHAPTER 2

Acute Abdominal Pain in Pregnancy

Richard Boothby

The pregnant patient with acute abdominal pain poses a difficult diagnostic challenge. In the United States approximately 0.2% to 2.2% of all pregnancies are complicated by surgical intervention other than cesarean section.[1] Approximately 50,000 pregnant women have surgery for nonobstetric causes each year.

Altered anatomy, physiology, and potential risk to mother and fetus contribute to confusion and delay in diagnosis of surgical disorders during pregnancy. It is important therefore to involve the obstetrician and general surgeon early in the evaluation of all pregnant patients with acute abdominal pain.

This chapter reviews the most frequent causes of abdominal pain during pregnancy. In general, the approaches to both the pregnant and nonpregnant patient with acute abdominal pain should be similar. When deciding which test to order, the risks to mother and fetus should be weighed against the obtainable information and whether that information will affect selection of treatment. Most radiographic or invasive diagnostic procedures carry little risk to mother or fetus and should be performed if they are necessary for the diagnosis.

Delay in diagnosis in pregnant women can occur because the normal anatomic and physiologic changes of pregnancy can obscure symptoms of disease.[2] The enlarging uterus can displace intra-abdominal organs, masking symptoms usually seen in the lower abdomen. Physical signs may be localized to altered locations. Pain from stretching uterine ligaments can be severe and confused with nonobstetric causes.

During normal pregnancy total circulating blood volume expands rapidly.[3]

Plasma expansion is more pronounced than red cell expansion, resulting in a mild dilutional decrease in hemoglobin and hematocrit. The total white blood cell (WBC) count increases from nonpregnant levels of 5000 to 6000 cells/mm^3 to 12,000 cells/mm^3. Other pregnancy-induced changes in the cardiovascular system include increases in cardiac output, pulse rate, and peripheral blood flow.

Renal function also undergoes major physiologic changes during pregnancy. Paralleling the increases in blood volume and cardiac output, there are increases in glomerular filtration rate (GFR) and renal plasma flow (RPF). This results in a decrease in blood urea nitrogen (BUN) and serum creatinine levels during pregnancy. Glucosuria can be seen during pregnancy despite normal blood glucose levels and is thought to be related to augmented GFR, which results in a filtered load of glucose that exceeds tubular resorption capacity. Anatomic changes of the urinary tract include enlargement of the kidneys and dilation of the ureters, which can be seen as early as 21 weeks of gestation.[4]

In the respiratory tract, pregnancy causes an elevation of the diaphragms. It does not affect the respiratory rate appreciably, but tidal volume, minute ventilatory volume, and minute oxygen uptake all increase as pregnancy advances.[5] These result in an overall decrease in partial pressure of carbon dioxide (PCO_2) to approximately 31 mmHg and a slight compensatory increase in pH to around 7.44.

Pathophysiology of Abdominal Pain

Before discussing some of the specific causes of abdominal pain in pregnancy it is important to have a basic understanding of the general mechanisms of abdominal pain. Pain perceived from the abdomen is caused by peritoneal irritation, mechanical stretching, or ischemia.[2] Both chemical and bacterial contact with the peritoneal lining lead to inflammation of the peritoneum and even adjacent organs, thus causing pain. Examples of chemical irritants include gastric or pancreatic juices, blood, urine, and amniotic fluid. Bacterial contamination of the abdomen can occur as the result of intestinal perforation or abscess rupture.

Mechanical stretching of a hollow viscus, such as the intestine or ureter when obstructed, causes abdominal pain. Distention of the capsules of solid organs, such as the ovary, liver, or spleen, from hemorrhage or inflammation causes mechanical stretching pain. This visceral abdominal pain is often poorly localized owing to the overlap of visceral sensory innervation.[2] Ischemia can cause severe abdominal pain and may be due to arterial or venous thrombosis, intrinsic vascular disease, or advanced intestinal obstruction.

Common Etiologies of Abdominal Pain

The differential diagnosis of acute abdominal pain in pregnancy is similar to that of the nonpregnant patient. The signs and symptoms of each entity may be altered by pregnancy. The following section reviews the major causes of abdominal pain during pregnancy. Each section discusses the pathophysiology in detail, with emphasis on the safest diagnostic evaluation for mother and fetus.

Appendicitis

Acute appendicitis is the most common nonobstetric surgical emergency that occurs during pregnancy.[6] The incidence of appendicitis is not altered by pregnancy and ranges from one in 1000 to one in 3000 pregnant patients. Appendicitis in pregnancy carries a higher risk of perforation, probably owing to delays in diagnosis and surgery.

The acute focal stage of appendicitis begins with obstruction of the appendiceal lumen. This is caused by hypertrophy of submucosal follicles following a viral infection, fecalith, foreign body, stricture, or tumor.[7] Distention and inflammation of the appendix follow, which produce colicky visceral pain, perceived in the periumbilical area. After several hours, local inflammation of the surrounding peritoneum occurs. The pain then becomes more constant and localizes to the area where the appendix is located. In the nonpregnant patient, the appendix is located in the right lower quadrant (65%), in the pelvis (30%), or retrocecally (5%).[8] As the uterus grows during pregnancy it gradually displaces the appendix upward, so that by the third trimester the patient's pain may be located in the right upper quadrant (Fig. 2-1).

Nausea and vomiting are frequently present and related to the degree of

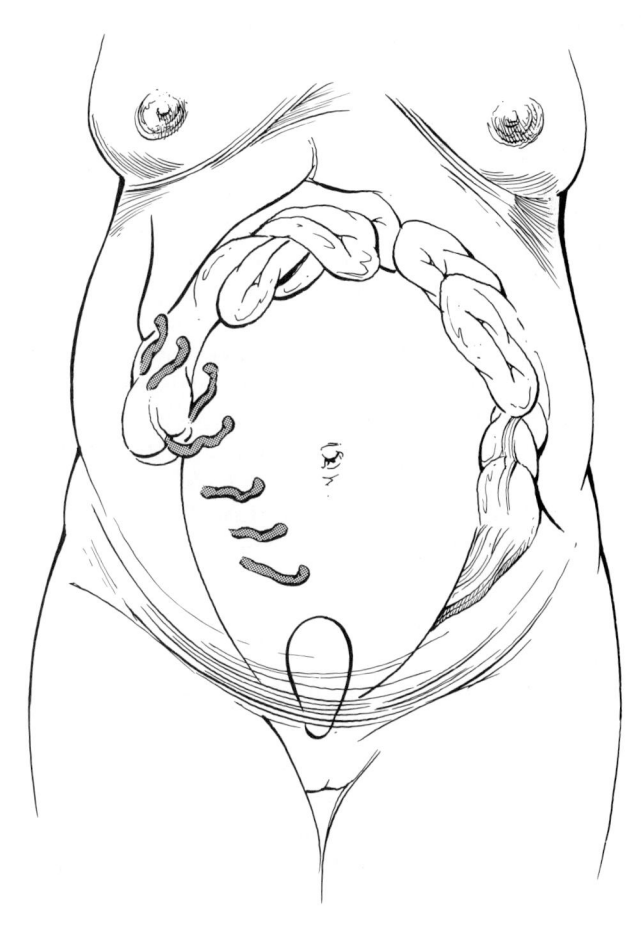

FIGURE 2-1
Changing position of appendix during pregnancy.

appendiceal distention and peritoneal irritation. Nausea is also a frequent complication of pregnancy, especially during the first trimester. The combination of abdominal pain and acute onset of nausea and vomiting in the pregnant patient must be viewed with caution.

If the inflamed appendix is in close proximity to the ureter or the urinary bladder, the patient may develop sterile pyuria or urinary frequency. Pyuria is rarely seen in nonpregnant patients with appendicitis. Anorexia, which is seen frequently in nonpregnant patients, may not always be present.

Because of the distention of the abdominal wall by the gravid uterus, it is difficult to elicit signs of rectus muscle spasm and rigidity. Auscultation of the abdomen will usually demonstrate normal active bowel sounds early in the course of acute appendicitis. As the inflammation increases, the bowel will quiet as an ileus develops. Examination of the abdomen prior to perforation generally demonstrates point tenderness over the area of the appendix. Early in gestation this is usually the right lower quadrant, but later in pregnancy it may be periumbilical or in the right upper quadrant. Pelvic examination may show cervical motion tenderness, especially on the right side. Rectovaginal examination may reveal a tender mass on the right side of the pelvis. Late in the course of appendicitis rebound tenderness can be elicited, and with rupture a true surgical abdomen may appear secondary to frank peritonitis. The physiologic leukocytosis seen in pregnancy (12,500 to 16,000/mm^3 with 80% bands) should not be confused with the leukocytosis associated with appendicitis in nonpregnant patients.

The treatment of appendicitis is always surgical. Early consultation with obstetric and surgical services in patients with suspected appendicitis is appropriate. Delay is associated with increased maternal and fetal morbidity. Diagnostic accuracy of appendicitis during pregnancy ranges from 50% to 65%.[9] Most surgeons recommend removal of the clinically normal-appearing appendix at the time of laparotomy, as very early appendicitis may not yet be grossly apparent.[10] Early exploratory laparotomy and appendectomy provide the best overall outcome. With the advent of modern anesthetic techniques, fluid and nutritional support, and antibiotics, maternal mortality has decreased substantially since the early part of this century. An early review of appendicitis in pregnancy reported a maternal mortality of 24%.[11] In recent series, occasional maternal deaths are reported and are due to delay in treatment and perforation.[12]

Modern obstetric management with the use of monitoring and tocolytic therapy has decreased the incidence of premature labor. The incidence of fetal morbidity and mortality is now quite low and is related to the severity of the appendicitis and not the surgical intervention.[2] Fetal morbidity and mortality rise sharply when perforation is present.[12]

Biliary Disease

During pregnancy the entire spectrum of biliary disease may be encountered, including acute and chronic cholecystitis, choledocholithiasis, and biliary pancreatitis. Cholecystitis and cholelithiasis occur more frequently in reproductive-age women than in men of comparable age. The incidence of acute cholecystitis during pregnancy is estimated to be approximately 0.08%.[13] In caring for pregnant patients with suspected biliary disease, the physician must choose diagnostic tests that will not harm the fetus, and operative intervention must be timed appropriately when deemed necessary.

Physiologic changes associated with pregnancy predispose to gallstone formation, which are associated with 90% of cases of cholecystitis. The other 10%, where no stones are present, are due to bile stasis and infection. There appears to be an increase in the incidence of cholecystitis during pregnancy. This is thought to be due to a combination of pregnancy-induced changes.[7] Theses changes include (1) delayed gallbladder emptying due to increased progesterone levels during gestation, (2) increased saturation of cholesterol in bile due to increased esterified and free blood cholesterol seen in pregnancy, and (3) a decrease in the bile salt pool. All these changes can predispose to new stone formation or accelerated growth of existing stones.

The incidence of acute cholecystitis increases during each trimester of pregnancy. The symptoms are similar in both the pregnant and nonpregnant state. The most characteristic symptom of acute cholecystitis in the pregnant patient is abdominal pain, which is usually abrupt in onset.[14] Pain generally begins in the midepigastrium and may radiate to the right upper quadrant, around the sides, or to the back in the region of the scapulas.[13] Nausea and vomiting may be present and can be accompanied by shaking chills.

Physical examination may show the patient's temperature to be elevated. She may have tenderness and guarding in the right upper quadrant. Generalized rebound tenderness can develop, reflecting perforation, or localized tenderness may result from abscess formation or pancreatitis.[7] The white blood count may be elevated. If there is biliary obstruction, bilirubin and liver enzymes may be elevated. Enzyme levels can be confusing during pregnancy because alkaline phosphatase of placental origin is elevated. The transaminases are usually not elevated in pregnancy. Because of the possibility of concomitant pancreatitis, an amylase level should be obtained with the initial diagnostic blood work.

An ultrasound of the gallbladder should be the first diagnostic test performed in pregnant patients with signs and symptoms of gallbladder disease. This test is 90% to 97% accurate in diagnosing gallstones and poses no risk to mother or fetus.[15] If the ultrasound is nondiagnostic, it may be necessary to perform an oral or intravenous cholecystogram. Endoscopic retrograde cholangiopancreatography and transhepatic cholangiography may be done if necessary.

Treatment for gallbladder disease during pregnancy should be conservative initially. Hospitalization with the use of intravenous fluids, nasogastric suction, and parenteral analgesics will lessen symptoms in most cases. Surgery, if contemplated electively, should be performed in the second trimester because there is less risk for spontaneous abortion and the size of the uterus does not yet pose technical difficulties with the surgery. The advent of laparoscopic cholecystectomy should prove even safer for mother and fetus. Surgery should be performed immediately if obstruction, perforation, or gangrene of the gallbladder is suspected.

A recent report suggests that for most patients conservative management is possible, and surgery can be delayed until after delivery.[14] On the other hand, others have pointed out that a conservative approach can be associated with multiple hospitalizations because of recurrent episodes of biliary tract disease, which can result in fetal loss.[16] Each case must be individualized, and management would depend on the gestational age at presentation, the frequency of repeat symptoms, and the severity of these symptoms.

Pancreatitis

Pancreatitis during pregnancy is not rare and should be considered in the differential diagnosis of any patient with hyperemesis gravidarum or those with acute abdominal pain. The incidence in pregnancy is generally lower than that in nonpregnant patients and ranges from approximately one in 1000 to one in 11,000.[17] Etiologic factors for pancreatitis in pregnancy are similar to those in nonpregnant women in that the majority of cases are secondary to gallstones. Other causes implicated include use of tetracyclines, infection, alcohol abuse, acute fatty liver, and preeclampsia.[18]

After inflammation of the pancreas develops enzymes are liberated, causing autodigestion of pancreatic tissues. A fulminating course can lead to circulatory collapse, renal compromise, and respiratory failure. Symptoms include epigastric pain, which is constant and radiates to the back. The patient may have persistent nausea and vomiting. An elevated temperature is present in approximately two thirds of patients.[19] Hypotension may be present secondary to fluid third-spacing, hemorrhage into retroperitoneum, or bowel vasodilation.

Laboratory data may demonstrate an elevated white blood cell count. Hemoglobin and hematocrit may be falsely elevated because of third-space fluid accumulation and resultant hemoconcentration. Serum amylase may be elevated and usually peaks within 6 to 12 hours of onset. The amylase/creatinine clearance ratio is accurate in the diagnosis of pancreatitis. DeVore has worked out the normal ratios expected during pregnancy.[20] The ratio ranges from 2.25% at the end of the first trimester to 2.8% at term. It is elevated in pregnancy complicated by pancreatitis and remains elevated even after the serum amylase returns to normal. Serum lipase may be elevated. Serum electrolytes and calcium should be obtained on admission to help guide fluid replacement therapy. Severe hypocalcemia can occur and is a grave prognostic sign. Hyperglycemia can be pronounced and may require insulin administration.

Clinically, the patient may appear quite ill. Examination of the abdomen may show distention. Bowel sounds may be hypoactive or absent. The patient may demonstrate tenderness or guarding in the upper abdomen. Peritoneal signs may be present.

Management of acute pancreatitis in pregnancy is supportive. Objectives of therapy include (1) prevention and treatment of shock, (2) suppression of pancreatic secretion, (3) relief of pain, (4) prevention and treatment of infection, and (5) diagnosis and treatment of surgical complications. To accomplish these objectives careful attention must be directed to fluid and electrolyte balance. Insulin is added to maintain a normal serum glucose. Invasive monitoring, including Swan-Ganz catheter placement, may be necessary, depending on the severity of the clinical situation. Suppression of pancreatic secretion is accomplished by nasogastric suction and stopping all oral intake. Appropriate analgesics are administered. Antibiotics are used to prevent infection, but tetracyclines should be avoided. Surgical complications include abscess formation, viscus perforation, acute biliary tract obstruction, rapidly enlarging pseudocyst, intestinal obstruction, spleen rupture, uncontrolled bleeding, and pulmonary effusion.[21] Each of these would require surgical intervention during pregnancy.

The severity of pancreatitis varies. Generally, it is self-limited and responds to medical management. The maternal morbidity rate is reported as 5 to 15%, but Wilkinson reported a rate of 37%.[21] Perinatal mortality correlates with the severity of maternal disease. In mild cases it should be unchanged from the normal population, but in severe cases perinatal morbidity approaches 40%.

Peptic Ulcer Disease

Peptic ulcer disease results in the formation of chronic ulcers of 1.0 mm to 1.0 cm in diameter in the duodenal bulb, postbulbar area, distal antrum, or pyloric channel of the upper gastrointestinal tract. Fortunately, active peptic ulcer disease is rare during pregnancy.[5] Pregnant patients with peptic ulcers often have a prior history of ulcer disease. Most women with peptic ulcer disease note improved symptoms during pregnancy. Two mechanisms contribute to this improvement: (1) Progesterone appears to lower gastric acid output and increases production of gastric mucus; (2) plasma histaminase synthesized by the placenta increases during pregnancy and inactivates histamine, which will decrease hydrogen ion secretion in the stomach.[7]

The most common symptom of peptic ulcer disease is midepigastric pain, described as moderate to severe cramping or burning that lasts 15 to 60 minutes. The pain is relieved by food or antacid and is exacerbated by ingestion of aspirin, coffee, or alcoholic beverages. Patients rarely experience nausea or vomiting. As erosion of vessels at the base of the ulcer occurs, patients may experience melena or hematemesis.

Physical examination is generally unremarkable except for tenderness in the midepigastrium. Laboratory data (complete blood count, serum electrolytes, and liver function tests) are generally in the normal range.

Uncomplicated peptic ulcer disease during pregnancy can be managed medically. Serious complications of peptic ulcer disease include hemorrhage from the base of the ulcer or perforation into the pancreatic bed or peritoneal cavity. Fortunately, these complications are rare in pregnancy. Diagnostic endoscopy is necessary to localize the site of bleeding and can be used to arrest blood loss with electrocoagulation. Surgery may be necessary when blood loss is massive. In such cases fetal mortality can reach 45%.[22] Obstruction can be treated conservatively with nasogastric suction for at least 72 hours, and surgery can be avoided in selected patients. Perforation may be life-threatening, and patients who present with perforation should be managed surgically. With prompt surgical management the outcome for both mother and fetus is favorable.

Intestinal Obstruction

Intestinal obstruction complicates pregnancy with a frequency of approximately one in 25,000.[23] There appear to be three periods during pregnancy when obstruction is likely. It is most common during the fourth and fifth months, when the uterus is enlarging and no longer a pelvic structure. In the third trimester, when the fetal head descends, obstruction can also occur. The immediate postpartum period, during rapid involution of the uterus, is the other likely period for obstruction to occur.

By far the most common cause of intestinal obstruction is adhesions from previous surgery.[24] Other causes in the pregnant patient are volvulus and intussusception. Incarcerated inguinal and femoral hernias are common causes in nonpregnant individuals but are rarely seen as causative factors in pregnant patients.

The symptoms of intestinal obstruction are the same in the gravid and nongravid patient: abdominal pain, vomiting, obstipation, and abdominal distention.[23] The entire symptom complex may not be present during pregnancy. Vomiting is quite common during the first trimester of pregnancy, but in the third trimester causes other than pregnancy must be considered. Constipation is common during the entire pregnancy, but obstipation should be viewed with suspicion. The degree of abdominal distention depends on the duration and level of the obstruction. Late in pregnancy, because of the overlying uterus, distention is difficult to assess.

Physical examination of the patient with intestinal obstruction may demonstrate abdominal tenderness and distention. When tenderness is present in the third trimester, early labor should be ruled out. The patient may demonstrate signs of hypovolemia secondary to vomiting or third-space losses into the intestinal lumen. Auscultation of the abdomen may reveal high-pitched hyperactive bowel sounds. Fever may be present if there is intestinal strangulation or perforation.

The leukocyte count may be elevated but may not be higher than that expected in normal pregnancy. Rapid elevation of the white blood count over a short period of time, however, is more ominous. Abdominal radiographs will show distended loops of bowel and air-fluid levels and should be performed when obstruction in pregnancy is suspected. Occasionally, a limited barium enema is necessary to clarify the site of obstruction to help plan appropriate surgical intervention.

Management of intestinal obstruction is the same in pregnant and nonpregnant patients. Their overall condition should be stabilized with adjustment of fluid and electrolyte balance. Tube decompression of the gastrointestinal tract is begun on admission. If there is evidence of intestinal perforation or strangulation, immediate surgery is indicated. In the absence of such severe complications more conservative measures are possible and surgery can be delayed while the patient is stabilized. Mechanical obstruction of the intestine may subside with conservative medical therapy. Endoscopic decompression can be attempted with large intestinal volvulus. If surgery is necessary to relieve the obstruction during pregnancy, data from available literature report a good outcome for mother and fetus.[23,24]

Urinary Tract Disorders

Acute pyelonephritis is one of the most common medical complications of pregnancy. Patients can present with a clinical picture of acute abdomen and, if unilateral, can have pain indistinguishable from that of appendicitis. Ascending bacterial infection from the urinary bladder appears to be the most common etiology.

Physiologic changes of pregnancy predispose to this condition. The enlarging uterus and enlarging ovarian veins increase pressure on the ureters at the pelvic brim. Higher circulating levels of progesterone have a relaxant effect on the smooth muscle of the ureter. These changes contribute to increased urinary stasis and predispose the pregnant patient to pyelonephritis.[5]

Symptoms of pyelonephritis in pregnancy include flank pain, urinary frequency, dysuria, and chills. When the infection is unilateral, it is more frequent on the right side. The left ureter is somewhat cushioned by the sigmoid colon, and the enlarged uterus will exert less pressure to the left collecting system. The patient may appear acutely ill and have a high fever. She may have nausea and vomiting. The clinical picture should make the diagnosis clear, but this condition can easily be confused with labor, appendicitis, placental abruption, infarction of a myoma, and, in the puerperium, an infection of the uterus or adnexa.

Physical examination of the patient with acute pyelonephritis generally demonstrates costovertebral angle tenderness on the affected side. Signs of abdominal tenderness or peritoneal irritation are generally absent except in extreme cases. The leukocyte count can be markedly elevated with a left shift. Urinalysis will demonstrate pyuria and bacteria. Urine culture will confirm the presence of bacteria.

There is general agreement that patients with acute pyelonephritis should have treatment initiated in the hospital with intravenous antibiotics. Ultimate choice of antibiotics is guided by the urine culture and sensitivity but initially should be directed at gram-negative enteric bacteria, with *E. coli* being a common isolate.

Patients may have recurrent episodes of pyelonephritis during pregnancy and, in that subgroup, consideration should be given to long-term antibiotic prophylaxis. Another group of patients that may be identified in the emergency department are those with asymptomatic bacteriuria. Twenty to 40% of these women will subsequently develop acute pyelonephritis. This risk can be almost eliminated by treating with antibiotics to eradicate the bacteria.[5]

Urinary calculi are uncommon during pregnancy. Women who have formed stones previously are at risk for forming them again. Pregnancy, however, does not appear to increase the risk.[25] Urolithiasis does not appear to have any ill effects on pregnancy except to increase the frequency of urinary tract infections.

The usual presenting symptom is flank pain, which can be intense. The pain can radiate to the groin or vulva, depending on the location of the stone. Patients may develop ureteral colic, with waves of nausea and vomiting following the pain. In the absence of infection the patient is usually afebrile.

The leukocyte count is generally normal. Examination of the abdomen is unremarkable except for flank pain in the involved side. Either microscopic or gross hematuria can be present on urinalysis. Complete radiologic work-up with an intravenous pyelogram is usually not required on initial presentation.

Treatment is usually medical and expectant, depending on the severity of symptoms. Oral fluid hydration and administration of analgesics are generally all that is required. Stones will usually pass spontaneously.[26] Antibiotics will be necessary if infection is present. Surgery during pregnancy is rarely indicated except in the presence of unilateral obstruction or refractory infection. The use of lithotripsy during pregnancy has not been reported.

Ovarian Tumors

Ovarian tumors may complicate pregnancy with a frequency of approximately one in 1000.[27] These masses are generally asymptomatic but can cause abdominal pain when torsion or rupture occurs or if they continue to enlarge during the second trimester. A mass greater than 6 cm or a symptomatic mass of any size should be considered significant and requires attention.

During the first trimester the most common cause of ovarian enlargement is the corpus luteum. Such enlargements usually remain smaller than 6 cm, are asymptomatic, and disappear by the second trimester. Occasionally, they may persist, enlarge, and produce symptoms.

Neoplastic ovarian masses can arise at any time during pregnancy. A large review of 164 ovarian neoplasms during pregnancy found that 27% were benign cystic teratomas, 23% were mucinous cystadenomas, and 18% were benign serous tumors. Only 2.4% of these ovarian neoplasms were malignant.[28]

During pregnancy adnexal torsion occurs in 10% to 15% of ovarian masses.[29] Most cases of torsion occur during early pregnancy, or the puerperium, when the uterus is changing size rapidly. Rupture of ovarian masses can occur at any time but is less common than torsion.

Acute abdominal pain is the usual presenting complaint of pregnant patients with torsion or rupture. Pain resulting from torsion is often crampy and intermittent and may radiate to the flank or thigh. Patients may experience nausea and vomiting. When rupture occurs the pain is usually sudden in onset and constant because of peritoneal irritation.

Physical examination may demonstrate a tender mass palpable in the lower quadrant, depending on the size of the mass and the gestational age. With rupture peritoneal signs may be present, especially in the case of dermoid cysts, which can produce a severe chemical peritonitis. Pelvic examination may show cervical motion tenderness.

The patient is usually afebrile. The white blood count can be normal or slightly elevated. If any bleeding from the cyst has occurred, the hemoglobin may be decreased. In extreme cases bleeding can be brisk and cause a hemoperitoneum and hypovolemic shock. Pelvic and abdominal ultrasound may be helpful in documenting the presence of an adnexal mass, especially in an advanced gestation, when the uterus is large. Laparoscopy can be helpful in distinguishing torsion or rupture from an ectopic pregnancy in the first trimester but should be discouraged in advanced pregnancy.

Treatment of ovarian torsion is surgical. When not treated promptly, torsion can result in ischemia, gangrene, and generalized peritonitis. Excision of the affected tube and ovary is generally required. Clamping of the ovarian vascular pedicle prior to untwisting the torsion is recommended to prevent embolization of thrombus from the ovarian veins (see Chap. 20).

In some cases, ovarian cyst rupture can be treated expectantly, depending upon the patient's clinical condition. Surgery can be avoided if the mass resolves after rupture and the patient is hemodynamically stable. Those patients that require surgery can often be managed conservatively with cystectomy and ovarian reconstruction when the histology is benign. With the advent of advanced pelviscopy, this can now be accomplished with the laparoscope in selected cases.

The outcome is generally good for both mother and fetus in all but the most severe cases. Maternal deaths, however, have been reported following rupture of dermoid cysts during pregnancy.[30]

History and Physical Examination

Although diagnosing the cause of abdominal pain during pregnancy can be perplexing, the physician in an emergency setting can formulate a working differential diagnosis with a careful history and physical examination. Then, with appropriate consultation from obstetric and surgical services, prompt and appropriate management can usually assure fetal and maternal well-being.

The pregnant patient, like any patient presenting to the emergency department, requires a rapid assessment of her overall condition to determine the pace of further diagnostic and, ultimately, therapeutic interventions. A patient in shock with abdominal pain must be stabilized and may require immediate exploratory surgery without an extensive diagnostic work-up. Shock during pregnancy is usually caused by hemorrhage or sepsis. The most common cause of hemorrhagic shock in pregnancy is a ruptured ectopic pregnancy.[2] Other causes of hemorrhage during pregnancy include rupture of an ovarian cyst, placenta percreta,[31] rupture of the spleen (usually secondary to trauma), or gastrointestinal hemorrhage due to ulcer disease or malignancy. Sepsis in pregnancy is usually due to untreated pyelonephritis, or chorioamnionitis.

Fortunately, most pregnant patients with abdominal pain do not present in shock. In these patients a careful history will be helpful to establish the cause of abdominal pain. The character and onset of the pain are important factors. Pain of sudden onset suggests rupture of an abdominal organ, such as perforation of an inflamed appendix, duodenal ulcer, or ovarian cyst. Acute abdominal pain can also be caused by the sudden torsion of an ovarian cyst. When abdominal pain has been building slowly over a period of time, obstruction of the intestine or ureter, or an inflammatory process may be the cause.

The character of the pain also helps determine the etiology. Sharp, stabbing pain suggests perforation of a viscus, torsion of an ovarian cyst, or a localized inflammatory process. Dull, periodic pain is more commonly seen with obstructive processes.

Location of the pain can be helpful but must be evaluated in light of the patient's stage of gestation. The pain from appendicitis will localize to the right lower quadrant early in pregnancy, but in the last trimester it may be seen in the upper quadrant (see Fig. 2-1). Generalized abdominal pain suggests diffuse peritonitis, as can be seen with a ruptured appendiceal abscess, a ruptured ovarian cyst, or intraabdominal hemorrhage. Pain that is perceived in the suprapubic area or pelvis is usually due to disease of the lower urinary tract or reproductive organs.[2]

The duration of the pain or a history of previous episodes can help diagnose an acute or chronic process and determine the urgency needed to proceed with further diagnostic tests and treatment.

A carefully collected history should also include any symptoms associated with the pain. Symptoms of nausea, vomiting, diarrhea, constipation, and anorexia can be associated with abdominal pain but may also be seen in normal pregnancy.

As the history is obtained, the physician should begin to formulate a differential diagnosis and thus be able to focus the physical examination and subsequent diagnostic tests. By the time the physical examination begins, the physician will have already assessed the overall status of the patient and know how urgently to proceed. A complete general physical examination is performed and in pregnancy in the second and third trimesters should include an attempt to auscultate fetal heart sounds and to establish how the fetus is reacting to these altered maternal events.

Examination of the abdomen should be performed carefully and begin with an overall inspection. The presence of abdominal scars indicates previous surgery, which raises the possibility of intestinal obstruction secondary to surgical adhesions. In early pregnancy the abdomen can be evaluated for distention, but in advanced pregnancy the enlarged uterus may obscure this sign.

Auscultation of the abdomen should generally be performed next, prior to palpation. Hypoactive bowel sounds can be indicative of an ileus, which can be caused by a diffuse inflammatory process or advanced obstruction. Hyperactive bowel sounds that come in rushes can be seen in early intestinal obstruction.

Palpation should be performed carefully and methodically. This part of the examination will usually yield the most diagnostic information. Diffuse peritonitis is manifested by pain with movement of the patient or movement of any intraabdominal organ, particularly the uterus. Patients with peritonitis usually lie very still and do not move, because this elicits pain. A rigid abdomen usually accompanies peritonitis and indicates a true surgical emergency. The patient will usually not allow the examination to proceed much beyond this point because of the extreme discomfort.

In patients without peritonitis the location of tenderness may help determine the etiology of the pain. It is usually best to begin at the least tender area and work to the area of greatest tenderness. Understanding the anatomic changes associated with pregnancy is important when evaluating point tenderness. Upper abdominal pain can be due to gallbladder disease, peptic ulcer disease, pancreatitis, or high-level intestinal obstruction. Upper abdominal pain can also reflect pulmonary disease, such as pneumonia or pleural irritation. Disease of the appendix, colon, urinary tract, or reproductive organs may all produce lower abdominal pain.

Palpation also allows the physician to estimate uterine size and gestational age. Early in pregnancy abdominal masses can be palpated, but as pregnancy advances, masses other than the uterus are difficult to assess.

A pelvic and rectovaginal examination should be performed in all pregnant patients with abdominal pain *except* those with third-trimester bleeding. In patients with third-trimester bleeding the location and status of the placenta must be established prior to any vaginal examination. Bimanual examination will help determine the presence of adnexal masses. A unilateral mass with tenderness could indicate torsion or rupture of an ovarian cyst. Cervical motion tenderness can be another sign of generalized peritonitis during pregnancy. It is not a sign of pelvic inflammatory disease. It is a sign of peritoneal inflammation regardless of cause. Rectovaginal exam allows the physician to evaluate the posterior cul-de-sac more fully.

Diagnostic Testing

Upon completion of the history and physical examination the physician should have a working differential diagnosis. With this information appropriate diagnostic tests are ordered. Baseline laboratory data useful in evaluating the pregnant patient with abdominal pain include a complete blood count, serum glucose and electrolytes, blood urea nitrogen, creatinine, and urinalysis. During pregnancy it is also important to obtain the patient's blood type and Rh factor. In patients with upper abdominal pain where a hepatobiliary or pancreatic etiology is suspected, liver enzymes and serum amylase levels would be helpful. Other laboratory tests should be individualized according to the specific clinical situation.

Conventional radiography, ultrasonography, and computerized tomography (CT) scanning can all be used when evaluating the pregnant patient. Plain flat and upright abdominal films can detect free air under the diaphragm, denoting a ruptured viscus. The intestinal gas pattern can show the presence or absence of obstruction. When pulmonary or thoracic disease is suspected, chest films can be obtained with abdominal shielding. The amount of radiation exposure to the fetus should be limited as much as possible, but a roentgenogram needed to make the diagnosis should be obtained.

Perhaps the most useful and safest imaging technique that can be used during pregnancy is ultrasonography. This is very useful in the diagnosis of gallstones. This technique allows the kidneys and ureters to be imaged quite clearly. Localized fluid collections in the abdominal cavity (abscess, hematoma, and ascites) can be readily identified. In the pelvis ultrasound can provide information on the age of gestation and status of the fetus. The character of adnexal masses (cystic or solid) can be determined.

CT scanning has limited indications when evaluating the pregnant patient with abdominal pain. In patients where an abscess is suspected it may be more accurate than sonography. In most instances a plain film will provide the diagnostic information necessary to make the diagnosis and exposes the mother and fetus to less irradiation.

It is a good policy to obtain consultation from an obstetrician on all pregnant patients with abdominal pain. Most patients will have obstetrically related pain, and the obstetrician can help identify that group. Further diagnostic testing can be streamlined with the help of the obstetric service. If the pregnancy is far enough along, the status of the fetus can be determined with ultrasound or fetal monitoring available from obstetrics. If there is no obstetric service in the hospital where the patient presents and she is past the first trimester and is stable, then consideration should be given to transfer the patient to a hospital with obstetric capabilities. In those patients with apparent surgical causes for their abdominal pain, early consultation from general surgery is also recommended. Because of the complexities involved in evaluating both mother and fetus and the potential for severe complications associated with delay in diagnosis and treatment, a multidisciplinary approach to the care of these patients is required.

The following are some key points:

Do not allow the presence of the fetus to delay the decision to perform necessary diagnostic testing and initiating therapy.
Do obtain early consultation from obstetric and surgical services when possible.
Do *not* perform a vaginal examination in a patient with third-trimester bleeding until the placenta is evaluated.
Do perform a bimanual rectovaginal examination on all other pregnant women with abdominal pain.

Do understand that morbidity and mortality for mother and fetus increase with delayed diagnosis.

REFERENCES

1. Brodsky JB, Cohen EN, Brown BW et al. Surgery during pregnancy and fetal outcome. Am J Obstet Gynecol 138:1165, 1980
2. Rubin S. Acute abdominal pain in pregnancy. In Benrubi G (ed): Obstetric Emergencies. New York: Churchill Livingstone, 1990
3. Brinkman CR. Biologic adaptation in pregnancy. In Creasy RK, Resnik R (eds): Maternal-Fetal Medicine: Principles and practice, p 734. Philadelphia: WB Saunders, 1989
4. Schulman A, Herlinger H. Urinary tract dilatation in pregnancy. Br J Radiol 48:638, 1975
5. Pritchard JA, MacDonald PC, Gant NF. Medical and surgical illness during pregnancy and the puerperium. In Williams Obstetrics, 17th ed. Norwalk, CT: Appleton & Lange, 1985
6. Gomez A, Wood W. Acute appendicitis during pregnancy. Am J Surg 137:180, 1979
7. DeVore GR. Acute abdominal pain in the pregnant patient due to pancreatitis, acute appendicitis, cholecystitis or peptic ulcer disease. Clin Perinatol 7:349, 1980
8. Babaknia A, Parsa M, Woodruff JD. Appendicitis during pregnancy. Obstet Gynecol 50:40, 1977
9. Frisenda R, Roty AR, Kilway JB, Brown AL, Pedlen M. Acute appendicitis during pregnancy. Am Surg 45:503, 1979
10. Cunningham GF, McCubbin JH. Appendicitis complicating pregnancy. Obstet Gynecol 45:415, 1975
11. Balbur EA. Perforative appendicitis complicating pregnancy. JAMA 51:1310, 1908
12. Horowitz MD, Gomez GA, Santiesteban R, Burkett G. Acute appendicitis during pregnancy. Arch Surg 120:1362, 1985
13. Hill LM, Johnson CE, Lee RA. Cholecystectomy in pregnancy. Obstet Gynecol 46:291, 1975
14. Hiatt JR, Hiatt JG, Williams RA, Klein SR. Biliary disease in pregnancy: strategy for surgical management. Am J Surg 151:263, 1986
15. Wengert PA, Metzger PP, Ecker HA et al. The use of ultrasonography in the diagnosis of calculus gallbladder disease. Am Surg 45:439, 1979
16. Dixon NP, Faddis DM, Silberman H. Aggressive management of cholecystitis during pregnancy. Am J Surg 154:292, 1987
17. Corlett RC, Mishell DR. Pancreatitis in pregnancy. Am J Obstet Gynecol 113:281, 1972
18. Berk JE, Smith BH, Akrawi MM. Pregnancy pancreatitis. Am J Gastroenterol 56:216, 1971
19. Jouppila P, Mokke R, Teuvo KI. Acute pancreatitis in pregnancy. Surg Gynecol Obstet 139:879, 1974
20. DeVore GR, Bracken M, Berkowitz RL. The amylase/creatinine clearance ratios in normal pregnancy and pregnancies complicated by pancreatitis, hyperemesis gravidarum, and toxemia. Am J Obstet Gynecol 136:747, 1980
21. Wilkinson EJ. Acute pancreatitis in pregnancy: a review of 98 cases and report of 8 new cases. Obstet Gynecol Surv 28:281, 1973
22. Becker-Anderson H, Husfeld V. Peptic ulcer in pregnancy. Acta Obstet Gynecol Scand 50:391, 1971
23. Hill LM, Symmonds RE. Small bowel obstruction in pregnancy: a review and report of four cases. Obstet Gynecol 49:170, 1977

24. Beck WW. Intestinal obstruction in pregnancy. Obstet Gynecol 43:374, 1973
25. Coi FL, Parks JH, Lindheimer MD. Nephrolithiasis during pregnancy. N Engl J Med 298:324, 1978
26. Strong DW, Murchison PJ, Lynch DF. The management of ureteral calculi during pregnancy. Surg Gynecol Obstet 146:604, 1978
27. Roberts JA. Management of gynecologic tumors during pregnancy. Clin Perinatol 10:369, 1983
28. Buttery BW, Beischer NA, Fortune DW et al. Ovarian tumors in pregnancy. Med J Aust 1:345, 1973
29. Disaia PJ, Creasman WT. Clinical Gynecologic Oncology. St Louis: CV Mosby, 1984
30. Mehra U, O'Conner T, Ostapowicz F et al. Pregnancy with bilateral ruptured benign cystic teratomas. Am J Obstet Gynecol 124:361, 1983
31. Archer GE, Furlong LA. Acute abdomen caused by placenta percreta in the second trimester. Am J Obstet Gynecol 157:146, 1987

CHAPTER 3

Ectopic Pregnancy

Hugh D. Wolcott, Richard J. Stock, and Andrew M. Kaunitz

Ectopic pregnancy is defined as implantation of the fertilized ovum or blastocyst anywhere other than in a normal uterine cavity. This includes tubal pregnancies in the ampullary, infundibular, isthmic, and interstitial portions of the oviduct as well as nontubal pregnancies involving the ovary; in the abdominal cavity, including peritoneal, omental, hepatic, and splenic pregnancies; in the rudimentary uterine horn; in the cervix; and in foci of adenomyosis or uterine surgical defects (Fig. 3-1). Ninety-five to 97% of ectopic pregnancies are tubal. The ampulla is the most common tubal site for implantation, followed by the isthmus, the fimbria, and the interstitial area.

Abdominal pregnancies are more a reflection of poor or unavailable care and are reported to constitute as high as 10% of ectopic pregnancies in Third World countries. In the United States they make up about 0.9% of ectopic pregnancies.[1] Ovarian pregnancies reportedly can constitute up to 10% of ectopic gestations and are associated with concurrent use of an intrauterine contraceptive device in most instances.[2] Heterotopic pregnancies, in which intra- and extrauterine gestations coexist, are thought to have an incidence of one in 30,000. However, abdominal and heterotopic pregnancies are increasing in frequency, especially in relation to the newer reproductive technologies of in vitro fertilization (IVF), gamete intratubal transfer (GIFT), and embryo transfer (ET).[3]

The incidence of ectopic pregnancy has been increasing worldwide. During the last few decades the rate has nearly quadrupled in the industrialized nations.[4] In

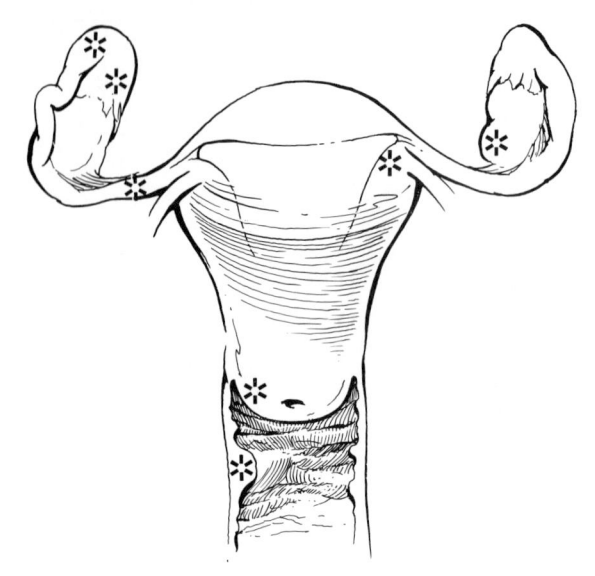

FIGURE 3–1
Sites of ectopic pregnancy.

1987 in the United States 1.7% of pregnancies were ectopic; however, complications of ectopic gestations accounted for 12% of the maternal mortality.[5] Despite the inordinate percentage of maternal deaths that ectopic gestations account for, the death rate had dropped by 1987 some 30% from 1986. Because the incidence has increased along with a shift in the population secondary to the postwar baby boom, the actual numbers have also risen. In 1970, 17,800 ectopic pregnancies were reported; this number increased to 88,000 cases in 1987.[5]

Women of minority races continue to be at greater risk for ectopic pregnancies, with the risk being 1.4 times that for white women. Although the mean age of 28 for a woman with an ectopic pregnancy has changed little since the 1930s, the risk for an ectopic gestation does increase with age. That risk is highest for those 35 to 44 years old. In contrast, the mortality rate is greatest for teenagers.[6] In this group the death rate for blacks and women of minority races was five times that of white teenagers. Eighty-five percent of deaths are secondary to hemorrhage.[1] Thirty percent of the women died at home, but about 77% had contacted a physician about their problem and 70% of those physicians were gynecologists.[1] One of the biggest problems was misdiagnosis, with the most common error being false diagnosis of gastrointestinal disorder, intrauterine pregnancy, and pelvic inflammatory disease. Seventy-five percent of the women died within 12 weeks of their last menstrual period. Of the 25% beyond 12 weeks, the ectopic sites were more often interstitial, cornual (in a rudimentary horn of a congenitally abnormal uterus), or abdominal.

Cause and Risk Factors

The fallopian tube serves a complex function in the process of fertilization and transport of the oocyte from the ovary to implantation of the blastocyst in the uterus. During the early stages of transport, the oocyte is fertilized by sperm that have ascended from the vagina through the cervix and uterus. Of the 200 to 300 million sperm deposited in the vagina, only about 200 survive for the fertilization process, which is believed to occur in the tube. At ovulation, the fimbriated end of the fallopian tube picks up the expelled oocyte with its cumulus mass of follicular cells. Entry into the tube is primarily due to a negative intraluminal pressure generated by tubal muscular contractions and ciliary flow dynamics. Conduction of the egg toward the uterus is thought to be primarily a function of muscle contractions, with a secondary contribution from ciliary beating. Completion of tubal transport takes about 3 days. Thirty hours are required to reach the ampullary-isthmic junction, where the fertilized ovum remains for an additional 30 hours. On completion of this period, the developing blastocyst begins rapid transport through the isthmus of the tube into the uterus.

Causes of ectopic implantation are unknown but may be related to the relatively aggressive nature of the human trophoblast.[7] Evidence of prior tubal disease is the single most common finding in patients with tubal ectopic pregnancies. This has been histopathologically identified in up to 95% of women with tubal gestations.

Sexually transmitted disease and pelvic inflammatory disease (PID) have also increased dramatically during the last 30 years.[8] One problem, however, has been the reliability of the nonoperative diagnosis of tubal infection. As a consequence, epidemiologic studies report very low relative risk numbers for PID in women who do have ectopic pregnancies. Conversely, for those women with laparoscopically documented salpingitis, the risk for a subsequent ectopic pregnancy is related both to the observed severity of the infection and to the number of episodes.[9] *Chlamydia trachomatis* is currently considered the most common etiologic agent in acute salpingitis. Patients with ectopic pregnancy have been found to have higher serum immunoglobulin G (IgG) titer specific for *C. trachomatis* than do controls.[10] In recent years some authors have tried to associate certain behavior with an increased risk for ectopic pregnancy, notably vaginal douching and the use of tobacco. A presumption about vaginal douching has been that it increases the risk for tubal infection. Stock could find no evidence to support that point of view.[11] In fact, vaginal douching is basically an American habit and would not explain the same increase in incidence of ectopic pregnancy identified in other industrialized nations.

Pregnancies that occur following tubal sterilization or with an intrauterine device (IUD) in place are at an increased risk for being extrauterine.[12] Following tubal sterilization, 15% to 20% of pregnancies are ectopic, with the highest incidence following tubal electrofulguration.[13] The IUD generally does not promote ectopic pregnancy, but it does prevent intrauterine pregnancy more effectively than ectopic pregnancy.[14] There is little evidence that it causes tubal infection, as was once believed. The most important factor is that if a pregnancy occurs with an IUD in place, the chance that it will be ectopic is considerably higher (about 5%) than if no intrauterine device were present. With the progesterone-containing IUD there is a significantly increased risk for an ectopic gestation.[12] Pregnancies occurring despite the use of postcoital estrogens for pregnancy interception or of progestin-only oral contraception are more likely to implant outside the uterus.[15,16] Likewise, pregnancies following the use of ovulation induction agents are at higher risk for ectopic pregnancy.[17,18] The risk of EP is also increased following tubal reconstructive surgery and the use of in vitro fertilization techniques.[19]

A host of other possible predisposing factors are linked to the occurrence of ectopic pregnancy (Table 3-1). However, up to 42% of women presenting with an ectopic pregnancy have none of these historical risk factors.[20]

TABLE 3-1
Risk Factors for Ectopic Pregnancy

Sexually transmitted disease/pelvic infection	Progesterone-only contraception
Previous surgery for ectopic pregnancy	Pelvic tuberculosis, schistosomiasis
Infertility	Intrauterine device
Tubal surgery	Tubal sterilization
Induced abortion	Ovulation induction
In vitro fertilization	Endometriosis

Clinical Presentation

The classic triad of pain, amenorrhea, and vaginal bleeding should raise a physician's suspicion of ectopic pregnancy.[21] Eighty to 100% of women later shown to have ectopic pregnancy will complain of pain.[21,22] The character of the pain is often nonspecific; it may be diffuse, unilateral, bilateral, or even contralateral to the side involved. In tubal pregnancies the pain may begin as vague lower abdominal discomfort that later becomes sharp and colicky as periodic tubal distention occurs. The pain may radiate toward the rectum or down the back of the thighs. Rupture of the tube may result in abrupt onset of sharp, shooting pain or, conversely, seeming resolution of pain because of decrease in tubal distention. Tubal rupture is often accompanied by a significant hemoperitoneum. Hemoperitoneum usually results in poorly localized abdominal pain. Shoulder pain is possible secondary to phrenic nerve irritation when blood contacts diaphragmatic surfaces. Hemoperitoneum usually results in orthostatic symptoms.

Amenorrhea is reported by 74 to 98% of patients with ectopic pregnancy. It is not unusual for a patient initially to deny having missed any periods. On careful review, however, the most recent period may be described as lighter and abnormally timed, perhaps representing pathologic bleeding from decidual slough.

Irregular vaginal bleeding seen in ectopic pregnancy is usually mild. Heavy bleeding or bleeding with clots is distinctly atypical and is more characteristic of imminent or incomplete abortion of an intrauterine pregnancy. The pain associated with an abortion is usually central and is likened to that of labor or a period. Symptoms referable to pregnancy, such as breast tenderness or nausea and vomiting, are reported in a minority of women with ectopic pregnancy. This is because most ectopic gestations are in the process of aborting and the human chorionic gonadotropin (hCG) titers are lower than that of a normal gestation of the same length of time.

The possibility of ectopic pregnancy should be considered whenever evaluating any woman of reproductive age with abdominal pain or abnormal bleeding. In the face of a prior history of an ectopic pregnancy every effort must be made to exclude a recurrence. Often the patient will volunteer the history that the symptoms are either similar to or different from those that she had with the prior ectopic gestation. If not, this line of inquiry is important.

Occasionally, a history of a recent induced abortion or assumed spontaneous abortion is given by the patient. Histopathologic diagnosis of the products of conception must be obtained if at all possible. The failure to identify placental or fetal tissues histologically may, in this setting, be the first sign that an ectopic pregnancy is present.

The physical examination of the patient with an ectopic pregnancy varies, depending on whether the gestation is early and unruptured or more advanced and ruptured with a hemoperitoneum. Orthostatic changes and narrowed pulse pressure are unusual except in the case of massive hemoperitoneum. Abdominal tenderness is the most common physical finding. The tenderness is classically unilateral and in the lower quadrant. Rebound tenderness, guarding, and rigidity are usually not present except in those cases with significant hemoperitoneum. However, absence of peritoneal signs should not be used to exclude the diagnosis of ectopic pregnancy. In one study, these were present in only 55% of ectopic gestations with hemoperitoneum.[23]

Pelvic examination reveals an adnexal mass in 50% of cases. In many patients the mass may be on the side contralateral to ectopic pregnancy, representing a corpus luteum. The uterus is usually normal or slightly enlarged in 97% of cases and is often noted to be soft secondary to the effects of placental hormones.[24] Cul-de-sac fullness may be found. This latter sign is usually associated with significant intraperitoneal bleeding. Bluish discoloration of the umbilicus (Cullen's sign) may be present with an extensive hemoperitoneum. It is not pathognomonic for ectopic gestation.

A minority of tubal pregnancies will occur with implantation in the interstitial portion of the oviduct or in the uterine cornu. These cases are often of more advanced gestational age and therefore are more likely to have the uterus enlarged to a degree consistent with an uncomplicated intrauterine pregnancy. These patients may have only vague pain and an unimpressive examination until rupture occurs, at which time they often present in shock with a massive hemoperitoneum.

Finally, it is important to appreciate that more sensitive pregnancy tests and refined imaging procedures allow physicians to diagnose ectopic pregnancy earlier. Because of this, surgical therapy has for many patients become elective rather than the acute surgical management of the past. An important distinction to be made, however, is that the patients that fall into the category of early diagnosis are usually those with high risk factors that are being closely followed by their physicians. They will most likely have had prior serum hCG titers. Patients usually presenting to emergency rooms have a spectrum of symptoms and findings.

Differential Diagnosis

The clinical presentation of a patient with ectopic pregnancy can mimic a number of other gynecologic and nongynecologic disorders (Table 3-2). Because most of these disorders are not immediately life-threatening, it is important that the clinician exclude ectopic pregnancy when considering these and other conditions in a woman of reproductive age with abdominal pain or abnormal bleeding. Conversely, ectopic pregnancy must be immediately suspected for the woman of reproductive age who presents in shock. Prompt surgical consultation is mandated under this condition.

Early confirmation of pregnancy is one of the keys to a timely diagnosis of ectopic

TABLE 3-2
Differential Diagnosis of Ectopic Pregnancy

Acute salpingitis
Threatened or incomplete abortion
Functional ovarian cyst
Ruptured corpus luteum cyst
Ovarian tumor
Appendicitis
Torsion of adnexal cyst
Endometriosis
Pelvic adhesions
Myomata uteri
Polycystic ovarian disease
Cystitis
Renal stone
Gastroenteritis

pregnancy. Confusion with other diagnostic entities, however, may occur in each of the following settings:

1. Pregnancy is not suspected in a woman with symptoms consistent with ectopic pregnancy. This can vary from ascribing the signs and symptoms to nonemergent diagnoses, such as dysfunctional uterine bleeding or salpingitis, to not considering ectopic pregnancy in a woman presenting in hemoperitoneal shock. Routine screening with a sensitive, reliable pregnancy test minimizes the risk of this type of oversight.
2. Pregnancy is confirmed in a symptomatic woman; the site of implantation, however, is not clear. As is discussed in the following section, errors in diagnosing extrauterine pregnancies as intrauterine can largely be precluded by judicious application of pelvic ultrasound, serial quantitative human chorionic gonadotropin titers, culdocentesis, and diagnostic laparoscopy. Although each of these tests has diagnostic utility, laparoscopy remains the definitive diagnostic technique today.
3. A false-negative pregnancy test is obtained in a woman with ectopic pregnancy. The confusion that often arose in this situation as recently as a few years ago has now been largely eliminated by replacing the less sensitive urine slide tests with the more sensitive urine enzyme-linked immunoabsorbent assay (ELISA) hCG tests. Some women with ectopic pregnancies, however, will have hCG titers below that which will be detected by even the sensitive urine screening tests. The likelihood of tubal rupture with a catastrophic outcome for these patients is very small. To exclude this remote possibility, a serum hCG should be obtained for the symptomatic female.

Salpingitis is one of the conditions most commonly confused with ectopic pregnancy. In differentiating between these two conditions, fever and leukocytosis are more consistent with the diagnosis of salpingitis. A negative quantitative serum hCG virtually excludes the presence of a gestation, whereas a sensitive urinary hCG in most instances excludes the diagnosis of an ectopic gestation.

Rupture or torsion of an ovarian cyst is the other condition most commonly mistaken for ectopic pregnancy. A negative sensitive pregnancy test again virtually excludes an ectopic gestation from the differential diagnosis. Intrauterine and ectopic gestations, however, may be present in the patient with a ruptured, hemorrhagic corpus luteum. To complicate this situation further, the pregnancy may be ovarian in origin. A serum hCG becomes an important element in the management of these patients.

A nonviable intrauterine pregnancy may be confused readily with ectopic gestation. Here the pregnancy test is usually positive. However, the bleeding with threatened or incomplete abortion is usually described as being much heavier than a menstrual period with clots, and the pain is often reported to be midline and crampy, usually like that of a period or labor. If the abortion is indeed inevitable or incomplete, the cervical os may be noticeably dilated with tissue and clot extruding. In five to 10% of ectopic pregnancies, a decidual cast may be shed and may be confused with products of conception associated with an incomplete abortion. All tissue passed by the patient should be examined. If the tissue is isolated from the blood clot and placed into saline, the presence of chorionic villi may be readily identified as fine, pale gray filamentous tissue. The presence of chronic villi virtually excludes the diagnosis of ectopic pregnancy. Serial quantitative serum hCG titers and vaginal sonography are used to distinguish aborting intrauterine pregnancies from ectopic pregnancy and will be discussed later.

It may be extremely difficult to distinguish between an ectopic pregnancy and a ruptured corpus luteum of pregnancy. The symptoms and signs can be similar, evidence of a hemoperitoneum can exist, and the pregnancy test will be positive. Although pelvic sonography may be able to demonstrate an intrauterine gestation, the clinical situation may mandate surgical intervention nonetheless.[25]

Other conditions commonly confused with ectopic pregnancy include appendicitis, dysfunctional uterine bleeding, and endometriosis. In the past, more tubal pregnancies were identified in the right tube than in the left. For the most part this was due to the fact that appendicitis was in the differential diagnosis. Appendicitis is also a potentially life-threatening situation. Today laparoscopy can be the definitive diagnostic tool for either of these conditions and even serve as the route for surgical treatment.

Ambulatory Evaluation and Management

Diagnostic modalities available to physicians in ambulatory settings can expedite the diagnosis of ectopic pregnancy, minimizing this condition's morbidity and mortality. Particularly distressing are findings that in more than two thirds of women dying from ectopic pregnancy, a physician had been consulted within 1 week of onset of symptoms.[26] Clearly, a high index of suspicion for ectopic pregnancy must be maintained to avoid catastrophic oversights. Therefore initial evaluation of any woman of reproductive age complaining of abdominal pain or abnormal vaginal bleeding should include a directed gynecologic history, a physical evaluation that includes a vaginal and bimanual pelvic examination, and a sensitive and rapid urine pregnancy test.

History

An appropriate interview in this setting focuses not only on the nature of the pain but also on menstrual history, sexual activity and contraceptive use, prior pregnancies, and gynecologic disease. Pain is almost a universal symptom for ectopic pregnancy, but it varies considerably in clinical presentation, owing to the duration of the gestation, the site of implantation, and the existence of rupture and hemoperitoneum. A history of amenorrhea or abnormal vaginal bleeding may be difficult to elicit in some patients. It is imperative that the timing and character of the last two to three menstrual periods be investigated through direct questioning. Often a patient will mistake the bleeding associated with endometrial sloughing secondary to a declining hCG levels, and no history of amenorrhea will be obtained. Finally, particular attention must be paid to the past obstetric and gynecologic history, particularly in regard to known risk factors for ectopic pregnancy.

Physical Examination

The physical findings in ectopic pregnancy will vary, depending on the site and duration of the gestation, on the degree of distention in a tubal pregnancy, and on whether a rupture has occurred. Orthostatic changes in pulse and blood pressure are seen only in those cases of acute hypovolemia due to significant hemoperitoneum. Abdominal tenderness is present in most patients. Rebound tenderness usually signifies hemoperitoneum, although its absence does not exclude a ruptured ectopic pregnancy.[23] Although an adnexal mass is appreciated in 38% of cases, this is contralateral to the side of ectopic implantation in 20 to 25% of cases. The uterus may be minimally enlarged, but the size is usually less than that expected for gestational age. Bluish discoloration of the cervix and vagina (Chadwick's sign) and softening of the uterus and lower segment (Hegar's sign) may be present. Fetal heart sounds may be detected in advanced ectopic gestations and should not be interpreted as being exclusive for an ectopic pregnancy.

Pregnancy Tests

A sensitive, rapid, and reliable pregnancy test is crucial in screening for ectopic pregnancy. There had been considerable confusion in the past relating to the need to identify the beta subunit of the hCG molecule and the standard of measurement.[26] The radioimmunoassay (RIA) technique served its purpose but has been replaced by the use of monoclonal antibodies and immunometric assays. These tests can be titrated against specific values of circulating hCG, so that the ratio of false-negative to false-positive values is ideal for the early diagnosis of pregnancy. The question of a unit of measurement was confusing because the first standards utilized were mixtures of biologically active hCG, free subunits, and other substances (World Health Organization's Second International Standard preparation). Subsequent standards used pure intact hCG molecules (First International Reference preparation). Although both preparations contained the same amount of intact hCG, the numerical results in terms of international units per liter were twice those of the RIA measurement against the Second International standard. It is important to understand these differences in interpreting serum titers for use of the so-called discriminatory hCG zone.

Regardless of the preceding difficulties, the newer urine tests are sensitive enough to identify pregnancy in more than 90% of women with ectopic pregnancies and require no special instrumentation or personnel training. Results are available in minutes.

Following the diagnosis of pregnancy, monitoring serial serum quantitative hCG levels in conjunction with pelvic ultrasound and clinical evaluation may in selected patients help distinguish intrauterine pregnancies from aborting intrauterine pregnancies or ectopic pregnancies. The usefulness of such monitoring follows from the observation that for a normal early intrauterine pregnancy, serum levels of hCG increase 66% or more each 48 hours.[27] In addition, for given quantitative levels a gestational sac should be detectable within the uterus by ultrasound. This was described by Kadar and colleagues and is referred to as the *discriminatory zone*.[27] Because of the previously mentioned confusion in the meaning of international units for hCG, the values used must be established by experience within a given institution.

Ultrasonography

Ultrasonography's main role in evaluating women suspected of having an ectopic pregnancy continues to be one of exclusion: visualizing an intrauterine pregnancy. With continually improved high-resolution ultrasound equipment and particularly the use of vaginal probes, intrauterine gestational sacs are being detected earlier and earlier. A sac is defined as a central sonolucency surrounded by an echogenic ring. At 5 weeks of gestation this sonolucency typically has a diameter of about 2 mm. Some authors emphasize the double decidual sac, thought to represent a distinct decidua vera and decidua capsularis, as a means of differentiating a true intrauterine gestational sac from a "pseudo-gestational sac," which has been associated with ectopic implantation.[28] Fetal heart motion should be apparent by 7 weeks gestational age.

Ultrasound is diagnostic of ectopic pregnancy only if a gestational sac can be identified and localized outside the uterus. This situation can occur in up to 62% of ectopic pregnancies when utilizing intravaginal probes with high-resolution ultrasound.[29] During the ultrasonographic evaluation of women suspected of having ectopic pregnancy, the cul-de-sac of Douglas and abdominal cavity should be evaluated. Although the presence of free blood in the cul-de-sac in the appropriate clinical setting suggests ectopic pregnancy, hemoperitoneum may also be encountered in women with a ruptured corpus luteum, spleen, or hepatic adenoma. Blood in the cul-de-sac may also be found during menses, with threatened or incomplete abortion, or after uterine curettage.

Culdocentesis

Culdocentesis, which can be performed readily in the emergency department setting, may expedite the evaluation of women suspected of having an ectopic pregnancy. This is especially true when an expeditious diagnosis is desired and sophisticated modalities such as vaginal probe ultrasound or sensitive hCG tests cannot be obtained in a timely fashion.[23] Culdocentesis entails puncturing the cul-de-sac of Douglas with a needle and aspirating its contents (Fig. 3-2). The aspirated results are usually classified into three categories: (1) positive—nonclotting blood with a hematocrit of greater than 12%; (2) negative—cul-de-sac fluid or blood-tinged fluid with a hematocrit of less than 5%; (3) nondiagnostic—no fluid or clotting blood. Culdocentesis is positive in 70% to 90% of patients with ectopic pregnancy and is negative in 2% to 17% of these cases. Even though the culdocentesis is negative or nonproductive, almost all these patients do have a hemoperitoneum at the time of surgery. Unfortunately, culdocentesis is also positive in up to 33% of those being evaluated for ectopic pregnancy who prove not to have an ectopic gestation. A nondiagnostic culdocentesis therefore should neither raise nor lower a clinician's suspicion of ectopic pregnancy.

In certain clinical situations culdocentesis may be deferred because more invasive intervention is already indicated. These situations would include patients (1) in whom extrauterine sonographic fetal heart motion is demonstrated, (2) with an acute surgical abdomen, (3) with a history of therapeutic abortion in which no chorionic villi could be demonstrated, (4) with no intrauterine gestational sac on ultrasound with a quantitative serum hCG above the discriminatory zone as determined in that institution, and (5) with an abnormal pattern of serial quantitative hCG.[30]

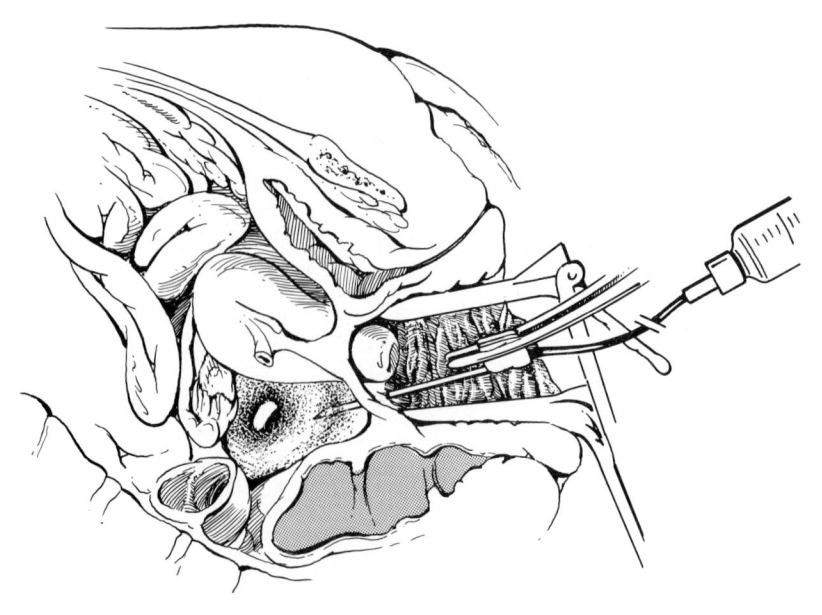

FIGURE 3-2
Technique of culdocentesi.

If clinically indicated, culdocentesis may be performed by a qualified emergency department physician without consultation from a gynecologist. The physician must be capable of performing an accurate pelvic examination and knowledgeable of the contraindications to culdocentesis. With proper precautions, culdocentesis is associated with few complications. The most common occur when the procedure is performed in the setting of a uterus adherent to the cul-de-sac or of a cul-de-sac mass. In the latter case, a remote risk exists of perforating a tubo-ovarian abscess, thereby possibly precipitating a generalized peritonitis. Concerns about contributing to peritonitis by large- or small-bowel perforation or introduction of vaginal flora are unfounded. Hemoperitoneum caused by laceration of the uterine artery or its branches can be avoided by directing the puncture downward in the midline. Before performing the procedure, the physician must discuss the technique and its indications, alternatives, benefits, and risks with the patient. The physician should allow the patient the opportunity to ask questions and answer them to her satisfaction. This should be documented in the medical record along with a procedure authorization signed by the patient and witnessed by another member of the emergency department team.

If the patient is not hypotensive, it may be useful to have her walk, stand, or sit to facilitate pooling of peritoneal fluid in the cul-de-sac. The patient is next placed in the dorsolithotomy position. A careful bimanual pelvic examination is conducted to ascertain the position of the uterus, to evaluate the adnexa for masses, and to exclude the presence of a mass in the cul-de-sac. A bivalve vaginal speculum is then inserted into the vagina to visualize the cervix and posterior fornix. With a large hemoperitoneum, the cul-de-sac occasionally will be noted to be bulging. The vaginal mucosa and cervix are then cleansed with an antiseptic solution such as povidone-iodine. At this point, consideration may be given to infiltrating the site on the cervix where the tenaculum will be placed for stabilization and traction. A solution of 1% lidocaine is adequate for this purpose. In most cases, the posterior lip of the cervix is grasped with a single-tooth tenaculum to allow visualization of the posterior aspect of the cervix and the reflection of the contiguous vaginal mucosa. If, on bimanual examination, the uterus is noted to be sharply retroverted, grasping the anterior lip of the cervix and application of gently axial traction may rotate the uterus anteriorly to allow access to the posterior cul-de-sac. On isolating the posterior reflection, a site approximately 1 cm posterior is selected and locally infiltrated with 2 to 3 mL of 1% lidocaine. A 20-gauge spinal needle is then attached to a 10- or 20-mL syringe into which 5 cc of air has been introduced. Alternatively, a "butterfly" needle can be used in conjunction with a uterine dressing forceps. This technique allows for adjustment to the pelvic curvature. At the previously infiltrated midline site, the needle is then directed downward 20° to 30° to a depth of 3 to 4 cm. Easy injection of air indicates entrance into the cul-de-sac. Once the needle is in the cul-de-sac, aspiration is performed while the needle is slowly withdrawn. It is often helpful to have the patient in a semi-Fowler's position at this time. If free-flowing fluid is encountered, a suitable sample is obtained for further studies. If no fluid at all is obtained, the cul-de-sac was not entered. After reassessing the anatomy, one or two more attempts should be made at an appropriate site using a new needle and syringe. Bloody fluid should be injected into a clot tube and into a second anticoagulated tube. Bloody fluid that clots may indicate that a vessel was inadvertently entered, whereas nonclotting blood usually indicates aspiration from an extravascular intraperitoneal source. A hematocrit of more than 15% implies hemoperitoneum; a hematocrit of less than 3% is likely to be associated with a ruptured functional ovarian cyst. Values between 3% and 15% do not exclude either condition. If the aspirated fluid appears purulent, a pelvic infection or appendicitis is likely. The fluid should then be sent for Gram stain and appropriate cultures. Mixed flora on Gram stain usually indicate the presence of a perforated bowel (appendicitis, diverticulitis).

As time and technology have progressed, the painful and invasive procedure of culdocentesis has become less important in diagnosing ectopic pregnancy. One exception to this trend is to analyze the hCG content of the aspirated peritoneal fluid. In contrast to aborting or failing intrauterine pregnancies, ectopic pregnancies are associated with quantitative values for hCG and progesterone that are almost always above the simultaneous serum values, whereas this is not seen with viable or aborting intrauterine pregnancies.

Suction Curettage

Some have recommended that uterine suction curettage be performed as an adjunct to diagnosis of ectopic pregnancy in those cases in which the pregnancy is not wanted by the patient. If chorionic villi are not present in the specimen, further investigation to exclude ectopic pregnancy might be appropriate. The value of this approach was suggested from a review of 272 patients with the initial diagnosis of spontaneous abortion who underwent suction curettage. Chorionic villi were found in 80% of the specimens. Of the 20% in whom chorionic villi could not be identified, one third proved to have ectopic pregnancy.[30]

Combining pregnancy testing and pelvic ultrasound expedites the diagnosis of ectopic pregnancy and allows the selection of those patients most likely to benefit from diagnostic laparoscopy. The concept of a discriminatory hCG zone was first described in 1981.[27] In that study the discriminatory hCG zone was defined as the level above which a normal intrauterine pregnancy should be sonographically evident. Conversely, it was postulated that the absence of an intrauterine gestational sac above this level signified ectopic pregnancy. The discriminatory zone in Kadar's series was determined to be between 6000 and 6500 mIU/mL (First International Reference Preparation). In Kadar's initial report, for those patients with values above 6000 to 6500 mIU and who were subsequently found to have an intrauterine pregnancy, an intrauterine gestational sac was noted by transabdominal sonographic examination in 94% of cases. In six of six patients with an hCG titer of more than 6500 mIU/mL and no intrauterine gestational sac, ectopic pregnancy was present. There are, however, several problems. First was the confusion regarding the units of measurement of hCG, as was explained previously; second was the fact that at least 75% of patients with ectopic gestations never attain these serum hCG levels. With the more recent introduction of vaginal probes and refined ultrasound technology, an intrauterine gestational sac can be identified much earlier when the serum titers fall more into that spectrum seen in patients with ectopic pregnancy. The concept of a "discriminatory zone" is a good one but must be defined for each institution based on the ultrasound equipment available, the experience of the physicians interpreting the ultrasound, and the correlative values of the quantitative serum hCG testing being used.[29]

As refinements continue in pelvic ultrasound technology, other pelvic anatomic changes can be defined that may lead one to a more accurate diagnosis even in lieu of quantitative hCG values. Needless to say an early intrauterine gestational sac virtually excludes an ectopic pregnancy. (An exception that constitutes a high risk for a heterotopic gestation would be a patient who underwent a form of in vitro fertilization.) On the other hand, Doppler examination of the uterotubal artery may be as diagnostic of a tubal gestation in the future as identification of the gestational sac in the tube is today.

Management

For the patient ectopic pregnancy may present as a continuum from that of minimal symptoms to irreversible shock preceding death. If the patient appears to have a surgical abdomen, blood should be drawn and sent to the blood bank and intravenous access should be assured with a large-bore cannula. If needed, fluid resuscitation should be commenced followed by appropriate blood-component therapy as indicated. Although hemodynamic stability is desirable before subjecting a patient to surgical anesthesia, it must be remembered that often the surgical intervention itself will be required to achieve stability by control of active hemorrhage.

Much more frequently, the patient suspected of ectopic pregnancy will have no, or only mild, abdominal pain, and tenderness and will be hemodynamically stable. Once the diagnosis of ectopic pregnancy is confirmed, immediate gynecologic consultation should be sought. Culdocentesis is appropriate, for it might expedite the decision for operative intervention, and is rapid, simple to perform, and has a good predicted value for hemoperitoneum.[31] If transfer to another facility was contemplated for a clinically stable patient, a positive culdocentesis would argue for prompt intervention instead. The algorithms depicted in Figures 3-3 and 3-4 suggest plans contingent on ultrasound availability for evaluation of suspected ectopic pregnancy before referring the patient for expectant management or more aggressive intervention.

A gynecologist should be consulted promptly, preferably one familiar with the newer evaluation modalities reviewed in this chapter and skilled in diagnostic and possibly operative laparoscopy. The earlier the diagnosis of ectopic pregnancy is made, the more likely it is that fallopian-tube-conserving measures will be successful. This is an extremely important point for the younger patient. For the patient presenting in shock, an emergency consultation should be obtained from any readily available physician with the surgical expertise to perform a laparotomy.

Transfer to another facility is appropriate in the clinically stable patient if it would facilitate performance of diagnostic studies not available within the referring ambulatory setting. In this instance, the patient would not require an ambulance or any other special support for transfer. Transfer to another facility is necessary for patients in whom ruptured ectopic pregnancy and/or hemoperitoneum is identified or suspected if the referring site does not have immediate access to an appropriate surgical facility. In this case, the most expeditious mode of transportation would be indicated with appropriate intravenous infusions, advanced cardiac life support, and even consideration for the use of mast trousers.

54 ♦ OBSTETRIC AND GYNECOLOGIC EMERGENCIES

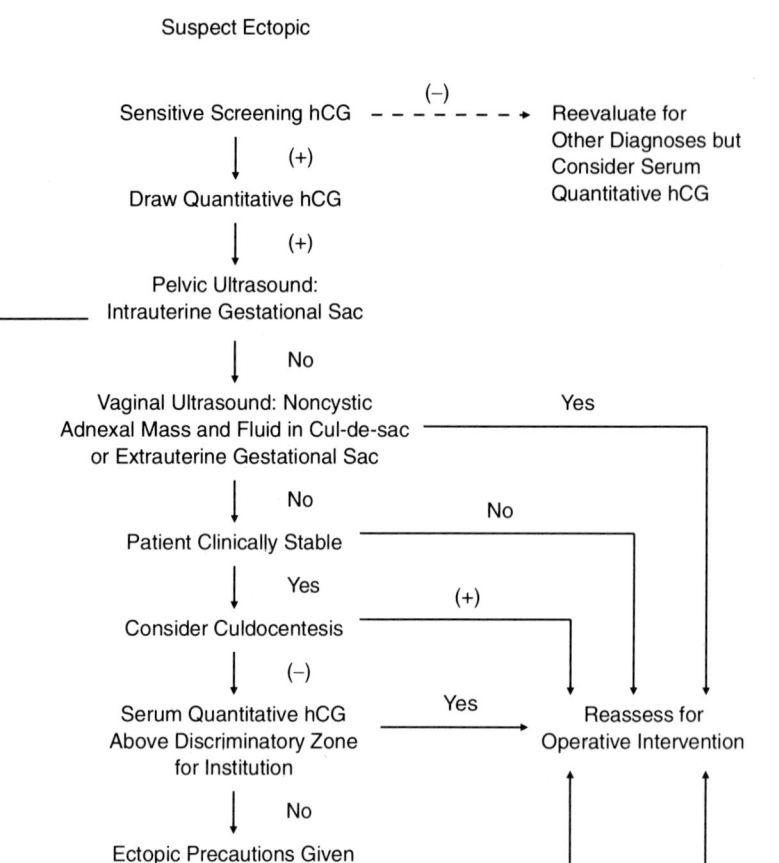

FIGURE 3–3
Algorithm for evaluation and management of suspected ectopic pregnancy when ultrasound is available.

ECTOPIC PREGNANCY ♦ 55

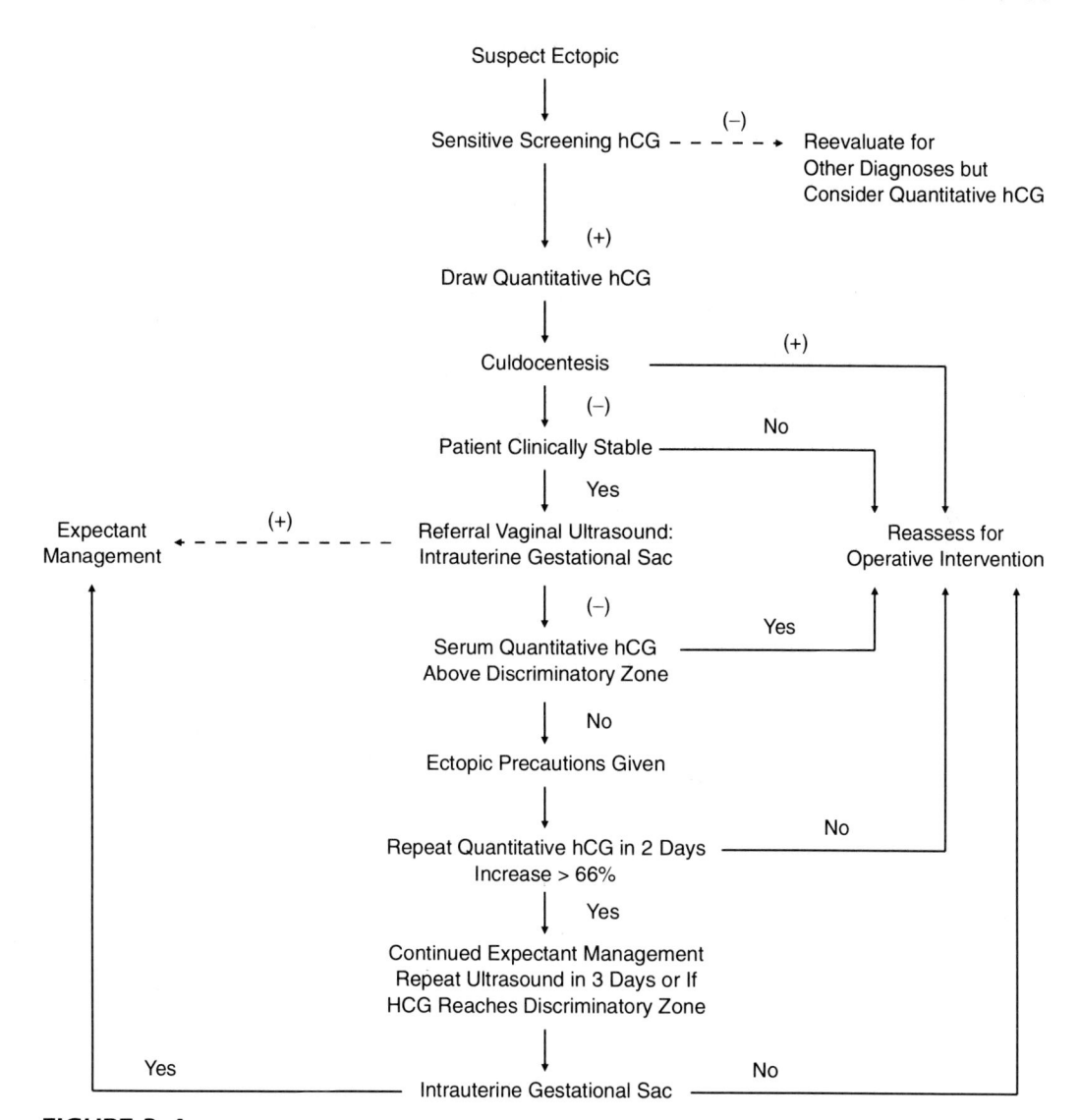

FIGURE 3-4
Algorithm for evaluation and management of suspected ectopic pregnancy when ultrasound is not readily available.

REFERENCES

1. Atrash HK, Friede A, Hogue CJ. Abdominal pregnancy in the United States: frequency and maternal mortality. Obstet Gynecol 69:333, 1987
2. Hallatt JG. Primary ovarian pregnancy: a report of twenty-five cases. Am J Obstet Gynecol 143:55, 1982
3. Dimitry ES, Margara R, Subak-Sharpe R. Nine cases of heterotopic pregnancies in 4 years of in vitro fertilization. Fertil Steril 53:107, 1990
4. Gorodeski IG, Bahary CM. Tubal pregnancy—reappraisal of incidence. Eur J Obstet Gynecol Reprod Biol 24:57, 1987

5. Nederlof KP, Lawson HW, Saftlas AF et al. Ectopic pregnancy surveillance, United States, 1970–1987. MMWR CDC Surveill Sum 39(4):9, 1990
6. Dorfman SF, Grimes DA, Cates W Jr et al. Ectopic pregnancy mortality, United States, 1979 to 1980: clinical aspects. Obstet Gynecol 64:386, 1984
7. Ramsey EM, Houston ML, Harris JWS. Interactions of the trophoblast and maternal tissues in three closely related primate species. Am J Obstet Gynecol 124:647, 1976
8. Westrom L. Incidence, prevalence, and trends of acute pelvic inflammatory disease and its consequences in industrialized countries. Am J Obstet Gynecol 138:880, 1980
9. Joesoef MR, Westrom L, Reynolds G, Marchbanks P, Cates W. Recurrence of ectopic pregnancy: the role of salpingitis. Am J Obstet Gynecol 165:46, 1991
10. Svensson L, Mardh PA, Ahlgren M et al. Ectopic pregnancy and antibodies from *Chlamydia trachomatis*. Fertil Steril 44:313, 1985
11. Stock RJ. A review of trends in vaginal douching: the relationship to changing incidences of PID and tubal ectopic pregnancy. Am J Gyn Health 3:22, 1990
12. Sivin I. Dose- and age-dependent ectopic pregnancy risks with intrauterine contraception. Obstet Gynecol 78:291, 1991
13. McCausland A. High rate of ectopic pregnancy following laparoscopic tubal coagulation failures. Am J Obstet Gynecol 136:97, 1980
14. Ory HW. Ectopic pregnancy and intrauterine contraceptive devices: new perspectives. Obstet Gynecol 57:137, 1981
15. Luikko P, Erkkola R, Laasko L. Ectopic pregnancies during the use of low-dose progesterones for oral contraception. Contraception 16:575, 1977
16. Morris JM, Wagenen G. Interception: the use of post-ovulatory estrogens to prevent implantation. Am J Obstet Gynecol 115:101, 1973
17. Gemzell L, Guillome J, Wang FC. Ectopic pregnancy following treatment with gonadotropins. Am J Obstet Gynecol 143:761, 1982
18. McBain JC, Evans JH, Pepperell RJ et al. An unexpectedly high rate of ectopic pregnancy following the induction of ovulation with human pituitary and chorionic gonadotropin. Br J Obstet Gynecol 87:5, 1980
19. Yovich JL, Turner SR, Murphy AJ. Embryo transfer technique as a cause of ectopic pregnancies in in vitro fertilization. Fertil Steril 44:318, 1985
20. Stock RJ. The changing spectrum of ectopic pregnancy. Obstet Gynecol 71:885, 1988
21. Kim DS, Chung SR, Park MI et al. Comparative review of diagnostic accuracy in tubal pregnancy: a 14-year survey of 1040 cases. Obstet Gynecol 70:547, 1987
22. Breen JL. A 21-year survey of 654 ectopic pregnancies. Am J Obstet Gynecol 106:1004, 1970
23. Romero R, Copel JA, Kadar N et al. Value of culdocentesis in the diagnosis of ectopic pregnancy. Obstet Gynecol 65:519, 1985
24. Brenner PF, Ray S, Mishell DR. Ectopic pregnancy: a study of 300 consecutive surgically treated cases. JAMA 243:673, 1980
25. Hallatt JG, Steele CH Jr, Snyder M. Ruptured corpus luteum with hemoperitoneum: a study of 173 surgical cases. Am J Obstet Gynecol 149:5, 1984
26. Bock JL. Editorial: HCG assays: a plea for uniformity. Clin Pathol 93:432, 1990
27. Kadar N, Caldwell BV, Romero R. A method of screening for ectopic pregnancy and its indications. Obstet Gynecol 58:162, 1981
28. Bradley WG, Fiske CE, Filly RA. The double decidual sac sign of early pregnancy: use in exclusion of ectopic pregnancy. Radiology 143:223, 1882
29. Timor-Tritsch IE, Yeh MN, Peisner DB et al. The use of transvaginal ultrasonography in the diagnosis of ectopic pregnancy. Am J Obstet Gynecol 161:157, 1989
30. Weckstein LN. Clinical diagnosis of ectopic pregnancy. Clin Obstet Gynecol 30:236, 1987
31. Stock RJ. Persistent tubal pregnancy. Obstet Gynecol 77:267, 1991

CHAPTER 4

Trauma in Pregnancy

Lynnette Doan-Wiggins

Obstetric and Gynecologic Emergencies, edited by Guy I. Benrubi. J.B. Lippincott Company, Philadelphia © 1994.

Trauma is the primary cause of death in women less than 35 years of age and is the leading nonobstetric cause of maternal mortality during pregnancy, accounting for up to 22% of such deaths.[1,2] Estimated to occur in 6% to 8% of all pregnancies, the incidence of accidental injury increases as pregnancy progresses until, by the end of the third trimester, minor trauma occurs more frequently than at any other time during female adulthood.[1-8] At this time an altered center of gravity caused by the enlarged uterus combined with pelvic ligamentous laxity produces a degree of gait instability that makes the pregnant woman particularly susceptible to injury by falls.[1,9] Although minor trauma is seldom associated with a poor pregnancy outcome, severe trauma requires a prompt and skilled team approach, including emergency medicine personnel, trauma surgeons, obstetricians, and pediatricians.[6]

Because the most common cause of fetal death is maternal death,[3,4,10] the overriding principle in the management of the pregnant trauma patient is that "maternal well-being is paramount. The best chance for fetal survival is to assure maternal survival."[3] Because the anatomic and physiologic alterations of pregnancy can alter the gravid woman's response to injury, an understanding of these changes is critical when approaching trauma management.

Anatomic and Physiologic Changes Associated With Pregnancy

During the first trimester of pregnancy the uterus is well protected by the bony pelvis, and the physiology of the mother is only moderately altered. As pregnancy progresses, however, increasing changes in maternal anatomy and physiology occur.

Cardiovascular System

Cardiopulmonary physiology is significantly altered throughout gestation. Cardiac output increases up to 40% during the first 10 weeks of gestation, reaching 6 to 7 L per minute and maintaining this level until term.[1,2,5,9,10] During the third trimester cardiac output may be transiently lowered because of aortocaval compression by the gravid uterus, resulting in decreased placental perfusion. This phenomenon, known as supine hypotension syndrome, may be observed clinically in otherwise normal pregnant patients.[6,11] Changing maternal position from supine to the left lateral decubitus position may increase cardiac output by as much as 25% at term.[11]

The average maternal heart rate accelerates during pregnancy such that by term normal maternal pulse rate is 80 to 95 beats per minute (normal is 60 to 80) in both awake and sleeping states, making borderline tachycardia difficult to evaluate.[2,9,11] Mean arterial blood pressure gradually decreases during the first two trimesters of pregnancy, reaching its nadir during the second trimester. Systolic arterial pressure declines by 0 to 15 mmHg, and diastolic pressure falls by 10 to 20 mmHg, creating a widened pulse pressure. These changes are the result of diminishing peripheral vascular resistance and should not be accepted as evidence of hypovolemia during the first two trimesters of pregnancy. During the third trimester blood pressure gradually rises, returning to normal levels near term.[2,5,9,11] True hypertension, systolic or diastolic, is never expected during pregnancy and, if present, may either be in response to pain, anxiety, or injury or be the result of a direct complication of pregnancy, such as pregnancy-induced hypertension.[9]

Associated with the underlying decreased peripheral vascular resistance of the first two trimesters of pregnancy is a paradoxical response to stimuli that would normally cause vasoconstriction. This altered response may mitigate the cool, clammy skin otherwise expected of a patient in hypovolemic shock, causing instead the skin to be warm and dry.[6,9] In addition, central venous pressure (CVP) gradually decreases throughout pregnancy until at term it reaches a level approximately one third that of nonpregnant controls.[5,12]

Total maternal blood volume increases by as much as 50% at 34 weeks of gestation, improving maternal response to hemorrhage. During periods of stress the mother will maintain homeostasis at the expense of the fetus. Acute maternal hemorrhage or maternal hypoxia induces uterine artery vasoconstriction, which can reduce uterine perfusion 10 to 20% before clinical evidence of maternal hypovolemia occurs.[1,3,9] Consequently, 30 to 35% of maternal blood volume may be lost before clinical signs of hypovolemia develop.[1,4,5,9,12] This, combined with the sensitivity of the placental vasculature to catecholamines, places the fetus at risk during maternal hemorrhage that may, upon clinical examination of the mother, appear minimally significant. Early and adequate maternal volume replacement and thorough fetal evaluation, including fetal monitoring, are therefore critical in managing the gravid trauma patient.

Electrocardiographic (ECG) changes in late pregnancy are not specific and reflect the leftward shift of the cardiac axis due to elevation of the diaphragm. The T waves may be flattened and inverted in lead III, and Q waves may appear in leads III and AVF. Supraventricular ectopic beats may also be seen.[9]

Respiratory System

Significant changes in the respiratory function occur due to changes in pulmonary anatomy, ventilation, lung volumes, and oxygen consumption. Diaphragmatic excursions increase as the diaphragm progressively rises an extra 4 cm during pregnancy, with compensatory flaring of the ribs. Landmarks used to evaluate thoracoabdominal wounds and thoracostomy tube placement therefore need to be correspondingly revised.

While respiratory rate generally remains unchanged, tidal volume increases, increasing minute ventilation by as much as 50%. The metabolic effect of this change is the production of a partially compensated respiratory alkalosis, with arterial blood gases showing a fall in pCO_2 to approximately 30 to 34 mmHg (normal is 35 to 40 mmHg) and a decrease in serum bicarbonate to an average of 19.5 mEq/L (normal is 22 to 28 mEq/L), leaving the pregnant woman with a decreased buffering capacity after trauma.[1,9] While cumulative respiratory changes cause a rise in maternal arterial pO_2 by 10 mmHg, oxygen consumption during pregnancy increases by as much as 20% at rest.[9] These alterations, combined with fetal oxygen demand and fetal sensitivity to hypoxia, place the pregnant trauma patient and her fetus at greater than normal risk of hypoxic insult. Prompt administration of supplemental oxygen in the awake trauma patient and early endotracheal intubation and mechanical ventilation, when required, may avert these deleterious effects.[6,9]

Gastrointestinal System

The major physiologic alterations of the gastrointestinal system are those of increasing compartmentalization of the small intestine into the upper abdomen and a progesterone-induced decrease in gastrointestinal motility (Fig. 4-1). Although the large uterus may, as pregnancy progresses, protect the abdominal viscera from injury to the lower abdomen, penetrating wounds to the upper abdomen may injure many loops of tightly crowded small intestine. In addition, stretching of the abdominal wall alters the normal response to peritoneal irritation, at times masking significant intra-abdominal organ injury. Decreased gastric emptying increases the possibility of aspiration during trauma and intubation.[1,5,7,9,12]

Urinary System

By the 10th week of gestation the urinary system has undergone important anatomic and physiologic alteration. Bilateral dilatation and diminished peristalsis of the ureters and renal calyces and pelves result from progesterone stimulation. This, combined with decreased bladder emptying from mechanical compression of the en-

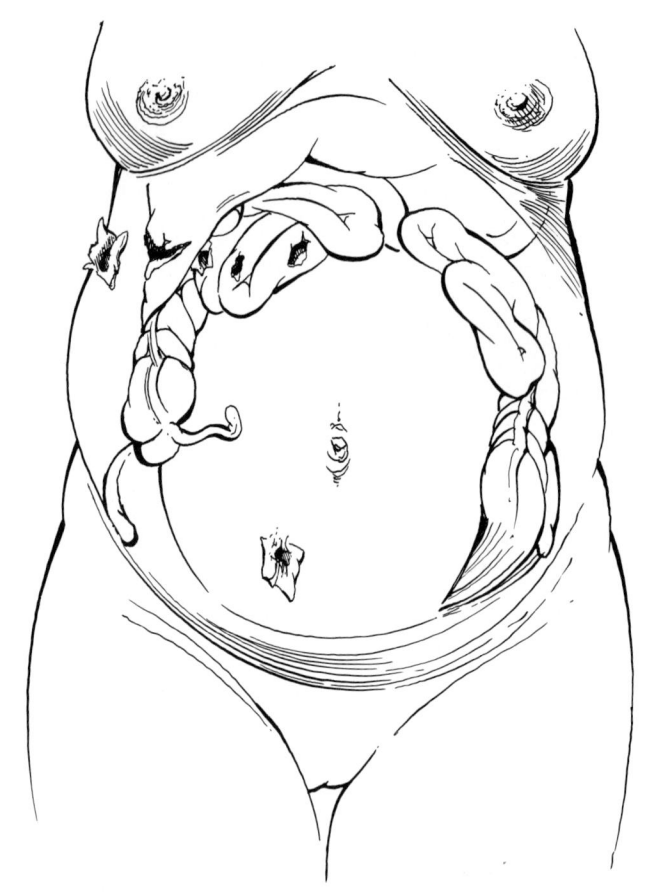

FIGURE 4–1
Compartmentalization of intestines during pregnancy, and sites of gunshot wounds above and below the umbilicus.

larging uterus, can lead to a picture resembling that of retroperitoneal hematoma on intravenous pyelography (IVP).[9] By the 12th week of gestation the urinary bladder is displaced anteriorly and superiorly by the enlarging uterus, making it increasingly vulnerable to injury.[2,11]

Reproductive System

The uterus itself changes dramatically during pregnancy, reaching 10 to 20 times its nonpregnant size at term. This alteration in the uterus causes increasing susceptibility to injury as pregnancy progresses. The vascular needs of the enlarging uterus create marked venous congestion in the pelvis and an increased potential for hemorrhage in patients with pelvic fractures.[1] Because the patient's entire blood volume circulates through the uterus every 8 to 11 minutes, major hemorrhage can result from seemingly minor abdominal wounds.[5] In addition, compression of the lower abdominal venous system by the gravid uterus increases peripheral venous pressure in the lower extremities, increasing potential blood loss from injury to the pelvis and legs.[5]

Hematology

Hematologic changes accompanying pregnancy may present a misleading picture during assessment and stabilization of the pregnant trauma patient. The increase in plasma volume that normally occurs during pregnancy is not paralleled by a proportional increase in red blood cell mass. This results in a physiologic dilutional anemia with average hematocrits of 32 to 34% by the 34th week of gestation.[1,5] A physiologic leukocytosis also occurs with white blood cell counts reaching 18,000/mm^3 during the second and third trimesters.[1,3,6,9]

Throughout pregnancy fibrinogen and coagulation factors VII, VIII, IX, and X generally increase and coagulation times decrease or remain unchanged.[1,6,9,11] Fibrinogen levels may reach 400 to 450 mg/dL by term, double those of the nonpregnant state. Thus at term a normal fibrinogen level may actually indicate disseminated intravascular coagulation (DIC), and levels below 150 mm/dL should be considered abnormal.[1,5,6] Although the hypercoaguable state of pregnancy is rarely a problem in the acute management of the trauma patient, it may increase the risk of thromboembolic events during the immobile, convalescent period.[6]

Table 4-1 outlines the physiologic, anatomic, and laboratory changes associated with pregnancy.

TABLE 4–1
Physiologic and Anatomic Changes of Pregnancy

System	Alteration	Effect
Cardiovascular	↑ cardiac output	↑ heart rate
	↑ blood volume	↑ maternal tolerance to hemorrhage
	↓ peripheral vascular resistance	↓ blood pressure; ↑ skin temperature
	Aortocaval compression	Supine hypotensive syndrome
	↓ uterine perfusion in response to hemorrhage	↑ fetal risk during hemorrhage
Pulmonary	↑ minute ventilation	↓ serum bicarbonate, ↓ tolerance to acidosis
	↑ oxygen consumption; ↑ fetal oxygen demand	↓ tolerance to hypoxia
Gastrointestinal	↓ motility, ↓ gastric emptying	↑ risk of aspiration
	Compartmentalization into upper abdomen	↑ risk of injury with upper abdominal trauma; ↓ risk with lower abdominal trauma
Genitourinary	Dilatation of kidneys and ureters, ↓ bladder emptying	Abnormal IVP
	Displacement of bladder	↑ risk of injury
Hematologic	↑ plasma volume without proportional ↑ in red cell mass	Dilutional anemia; mean hematocrit of 32% to 34% during late pregnancy
	Leukocytosis	WBC up to 18,000/mm^3 during 2nd and 3rd trimesters
	Hypercoagulability	↑ risk of deep vein thrombosis during immobilization

Patterns of Fetal and Maternal Injury

Among pregnant women who die as a result of trauma, head injury and hemorrhagic shock account for the majority of deaths.[3,11] There are no data to suggest that serious injuries result in a higher mortality rate in pregnant women than in those who are not pregnant. However, increased risks of splenic rupture and retroperitoneal hemorrhage due to blunt abdominal trauma have been reported. Conversely, the bowel is reported to be less frequently injured when the victim is pregnant.[11]

Early studies showed that minor maternal trauma was not associated with an increased incidence of abortions, stillbirths, and neonatal deaths.[5,7] More recent reports have demonstrated fetal loss, although still infrequent, due to placental abruption associated with apparently insignificant maternal trauma.[8,13-16] Unsuccessful pregnancy outcome following more significant maternal trauma is typically related to maternal death, maternal hypotension, fetal injury, and injuries to the pelvic viscera, uterus, and placenta.[3]

During the first trimester of pregnancy the uterus sits well within the bony pelvis and the fetus is further protected by the amniotic fluid, which is proportionally greater in early pregnancy and acts as a natural buffer to injury.[5,16,17] During early pregnancy direct fetal injury is uncommon and usually results from pelvic fractures and penetrating injuries to the lower abdomen or perineum.[16] Indirect fetal injury and loss are more commonly due to maternal shock or infection, which compromise uteroplacental perfusion.[4] Because the expected rate of spontaneous abortion during the first trimester is approximately 15 to 25% and abortion due to embryonic injury from trauma may not occur until several weeks or months after an accident, exact figures describing fetal wastage following first-trimester trauma are unavailable.[18]

As pregnancy progresses, the uterus rises out of the pelvis, becoming more vulnerable to direct injury.[4] In penetrating trauma it is rare for a projectile wound to the abdomen to spare the gravid uterus. The uterine musculature absorbs a great amount of the projectile's force and diminishes its ability to damage other abdominal viscera.[12,19,20] The incidence of fetal injury following penetrating trauma to the uterus ranges from 59 to 78%; fetal mortality ranges from 41 to 71%.[1,6,12,19]

Fetal and Placental Injury Following Blunt Abdominal Trauma

Following blunt abdominal trauma during the latter part of pregnancy, the gravid uterus is subject to direct injury as well as to the shearing forces resulting from sudden deceleration. In victims of severe automobile accidents the most common cause of fetal death is maternal death; with maternal survival the most common cause of fetal death is *placental abruption*.[5,18,21,22] Although trauma is implicated as a cause of abruption in less than 2% of all cases of abruption, when severely traumatized pregnant patients alone are considered, the incidence of abruption is quite high, ranging from 6 to 66%.[15,23,24] Maternal death from abruption is 1%; the incidence of fetal death ranges from 30 to 68%.[5] Although cases of abruptio placentae have been reported up to 5 days after severe trauma,[25,26] abruption large enough to cause fetal death usually becomes evident within 48 hours of the traumatic episode.[5,17,26] Signs and symptoms suggestive of placental abruption include vaginal bleeding, abdominal pain or cramping, uterine tenderness, and amniotic fluid leak. If the placenta is posteriorly implanted, the patient may complain only of backache.[5] Although the presence of these symptoms is significant, the absence of symptoms following trauma does not exclude the possibility of placental abruption.[7,21,24,26]

Less common than placental abruption, direct injury to the uterus may result from blunt trauma. Unique to pregnancy, *uterine rupture* complicates about 0.6% of traumatic events during pregnancy and usually occurs only with major blunt abdominal trauma.[11] Uterine rupture usually presents as an acute surgical emergency with signs of an acute abdomen and maternal hypotension. Fetal mortality approaches 100%;[11,21] maternal mortality is usually due to concurrent injury.[11]

Preterm labor is another sequel of maternal trauma.[1,15,22,27] Up to 41% of traumatized gravidas experience frequent contractions during the initial 4 hours of monitoring.[15] Postulated etiologies include placental abruption, uterine contusion, membrane ischemia, and membrane rupture.[1] The use of tocolytics to halt premature contractions associated with trauma is controversial. Although some authors report successful cessation of preterm contractions with these agents,[22,27,28] others discourage their use, believing that regular uterine activity after trauma is a result of placental abruption until proved otherwise.[15]

Direct injury to the fetus resulting from blunt maternal trauma is not as common as might be expected because of the buffering effects of the amniotic fluid.[16] Most fetal injuries occur late in pregnancy, when the amniotic fluid/fetus ratio is reduced and the fetal head is fixed in the pelvis, with the remainder of the fetus lying above the protective confines of the bony pelvis. The most common fetal injuries after blunt trauma are skull fractures and intracranial hemorrhage; these injuries are frequently fatal.[3,4]

Fetomaternal Hemorrhage

Fetomaternal hemorrhage (ie, the transplacental passage of fetal blood into the maternal circulation) is reported in 8.8 to 30.6% of victims of blunt abdominal trauma.[15,29,27] The volume of blood lost from the fetus varies from 5 to 69 mL, with the average volume of transfusion ranging from 12 to 16 mL.[15,29,30] Although neither the nature of the trauma nor the gestational age of the infant is related to the frequency or volume of fetomaternal hemorrhage, fetomaternal hemorrhage has been found to be more common when there is uterine tenderness after trauma or the placenta is anteriorly located.[15,27] Complications of fetomaternal hemorrhage include Rh sensitization of the mother, neonatal anemia, and fetal death from exsanguination.[11] Because as little as 0.01 to 0.03 mL of fetal blood may sensitize Rh-negative patients and Rh sensitization can be prevented by the administration of $Rh_o(D)$ immune globulin (RhIG), early detection of fetomaternal transfusion is critical.[11,29] Testing is recommended for all women with abdominal trauma beyond 12 weeks of gestation.[15]

Detection of fetomaternal hemorrhage is made using the Kleihauer-Betke test, which tests the resistance of fetal red blood cells to acid. A sample of maternal blood is mixed with acid and the ratio of fetal cells to lysed maternal cells is recorded, enabling prediction of the volume of fetal blood transfused into the maternal circulation.[5,29] Because sensitivity of the Kleihauer-Betke test varies among laboratories and may not be sufficient to detect small hemorrhages capable of sensitizing certain Rh-negative mothers, some authors recommend that full-dose RhIG (300 μg) be given to all Rh-negative mothers sustaining blunt abdominal trauma. Fetomaternal hemorrhage is then quantified in those patients with clinical evidence of significant trauma or associated obstetric findings to detect rare, massive hemorrhage or hemorrhage in excess of the amount covered by the standard dose of RhIG.[27]

Use of Restraints

Because blunt vehicular trauma is the most common mechanism of injury among pregnant women,[28,31,32] the use of automobile restraints deserves special mention. Seat belts decrease the frequency of maternal injury and death by preventing ejection of the occupant.[18] When used alone during rapid deceleration, however, lap belts allow enough forward flexion of the maternal abdomen and uterus over the belt that resultant compression elevates intrauterine pressure and distorts the size and shape of the uterus (Fig. 4-2).[18,33,34] This distortion predisposes to placental abruption and less frequently to uterine rupture and direct fetal injury.[18,33] To minimize abdominal compression during impact, seat belts should be placed securely across the pelvis below the protuberant abdomen rather than high on the abdomen over the uterine fundus (Fig. 4-3).[23,33] The addition of a shoulder harness has been shown to improve fetal outcome, presumably by dissipating the deceleration force over a greater surface and preventing forward flexion of the mother.[32,34] Routine use of a lap/shoulder belt reduces the chance of serious injury and death in the adult by 50% without increasing the risk of fetal loss.[32]

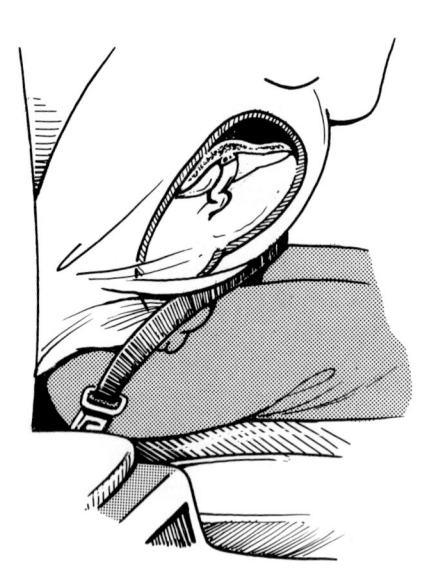

FIGURE 4-2
Seat belt use without shoulder belt.

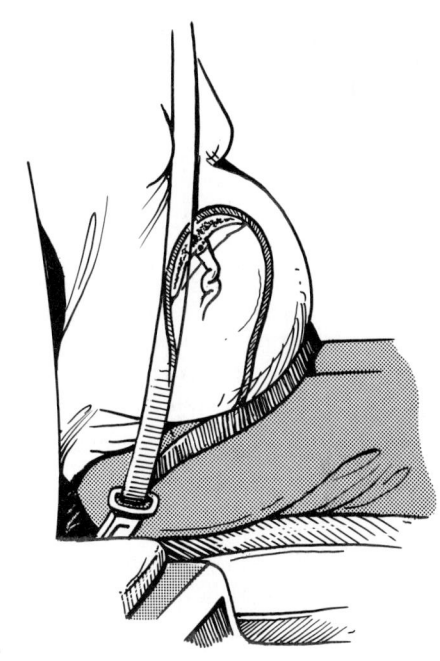

FIGURE 4–3
Shoulder and lap belt.

Evaluation and Management

Because the most common cause of fetal death is maternal death, initial evaluation and resuscitative efforts should be directed toward the mother. Although the initial approach to the trauma patient is similar to that of her nongravid counterpart, once maternal hemodynamic stability is assured, attention must be immediately directed to assessment and assurance of fetal health.

Prehospital Management

When possible, injured pregnant women, particularly those in the latter half of pregnancy, should be transported to an appropriately designated trauma center with facilities for adequate maternal and specialized neonatal care. During the second and third trimester transport should be performed with the patient in the left lateral decubitus position, or when the spine must be immobilized, with the backboard tilted 15° to the left.[1,5,9] Listening for fetal heart tones may be performed en route but should not delay transport.[5] Although no prospective studies have evaluated the use of the military antishock trousers (MAST) during pregnancy, it is generally believed that pregnancy is a relative contraindication to inflation of the abdominal compartment.[1,5,9,11] Use of the lower-extremity sections alone is of questionable benefit.[9]

In both the prehospital setting and the emergency department, oxygen therapy provides special benefit for the fetus. Although arterial maternal blood is usually well saturated at room air, the oxygen/hemoglobin dissociation curve of fetal blood is shifted, such that increasing alveolar oxygen tension continues to improve fetal saturation and thereby fetal outcome.[5]

Maternal hemorrhage can reduce uterine blood flow 10% to 20% before signs of maternal hypovolemia appear, and maternal catecholamines can further reduce uterine blood flow. Therefore early intravenous access and volume resuscitation are important for both the mother and fetus. Because they can further decrease uterine blood flow, vasopressors should be avoided.[5]

Evaluation of Mother and Fetus

When available, prehospital information is critical in ascertaining the mechanism of injury, vital signs, and patient condition in the field. Prenatal history is of particular importance, especially in ascertaining gestational age of the fetus and the presence of complicating medical conditions. Maternal perception of fetal movement may give a *very cursory* indication of fetal health. The time of the last meal is more significant than in the nonpregnant patient because of the prolonged gastric emptying time associated with pregnancy.[5,9] Initial physical assessment of the mother is, as in the nongravid patient, focused on the stability of the airway and circulation and evaluation for occult injuries. As noted earlier, the expanded maternal intravascular volume may delay the onset of clinical signs of shock.

Once maternal hemodynamic stability has been assured and assessment of maternal injuries begun, the condition of the fetus should be ascertained. Fetal evaluation includes determining fetal heart rate and fetal movement, evaluating uterine size and irritability, and examining the vagina for vaginal bleeding or leakage of amniotic fluid. The earliest sign of fetal distress is fetal bradycardia, defined as a heart rate of 110 beats per minute or less. Although optimally fetal heart rate and maternal contractions should be continuously monitored using external tococardiography, when this is not available fetal heart tones should be auscultated at intervals of 10 minutes or less. Persistent bradycardia after trauma, even in the absence of vaginal bleeding and uterine tenderness or irritability, is highly suggestive of placental abruption.

Determination of fetal age and maturity may be critical in management decisions for the fetus. The quickest means of estimating gestational age is by palpation of fundal height. At 12 weeks of gestation the uterine fundus rises just above the symphysis pubis, at 20 weeks it reaches the level of the umbilicus, and by 36 weeks it lies just below the xiphoid process. The age of fetal viability is generally considered to be 24 to 26 weeks of gestation and is dependent in part on the neonatal facilities available.[1,2,5]

Routine Laboratory Studies

In addition to routine laboratory studies, the following tests are generally recommended in any gravid patient with significant trauma: type and cross-match; complete blood count with platelet count; coagulation panel, including prothrombin

(PT), partial thromboplastin (PTT), fibrinogen level, and fibrin degradation products; and Kleihauer-Betke test for the detection of fetal hemorrhage. Baseline coagulation studies are of particular importance because of potential placental injuries with associated DIC.[1,6,9,11]

Radiographic Procedures

The greatest embryonic and fetal sensitivity to radiation occurs during the first trimester of pregnancy.[35] In the preimplantation period (first week after conception), the embryo is particularly sensitive to the lethal effects of radiation but has a low probability of sustaining teratogenic effects if implantation and continued development occur. During the period of major organogenesis (2 to 7 weeks after conception) the embryo is sensitive to the growth-retarding, teratogenic, and postnatal neoplastic effects of radiation. During the fetal period (8 to 40 weeks after conception) there is decreased sensitivity for organ teratogenesis but postnatal neoplastic effects, growth retardation, and functional abnormalities, particularly of the central nervous system, may occur.[36,37] Determining the exact incidence of adverse effects due to radiation exposure is difficult because of the prevalence of congenital malformations in the general population and the frequent other biomedical and social factors that may influence the outcome of pregnancy.[35–37] It is generally accepted that a teratogenic risk exists with cumulative radiation exposures of greater than 5 to 10 rad; and increased risk of childhood cancers has been suggested at slightly lower doses.[9,35–37]

The dose of radiation absorbed by the fetus depends on several factors, including the (1) energy and intensity of the x-rays, (2) proximity of the uterus to the anatomic area exposed, (3) extent of the area exposed, (4) patient positioning, (5) depth of the fetus, and (6) number of films required.[38] If the uterus is outside the area radiographed, the dose of radiation to the conceptus is limited to that delivered by scatter and leakage radiation and drops off rapidly the farther the uterus is from the radiographed area. Scatter effects can be limited by using the smallest reasonable field size, appropriate choice of grid, and proper collimation. Pelvic shielding should be used whenever possible.[9] Table 4-2 lists estimates of fetal radiation exposure from commonly used procedures. As can be seen, routine diagnostic radiographs seldom result in significant radiation exposure to the fetus. Therefore although unnecessary radiography should be avoided, necessary diagnostic studies should never be withheld out of concern for fetal radiation.[1,3,9] When possible, effective alternative imaging modalities, such as ultrasonography, should be used in evaluating the pregnant trauma patient.

Abdominal computerized tomography is not commonly recommended for evaluation of the traumatized pregnant patient.[1] Its use, however, has recently been recommended by some authors as a potentially effective means for diagnosing maternal, uteroplacental, and fetal injury in near-term gravidas.[31,39] The radiation dose is estimated to be half that of traditional pelvimetry.[39] Although magnetic resonance imaging may provide a safe and effective alternative to conventional x-ray use during pregnancy, data are currently insufficient to justify its routine use.[9,38,40]

TABLE 4-2
Estimated Radiation Dose to the Uterus From Commonly Used Radiographic Examinations*

Examination	Estimated Mean Dose[†]	Reported Range[§]
Cervical spine	<0.5	<0.5–3.0
Extremities (excluding femur)	<0.5	<0.5–18.0
Chest	1	0.2–43
Thoracic spine	11	<1.0–55
Hips and proximal femur	170	73–1370
Pelvis	290	55–2190
Abdomen	300	25–1920
Lumbar spine	990	27–3970
Intravenous urography	960[‡]	70–5480
Urethrocystography	2060[‡]	275–4110

*Dose estimates are expressed in millirads per radiographic examination and do not include fluoroscopy.
[†]Figures are from the Bureau of Radiological Health, FDA (1976), except as noted.
[‡]Figures are from the International Commission on Radiological Protection (1970).
[§]Range is that reported by Wagner LK, Lester RG, Saldana LR: Prenatal risks from ionizing radiations, ultrasound, magnetic files, and radiofrequency waves. In: Exposure of the pregnant patient to diagnostic radiations, p. 61. Philadelphia: JB Lippincott, 1985.

Ultrasonography

Ultrasonography is indicated in all cases of significant maternal trauma.[1,2,8,15,28] An accurate modality for assessing fetal status, sonography is a sensitive indicator of gestational age, presentation, amniotic fluid volume, and fetal movement and may be useful in identifying intra-abdominal bleeding.[1,15] Although small abruptions are not easily seen, large abruptions, retroplacental clots, and some fetal fractures may be identified.[1,2] Mobile units can be used effectively in the emergency department to assess fetal status and gestational age acutely.[4]

Peritoneal Lavage

Although pregnancy was once considered a relative contraindication to peritoneal lavage, it is now generally felt to be a safe and accurate procedure for diagnosing intra-abdominal injuries in blunt abdominal trauma and may be particularly useful because pregnancy may mask the usual clinical criteria for making operative decisions.[3,5,31,41]

Indications for lavage are similar to those for the nonpregnant patient and include an equivocal abdominal examination, altered sensorium, and unexplained hypotension. Open lavage, which allows direct visualization of the peritoneum, at a site in the midline just above the uterine fundus is usually recommended.[3,5] Unless gross blood is obtained from the initial aspirate, a peritoneal dialysis catheter should be gently directed toward the pelvis and a liter of crystalloid infused through it. Fluid is returned by gravity drainage. Criteria for a positive lavage are identical to those in a nonpregnant patient.[3,41]

External Tocacardiography

Continuous external tococardiography (i.e., monitoring fetal heart rate and uterine contractions) has proved a valuable tool in the evaluation of fetal status after injury, particularly in identifying preterm labor and placental abruption. External fetal monitoring should be instituted as soon as feasible in all pregnancies beyond 20 to 24 weeks of gestation.[15,30,31] Although all authorities agree on the value of tococardiography, the recommended duration for routine monitoring varies considerably, from a minimum of 30 minutes for uncomplicated cases of maternal trauma[27] to at least 24 hours following the incident.[8,30,31] Although placental abruption has been shown to occur up to 5 days following injury,[25,26] most trauma-related pregnancy complications become evident within 6 hours of injury.[8,13,15,27] Therefore a period of routine monitoring for 2 to 6 hours following injury seems reasonable, with more prolonged observation for women with severe trauma and for those demonstrating obstetric findings such as uterine contractions, vaginal bleeding, rupture of membranes, uterine tenderness, or abnormalities during initial tococardiography.[22,27]

Management of Maternal and Fetal Trauma

To ensure maternal survival and thereby fetal survival, initial resuscitative efforts should be directed to the mother followed by prompt attention to the fetus. Initial management priorities are the same as those in the nonpregnant population (ie, ensuring an adequate airway and ventilation and maintaining adequate blood pressure and perfusion). Certain modifications of standard therapy are necessitated by the anatomic and physiologic changes that occur during pregnancy.

General Considerations

As noted earlier, oxygen therapy provides special benefit to the fetus and should be administered to the mother immediately upon arrival at the hospital. Early intubation should be considered for evidence of airway compromise or poor oxygenation.

Similarly, aggressive volume resuscitation begun in the prehospital phase should be continued or initiated once the patient arrives in the emergency department. Because large volumes of crystalloid will not prevent fetal hypoxia, early replacement of red cells after proper cross-matching of blood to avoid Rh incompatibility is indicated. When massive hemorrhage affects maternal hemodynamic stability and time precludes proper cross-matching, type-specific blood may be used. Un-cross-matched type O, Rh-negative blood can be used if type-specific blood is not immediately available.[11] Because most vasopressors induce uterine vasoconstriction, further compromising the fetus, their use should be avoided.[5]

Because of the delay in gastric emptying associated with pregnancy, decompression of the stomach with a nasogastric tube should be considered in all seriously injured patients. In addition, prompt placement of an indwelling urinary catheter is essential for both monitoring renal function and fluid replacement and testing the urine for blood and protein.[6]

Tetanus prophylaxis. Because the mortality rate from maternal and neonatal tetanus approaches 60%, postexposure immunization with tetanus toxoid is recommended during pregnancy, as is passive immunization with tetanus immune globulin (TIG) when indicated.[42,43] Indications, dosage, and timing for postexposure tetanus prophylaxis are identical to those in the nongravid female. Although there is no evidence that tetanus or diphtheria toxoids are teratogenic, routine administration of tetanus immunization should be performed during the second or third trimester to minimize concerns over teratogenicity.[42,43]

Specific Trauma Episodes

Blunt Abdominal Trauma

Mild abdominal trauma, usually the result of minor falls, is common during pregnancy. Although fetal and maternal outcome is frequently satisfactory,[5,7] cases of placental abruption associated with apparently insignificant maternal trauma have been reported.[8,13–16] Pregnant patients who are beyond 20 weeks of gestation and have minor and insignificant injuries should be monitored with external tococardiography and observed for several hours. Clinical signs of placental abruption and premature labor include vaginal bleeding; uterine irritability; abdominal pain, cramps, or tenderness; and leakage of amniotic fluid. Fetal bradycardia or tachycardia, the absence of variability between beats, persistent decelerations, or the presence of uterine contractions on tococardiography may indicate placental abruption and require emergency obstetric evaluation.[11] If the patient remains asymptomatic without abnormalities on tococardiography throughout the observation period, she may be discharged with instructions to return if symptoms occur.[3,6,25] Obviously, patients with more severe forms of blunt abdominal trauma should be admitted to the hospital and managed as inpatients.[6] Because placental injury can produce a consumptive coagulopathy through the release of thromboplastin stores, patients with evidence of placental injury should also receive serial evaluation of coagulation profiles.[5,6]

The management of mild degrees of placental abruption remains controversial and depends in part upon fetal age and maternal condition. It is generally agreed that fetal distress, heavy vaginal bleeding, and coagulopathy are indications for delivery, usually by cesarean section.[6] The management of abruption is, of course, left to the expertise of the obstetrician.

As noted earlier, *fetomaternal hemorrhage* may be detected by Kleihauer-Betke test. A positive test is an indication for prolonged fetal monitoring. When fetomaternal hemorrhage is detected in the Rh-negative mother, RhIG should be administered to prevent sensitization.[6,44] Standard-dose RhIG (approximately 300 μg) administered within 72 hours of antigenic stimulus is adequate to prevent sensitization in the majority of women with fetomaternal hemorrhage. When the volume of transfusion of Rh-positive red cells is determined to be above 15 mL, however, an additional dose (≈ 300 μg) of RhIG should be administered for each 15 mL of Rh-positive cells transfused.[44]

Intra-abdominal hemorrhage must be considered in all gravid patients with significant abdominal trauma. As noted earlier, indications for lavage in the pregnant patient are similar to those of the general population. When evidence of serious or life-threatening hemorrhage is found, laparotomy should not be delayed because of pregnancy.[16,28,31] Although fetal and neonatal loss frequently occurs in association with maternal trauma severe enough to require laparotomy, it appears to be directly related to fetal injury and not to maternal surgery or anesthesia.[28,31]

In summary, asymptomatic patients with minor or insignificant abdominal trauma may be discharged with reassurance after a brief period of fetal and maternal monitoring. In patients with more significant trauma abruptio placentae, fetomaternal hemorrhage, and intra-abdominal hemorrhage are the principal considerations. The evaluation and management of intra-abdominal injury are similar to those of the nonpregnant population. Fetal monitoring for at least 24 hours is indicated in severely traumatized patients and in those with obstetric complications to detect placental abruption and, less commonly, direct fetal injury.

Penetrating Abdominal Trauma

In late pregnancy the enlarged gravid uterus is the intraperitoneal organ most commonly injured by penetrating wounds. Gunshot and stab wounds are the most common form of injuries sustained.[6] When a bullet, particularly one of low velocity, such as that commonly found in civilian injuries, strikes the pregnant uterus, much of its energy is dissipated in the dense uterine musculature, diminishing its velocity and ability to penetrate other abdominal organs. Gunshot wounds to the pregnant abdomen are therefore associated with low maternal morbidity and mortality.[12,19] Fetal outcome, however, is generally poor, with reported fetal injury varying from 59 to 78% and perinatal mortality ranging from 41 to 71%.[1,6,12,19] Fetal mortality is due to both prematurity and direct fetal injury.[12] Although direct fetal injury carries a poor prognosis, cases have been reported in which a fetus, having sustained a nonfatal injury, was successfully later delivered alive.[5,12,20]

The approach to the management of penetrating wounds to the pregnant abdomen must be individualized and is based upon the type and location of injury, fetal and maternal status, and gestational age.[5,20,45] Although aggressive management of *gunshot* wounds is frequently recommended for the nongravid patient, more conservative therapy may be indicated during pregnancy. If maternal vital signs and fetal heart rate tracings are stable, there is no evidence of maternal compromise or intra-abdominal hemorrhage, and the entry wound is below the level of the fundus, observation is recommended with radiographic evaluation of projectile location. If the bullet is found to lie within the uterus, continued observation is recommended.[20,45] If the entry wound is above the level of the uterine fundus, there is evidence of fetal or maternal compromise, or intraperitoneal violation is suspected, immediate exploratory laparotomy should be performed. Cesarean delivery is not necessary at the time of surgery unless there is evidence of fetal compromise or infection.[20,45] If the fetus is dead, conservative measures are followed, with surgery reserved for maternal compromise or entry wounds above the fundus. Cesarean delivery is almost always contraindicated in such circumstances, and spontaneous vaginal delivery is anticipated or induced.[19,20,45] As with blunt trauma, the risk of precipitating labor or inducing fetal injury with laparotomy is negligible.[20]

In both the pregnant and nonpregnant patient, *stab wounds* to the abdomen are associated with a lower mortality than gunshot wounds. As with gunshot wounds, the gravid uterus may protect the victim of a lower abdominal stab wound by shielding abdominal contents. Penetrating stab wounds to the upper abdomen during pregnancy, however, carry a high incidence of visceral injury because of upper abdominal crowding and compartmentalization of the intestine by the gravid uterus (see Fig. 4-1).[5,6]

The trend toward conservative management of abdominal stab wounds extends to the pregnant patient. Local wound exploration can frequently differentiate superficial injury from those that penetrate the peritoneal cavity. In those cases where peritoneal penetration cannot be excluded by local exploration, peritoneal lavage may be helpful in ruling out intraperitoneal bleeding or bowel injury. In lower abdominal injuries, retrograde cystography will rule out bladder injury, and external fetal monitoring will establish fetal stability. When full evaluation rules out life-threatening maternal and fetal injuries, patients with lower abdominal stab wounds can be managed with careful observation.[5,45] Because of crowding of abdominal contents resulting from the gravid uterus and an associated increased risk of injury, management of upper abdominal stab wounds is more controversial, with some authorities recommending laparotomy if peritoneal entry cannot be excluded by local exploration.[45]

Thoracic Injuries

Management of chest injuries in the gravid and nongravid patient is essentially the same. Early management of the airway and prompt treatment of pneumothorax and hemothorax is particularly important because of the increased risk of fetal hypoxia with maternal airway compromise. Because of the elevation of diaphragm by the gravid uterus, thoracostomy tubes should be inserted one or two interspaces above the usual site with careful digital exploration of the pleural space before insertion of the tube.

Head Injuries

Management of the pregnant head-injured patient is similar to that of the nonpregnant patient. Cervical spine films and head CT should be performed with abdominal shielding. Increased intracranial pressure is treated with hyperventilation and osmotic diuresis with mannitol in the usual doses. Corticosteroids, although controversial in the management of head trauma, can be given without adverse fetal effects.[6]

Despite the possibility of traumatically induced seizures or coma, any patient beyond 20 weeks of gestation presenting with these symptoms should be suspected of having eclampsia and treated as such while undergoing evaluation and management for suspected head injury. Although hypertension, edema, proteinuria, and hyperactive reflexes are frequently present, they may not be prominent. When eclampsia is suspected, treatment should be initiated immediately with magnesium sulfate ($MgSO_4$). A loading dose of 4 g as a 20% solution is given intravenously at a rate of 1 g per minute followed by a continuous intravenous infusion of 1 to 3 g per minute.[46] Urinary output, respiratory status, and the presence of patellar reflexes should be monitored during MgSO$_4$ infusion.

Burns

Thermal Burns

Although thermal burns uncommonly complicate pregnancy, it is estimated that between 5% and 10% of women of reproductive age admitted to burn units with significant burns are pregnant.[45,46] Several observations have emerged from published studies of gravid patients who have sustained thermal injury.[47-50] First, pregnancy does not appear to alter maternal outcome after thermal injury.[47] In addition, as might be expected, maternal and fetal survival are inversely related to the extent of the mother's burn,[47-50] with burns covering more than 50% of total body surface area portending a poor prognosis for both mother and fetus.[45] Premature labor or fetal death generally occur within the first week after burn injury and are often preceded by episodes of maternal hypotension, sepsis, or respiratory failure.[48,49]

Because maternal survival is usually accompanied by fetal survival,[48,49] the basic principles of burn management that apply to the general population also apply to the gravid patient. Because of the uterine vasoconstriction that accompanies maternal hypoxia and hypovolemia, adequate oxygenation, including intubation at the first sign of respiratory compromise, and aggressive fluid replacement are essential to ensure satisfactory outcome for mother and fetus.[45,47,48] When possible, major burns should be treated in specialized burn units with obstetric consultation.

Electrical Injury

Electrical injury during pregnancy is uncommon. From 1833 to 1987 there were 15 cases documented in the literature; electrical sources ranged from household appliances to lightning. Nine of these cases resulted in intrauterine or perinatal death.[51] From the limited number of cases reported, it appears that there are no specific clinical or pathologic signs of fetal damage from electrical injury. It seems reasonable to assume that the fetus is subject to the same pathophysiologic effects as the mother and may be at even greater risk because of its immersion in amniotic fluid, an excellent conductor.[52] The severity of fetal injury does not directly correlate with that of the mother, with apparently minor maternal injury associated with fetal death.[53] When fetal demise occurs, it may be due to changes in fetal cardiac conduction or to lesions in the uteroplacental bed. Early signs associated with fetal death are cessation of fetal movement and changes in fetal heart rate. If shock occurs early in gestation and the infant survives, intrauterine growth retardation and oligohydramnios are common. Precipitation of labor and rupture of the uterus following electrical injury have also been reported.[51-53]

Obstetric consultation should be obtained following even minor electrical shock during pregnancy. In patients of at least 24 to 26 weeks of gestation, fetal monitoring should be performed to detect fetal distress. In the previable fetus simple auscultation of fetal heart tones will probably suffice.[51] Ultrasonography should be performed in all patients for assessment of gestational age and amniotic fluid volume to provide baseline parameters for following fetal growth.[51]

Perimortem Cesarean Section

If massive trauma has resulted in maternal death and there is a chance of fetal viability, perimortem cesarean delivery is appropriate. Perinatal outcome following this procedure is directly related to the maturity of the fetus, the lapsed time from maternal death, the performance of cardiopulmonary resuscitation on the mother, and to some extent, the availability of neonatal intensive-care facilities.[54–56] The fetus is most likely to survive if cesarean delivery is performed within 5 minutes of maternal arrest, but the procedure is justified regardless of elapsed time if fetal vital signs are present.[11] In some cases perimortem cesarean delivery has been shown to improve maternal hemodynamics by relieving aortocaval compression, resulting in maternal survival.[11,55]

Summary

The leading nonobstetric cause of death in women of reproductive age, significant trauma in the gravid female, requires an intense and highly specialized management approach involving emergency medicine personnel, trauma surgeons, obstetricians, and pediatricians. Because of the anatomic and physiologic changes that accompany pregnancy, ensuring adequate oxygenation and recognition of increased fluid requirements becomes the mainstay of initial resuscitative efforts. Once maternal stabilization is achieved, attention is rapidly directed to the fetus. For the previable fetus, assessment of fetal heart tones and observation for maternal complications of pregnancy may be all that is necessary. Once fetal age approaches that of viability, however, assessment of fetal health through ultrasonography, continuous external tococardiography, and testing for fetomaternal hemorrhage becomes mandatory. Because fetal prognosis can be improved in hospitals with advanced neonatal and obstetric facilities, transport to such a center is frequently appropriate. Such transport should not, however, take precedence over efforts directed toward maternal resuscitation and stabilization.

REFERENCES

1. Pimentel L. Mother and child: Trauma in pregnancy. Emerg Med Clin North Am 9:549, 1991
2. Bocka J, Courtney J, Pearlman M et al. Trauma in pregnancy. Ann Emerg Med 17:829, 1988
3. Rothenberger D, Quattlebaum FW, Perry JF, Zabel J, Fischer RP. Blunt maternal trauma: a review of 103 cases. J Trauma 18:173, 1978
4. Baker DP. Trauma in the pregnant patient. Surg Clin North Am 62:275, 1982
5. Neufeld JDG, Moore EE, Marx JA, Rosen P. Trauma in pregnancy. Emerg Med Clin North Am 5:623, 1987

6. Smith CV, Phelan JP. Trauma in pregnancy. In Clark SL, Phelan JP, Cotton DB (eds): Critical Care Obstetrics, p 382. Oradell, NJ: Medical Economics Books, 1987
7. Fort AT, Harlin RS. Pregnancy outcome after noncatastrophic maternal trauma during pregnancy. Obstet Gynecol 35:912, 1970
8. Farmer DL, Adzick NS, Crombleholme WR, Crombleholme TM, Longaker MT, Harrison MR. Fetal trauma: relation to maternal injury. J Pediatr Surg 25:711, 1990
9. Sherman HF, Scott LM, Rosemurgy AS. Changes affecting the initial evaluation and care of the pregnant trauma victim. J Emerg Med 8:575, 1990
10. McAnena OJ, Moore EE, Marx JA. Initial evaluation of the patient with blunt abdominal trauma. Surg Clin North Am 70:495, 1990
11. Pearlman MD, Tintinalli JE, Lorenz RP. Blunt trauma during pregnancy. N Engl J Med 323:1609, 1990
12. Buschbaum HJ. Diagnosis and management of abdominal gunshot wounds during pregnancy. J Trauma 15:425, 1975
13. Agran PF, Dunkle DE, Winn DG, Kent D. Fetal death in motor vehicle accidents. Ann Emerg Med 16:1355, 1987
14. Fries MH, Hankins GDV. Motor vehicle accident associated with minimal maternal trauma but subsequent fetal demise. Ann Emerg 18:301, 1989
15. Pearlman MD, Tintinalli JE, Lorenz RP. A prospective controlled study of outcome after trauma during pregnancy. Am J Obstet Gynecol 162:1502, 1990
16. Stuart GCE, Harding PGR, Davies EM. Blunt abdominal trauma in pregnancy. Can Med Assoc J 122:901, 1980
17. Golan A, Sandbank O, Teare AJ. Trauma in late pregnancy: a report of 15 cases. S Afr Med J 57:161, 1980
18. Crosby WM, Costiloe JP. Safety of lap-belt restraint for pregnant victims of automobile collisions. N Engl J Med 284:632, 1971
19. Iliya FA, Hajj SN, Buschbaum HJ. Gunshot wounds of the pregnant uterus: report of two cases. J Trauma 20:90, 1980
20. Pierson R, Mihalovitis H, Thomas L, Beatty R. Penetrating abdominal wounds in pregnancy. Ann Emerg Med 15:1232, 1986
21. Pepperell RJ, Rubinstein E, MacIsaac IA. Motor-car accidents during pregnancy. Med J Aust 1:203, 1977
22. Williams JK, McClain L, Rosemurgy AS, Colorado NM. Evaluation of blunt abdominal trauma in the third trimester of pregnancy: maternal and fetal considerations. Obstet Gynecol 75:33, 1990
23. Rosenfeld JA. Abdominal trauma in pregnancy: when is fetal monitoring necessary? Postgrad Med 88:89, 1990
24. Kettel LM, Branch W, Scott JR. Occult placental abruption after maternal trauma. Obstet Gynecol 71:449, 1988
25. Higgins SD, Garite TJ. Late abruptio placenta in trauma patients: implications for monitoring. Obstet Gynecol 63:10S, 1984
26. Lavin JP, Miodovnik M. Delayed abruption after maternal trauma as a result of an automobile accident. J Reprod Med 26:621, 1981
27. Goodwin TM, Breen MT. Pregnancy outcome and fetomaternal hemorrhage after noncatastrophic trauma. Am J Obstet Gynecol 162:665, 1990
28. Drost TF, Rosemurgy AS, Sherman HF, Scott LM, Williams JK. Major trauma in pregnant women: maternal/fetal outcome. J Trauma 30:574, 1990
29. Rose PG, Strohm PL, Zuspan FP. Fetomaternal hemorrhage following trauma. Am J Obstet Gynecol 153:844, 1985
30. Bickers RG, Wennberg RP. Fetomaternal transfusion following trauma. Obstet Gynecol 61:258, 1983

31. Esposito TJ, Gens Dr, Smith LG, Scorpio R. Evaluation of blunt abdominal trauma occurring during pregnancy. J Trauma 29:1628, 1989
32. Attico NB, Smith RJ, FitzPatrick MB, Keneally M. Automobile safety restraints for pregnant women and children. J Reprod Med 31:187, 1986
33. Crosby WM, Snyder RG, Snow CC, Hanson PG. Impact injuries in pregnancy. Am J Obstet Gynecol 101:100, 1968
34. Crosby WM, King AI, Stout LC. Fetal survival following impact: improvement with shoulder harness restraint. Am J Obstet Gynecol 112:1101, 1972
35. Swartz HM, Reichling BA. Hazards of radiation exposure for pregnant women. JAMA 239:1907, 1978
36. Wagner LK, Lester RG, Saldana LR: Prenatal risks from ionizing radiations, ultrasound, magnetic files, and radiofrequency waves. In: Exposure of the pregnant patient to diagnostic radiations, p 61. Philadelphia: JB Lippincott, 1985
37. Mossman KL, Hill LT. Radiation risks in pregnancy. Obstet Gynecol 60:239, 1982
38. The amount of radiation absorbed by the conceptus. In Wagner LK, Lester RG, Saldana LR (eds): Exposure of the pregnant patient to diagnostic radiations, p 40. Philadelphia: JB Lippincott, 1985
39. Civil ID, Talucci RC, Schwab CW. Placental laceration and fetal death as a result of blunt abdominal trauma. J Trauma 28:708, 1988
40. Lowe TW, Weinreb J, Santos-Ramos R, Cunningham FG. Magnetic resonance imaging in human pregnancy. Obstet Gynecol 66:629, 1985
41. Rothenberger DA, Quattlebaum FW, Zabel J, Fishcer RP. Diagnostic peritoneal lavage for blunt trauma in pregnant women. Am J Obstet Gynecol 129:479, 1977
42. Adult immunizations: recommendations of the immunization practices advisory committee (ACIP). MMWR 33:8S, 1984
43. General recommendations on immunization. MMWR 38:205, 1989
44. Doan-Wiggins L. Obstetric and gynecologic emergency drug therapy. In Barsan WG, Jastremski MS, Syverud SA (eds): Emergency drug therapy, p 500. Philadelphia: WB Saunders, 1991
45. Dudley DJ, Cruikshank DP. Trauma and acute surgical emergencies in pregnancy. Sem Perinatol 14:42, 1990
46. Doan-Wiggins L. Hypertensive disorders of pregnancy. Emerg Med Clin North Am 5:495, 1987
47. Amy BW, McManus WF, Goodwin CW, Mason A, Pruitt BA. Thermal injury in the pregnant patient. Surg Gynecol Obstet 161:209, 1985
48. Rayburn W, Smith B, Feller I, Varner M, Cruikshank D. Major burns during pregnancy: effects on fetal well-being. Obstet Gynecol 63:392, 1984
49. Taylor JW, Plunkett GD, McManus WF, Pruitt BA. Thermal injury during pregnancy. Obstet Gynecol 47:434, 1976
50. Deittch EA, Rightmire DA, Clothier J, Blass N. Management of burns in pregnant women. Surg Gynecol Obstet 161:1, 1985
51. Strong TH, Gocke SE, Levy AV, Newel GJ. Electrical shock in pregnancy: a case report. J Emerg Med 5:381, 1987
52. Pierce MR, Henderson RA, Mitchell JM. Cardiopulmonary arrest secondary to lightning in a pregnant woman. Ann Emerg Med 15:597, 1986
53. Lieberman JR, Mazor M, Molcho J, Haiam E, Maor E, Insler V. Electrical accidents during pregnancy. Obstet Gynecol 67:861, 1986
54. Katz VL, Dotters DJ, Droegemueller W. Perimortem cesarean delivery. Obstet Gynecol 68:571, 1986
55. DePace NL, Betesh JS, Kotler MN. "Postmortem" cesarean section with recovery of both mother and offspring. JAMA 248:971, 1982
56. Weber CE. Postmortem cesarean section: review of the literature and case reports. Am J Obstet Gynecol 110:158, 1971

CHAPTER 5

Cardiopulmonary Resuscitation During Pregnancy

Lynnette Doan-Wiggins

Although uncommon, the incidence of maternal cardiac arrest during pregnancy has risen in recent years. This increase is due to (1) the social trends and medical progress that have expanded the number of pregnant women with preexisting medical illness and (2) the increased number of surgical, anesthetic, and medical procedures used in the care of pregnant women.[1] Events leading to cardiac arrest in the gravida include those found in the general population (eg, congenital heart disease, myocardial infarction, pulmonary embolism, and trauma) and those related specifically to pregnancy (eg, pregnancy-induced hypertension, iatrogenic hypermagnesemia, amniotic fluid embolism, and anesthetic agents used during delivery).[1-8] A more complete list of etiologies of maternal cardiac arrest is found in Table 5-1.

As with many diseases that complicate pregnancy, the dramatic alterations in cardiopulmonary physiology that accompany pregnancy and the unique fetal effects associated with maternal cardiac arrest and resuscitation deserve special mention.

Anatomic and Physiologic Considerations in the Mother and Fetus

Cardiovascular System

Maternal cardiovascular physiology undergoes profound alterations throughout pregnancy. During the first trimester blood volume begins to increase, and by the 30th week of gestation it reaches a level 40% above that of the nongravid woman.

TABLE 5-1
Some Common Etiologies of Cardiac Arrest During Pregnancy

Specifically Associated With Pregnancy
    Pregnancy-induced cardiomyopathy
    Pregnancy-induced hypertension (preeclampsia/eclampsia)
    Obstetric hemorrhage
    Amniotic fluid embolism
    Iatrogenic
        Hypermagnesemia
        Anesthesia during delivery
Not Specific to Pregnancy
    Preexisting cardiovascular disease
        Myocardial infarction
        Congenital heart disease
        Acquired valvular disease
        Arrhythmia
    Pulmonary disease
        Pulmonary embolism
        Asthma
        Aspiration pneumonia
    Anaphylaxis/angioedema
    Intracranial hemorrhage
    Sepsis
    Trauma
    Electrical injury

This increase in volume results in part from a 20 to 40% rise in the number of erythrocytes but to a larger extent from an expansion of plasma volume that increases up to 50% by the 32nd week of gestation. This difference in the expansion of red cell mass relative to that of plasma volume results in the dilutional anemia seen during normal pregnancy.[9,10]

Beginning during the first 10 weeks of pregnancy, cardiac output also rises, reaching a peak 30 to 45% above resting, nonpregnancy levels around the 20th week of gestation and maintaining this level until term. Coincident with this rise in cardiac output is a decrease in systemic vascular resistance (SVR) that results primarily from decreased resistance in the uteroplacental and pulmonary circulations. Reaching a nadir from the 14th to 24th week of gestation, this decrease in SVR results in a gradual lowering of mean arterial blood pressure during the first two trimesters of pregnancy and in a return to nonpregnant levels by term.[1,9,10]

In addition to the low vascular resistance of the uteroplacental bed, redistribution of blood volume occurs because of growth of the uteroplacental mass. In the nonpregnant state the uterus receives less than 2% of cardiac output.[1] As pregnancy progresses, this proportion increases until at term uterine blood flow reaches 500 mL per minute, representing more than 10% of systemic cardiac output.[10] By the end of the first half of pregnancy, the uteroplacental vascular bed functions as a maximally dilated, passive, low-resistance system such that uterine blood flow is principally determined by maternal perfusion pressure. During maternal hypoxia or hypotension, therapeutic doses of vasopressors, especially alpha-adrenergic or combined alpha- and beta-adrenergic agents, may produce uteroplacental vasoconstriction when the maternal cardiovascular system has enhanced sensitivity to their action, thereby further compromising already diminished uteroplacental blood flow.[1]

In addition to the redistribution of blood flow that results from the enlarging uteroplacental bed, during the second half of pregnancy the gravid uterus can exert profound mechanical effects on the maternal cardiovascular system by virtue of its weight and size. Compression of the inferior vena cava, particularly in the supine position, results in significant obstruction of caval blood flow in approximately 90% of women. This compression leads to decreased venous return to the heart and a corresponding reduction in cardiac output of 10 to 25% during spontaneous circulation[11] and can further compromise the already poor venous return that exists during cardiopulmonary resuscitation (CPR).[12] Correspondingly, poor venous return from infradiaphragmatic vessels makes the femoral and saphenous sites poor choices for administering drugs and fluids during CPR.[12]

In addition to obstruction of the inferior vena cava, the gravid uterus exerts pressure on the abdominal aorta, reducing arterial flow distal to the obstruction and placing uteroplacental blood flow in jeopardy both by decreasing arterial blood flow and by raising venous pressure.[13] Maternal hypotension and uterine contractions markedly enhance these obstructive effects.[13] Changing the late gravida from the supine to left lateral decubitus position or manually displacing the uterus in a leftward and cephalad direction will minimize aortocaval compression and improve decreased venous return.[11–13]

Respiratory System

The maternal respiratory system also undergoes significant changes during pregnancy. A progesterone-induced hyperventilation begins during the first trimester with minute ventilation increasing by as much as 48% over control values at term. The metabolic effect of this hyperventilation is the production of a partially compensated respiratory alkalosis with arterial blood gases showing a fall in pCO_2 to approximately 30 to 34 mmHg and a compensatory decrease in serum bicarbonate to 19.5 mEq/L. These changes leave the pregnant woman with a decreased buffering capacity during periods of hypotension and cardiac arrest.

During pregnancy maternal oxygen consumption and basal metabolic rate increase 20 and 14%, respectively.[10,14] Although the progesterone-induced hyperventilation causes a rise in maternal arterial pO_2 of about 10 mmHg,[15] the increase in maternal oxygen consumption and metabolic rate as well as a decrease in functional residual capacity make the parturient particularly susceptible to hypoxia during periods of apnea.[14] In addition, enlargement of the uterus with upward displacement of the viscera and diaphragm decrease compliance for both artificial ventilation and external cardiac compression in the arrest victim.[1,13]

Fetal Considerations

Critical to the concept of maternal cardiac arrest is the effect that the resulting hypoperfusion and hypoxia have on the fetus. Experience with perimortem cesarean section indicates that fetal survival and neurologic outcome are best if delivery is performed within 5 minutes of maternal arrest, suggesting that neuronal damage occurs within this time.[3] Several physiologic fetal adaptations and reflexes in response to the hypoxic state, however, protect the fetus from severe hypoxia and may account for the occasional survival of infants delivered more than 20 minutes after the initiation of maternal CPR.[3]

First, the oxyhemoglobin dissociation curve of fetal hemoglobin is shifted to the left when compared to maternal hemoglobin, yielding a greater oxygen saturation of fetal hemoglobin at any given partial pressure of oxygen.[12,16] In addition, the physiologic acidosis of the fetus compared with that of the mother favors placental oxygen transfer by the Bohr effect.[12] These factors, combined with the higher concentration of fetal hemoglobin in fetal erythrocytes, enable the fetus to extract and carry a larger amount of oxygen at lower oxygen tension than the mother. The net effect of this higher oxygen saturation of fetal blood is to provide a greater amount of oxygen to fetal tissues.[12,16]

In addition to the benefit of increased oxygen-carrying capacity of fetal blood, fetal cardiac output under both normal and hypoxic conditions optimizes oxygenation of vital fetal tissues. Under normal conditions, fetal cardiac output is distributed so that the highest oxygen concentration is delivered to vital structures and less is sent to the abdominal organs and lower body.[16] In response to fetal asphyxia, an even more beneficial redistribution of fetal blood occurs. As fetal blood pressure and heart rate rise in response to hypoxia, umbilical blood flow increases, causing an increase in placental exchange.[16] In addition, a reflex-selective peripheral vasoconstriction causes a redistribution of blood flow to the fetal brain, heart, and adrenals, with the brainstem and heart being the best protected.[12,16,17] Although the integrity of vital organs can be preserved for a limited period of time with this central redistribution of blood flow, if asphyxia persists, such physiologic adjustments become inadequate, and neurologic damage or death of the fetus will occur.[16]

It appears that the survivors of intrauterine asphyxia generally do well with the majority of even severely asphyxiated neonates suffering little or no detectable neurologic or intellectual sequelae.[12,18,19] Hypoxic injury to the fetus seems to follow an "all-or-nothing" pattern, with a hypoxic insult of sufficient magnitude to cause brain damage frequently causing fetal death. In those who survive with chronic brain damage, the hypoxic insult is likely to have been very severe and prolonged, and brain damage is usually associated with major motor disorders, severe retardation, chronic seizure disorders, and difficulty with respiratory control during the neonatal period.[12,18]

Cardiopulmonary Resuscitation

When cardiac arrest occurs before the onset of fetal viability, about the 24th week of gestation, the objectives of cardiopulmonary resuscitation should be directed almost exclusively to maternal considerations. Successful recovery of maternal physiologic function at this gestational age provides the best chance of fetal survival. Beyond the 24th week of gestation, the life of the potentially viable fetus must be considered in addition to that of the mother.[1,2]

Resuscitation Technique

Most of the standard resuscitation procedures can and should be applied during pregnancy, with some requiring modification because of the anatomic and physiologic changes that accompany pregnancy.[2,12] As in the nonpregnant woman, intubation and airway support should be instituted early. This is particularly important in the gravida because of her decreased tolerance to hypoxia secondary to both a reduction in the functional residual capacity of the lung and the increased oxygen demands and higher basal metabolic rate associated with pregnancy.[3] Closed-chest compressions and ventilatory support may be done using conventional technique.[2] During the latter half of pregnancy, displacement of the gravid uterus becomes necessary to minimize aortocaval compression and improve venous return. This may be accomplished by having a member of the resuscitation team manually deflect the uterus to a leftward and cephalad position or by placing a wedge, such as a pillow, under the patient's right flank and hip. Although placing the patient in the true left lateral decubitus position will make manual chest compressions clumsy and ineffective, placing the patient in a 15° left lateral tilt position through the use of either a backboard or a tiltable table may provide an acceptable alternative to manual uterine displacement without significantly compromising chest compressions.[1,12]

If the patient has suffered cardiac arrest from ventricular fibrillation, prompt electrical countershock using current Advanced Cardiac Life Support (ACLS) guidelines is indicated.[1,2] There is no contraindication to external defibrillation during pregnancy, and direct current (DC) countershocks of up to 300 J have been used in pregnant patients without adverse fetal effect.[5,6,12]

Thoracotomy and open-chest cardiac massage are advocated by some authorities if standard CPR with patient positioning, airway support, and defibrillation fail to result in spontaneous circulation within 15 minutes; thoracotomy may be indicated even earlier if closed-chest compressions fail to generate adequate pulses. Increased cardiac output resulting from open cardiac massage and a decreased need for epinephrine, with its attendant negative effects on uteroplacental circulation, are cited as the principal reasons for employing this procedure.[1,2,12]

When fetal viability has been reached, between 24 and 26 weeks of gestation, the decision to expedite delivery in the face of maternal cardiac arrest must be made. Because delivery of the fetus may improve maternal hemodynamics such that successful resuscitation of the mother is possible, and because infant prognosis improves as the time from maternal arrest decreases, the decision to perform perimortem cesarean section should be made expeditiously.[1,2,3,8,20] Although infant prognosis is best when delivery is accomplished within 5 minutes of maternal arrest, cesarean delivery should be attempted up to 25 minutes after maternal death, the longest interval for which fetal survival has been reported.[3] CPR should be continued, of course, during and after delivery.

Drugs Used in Resuscitation

The standard medications used during cardiopulmonary resuscitation have generally not been found to be harmful to the fetus, and their use in the arrest situation is certainly justified.[12] Although lidocaine crosses the placenta, when used in standard doses it appears to cause little harm to the fetus.[2] Vasopressors, such as epinephrine and dopamine, should be avoided if possible during pregnancy, since they induce uteroplacental vasoconstriction, especially when maternal hypoxemia or hypotension is present.[1,2] Although sodium bicarbonate is not recommended for the treatment of cardiac arrest in the nonpregnant patient, it may be considered in the gravida when arterial blood gases indicate that the pH is below 7.3 and the partial pressures of oxygen and carbon dioxide are acceptable. In this situation bicarbonate may help correct maternal metabolic acidosis and the resulting increased reactivity of the uteroplacental vasculature to alpha-adrenergic agents.[1] Table 5-2 lists the drugs commonly used during CPR and their application during pregnancy.

Complications of Cardiopulmonary Resuscitation

Maternal complications of CPR include laceration of the liver, uterine rupture, hemothorax, and hemopericardium. Fetal complications include cardiac arrhythmia or standstill from maternal defibrillation and drug therapy, central nervous system toxicity from antiarrhythmic drugs, and altered uteroplacental perfusion from maternal hypoxemia, acidosis, and vasoconstriction.[1,2] In the patient suffering cardiopulmonary arrest associated with eclampsia, spontaneous intrahepatic hemorrhage

TABLE 5-2
Medications Used During Cardiopulmonary Resuscitation—Considerations in Pregnancy*

Drug	Indications	Considerations in Pregnancy
Epinephrine	Potentially beneficial in all forms of cardiac arrest	Category C. Has been shown to be teratogenic in animals in large doses; may induce uteroplacental vasoconstriction.
Lidocaine	Ventricular ectopy, tachycardia and fibrillation	Category C. Use during pregnancy is not well studied; crosses the placenta but in therapeutic doses has no teratogenic effect on the fetus; may cause fetal bradycardia.
Bretylium	Ventricular fibrillation and tachycardia unresponsive to other therapy	Category C. Safety has not been established in human pregnancy; use only if clearly indicated.
Atropine	Symptomatic bradycardia, asystole	Category B. Crosses placenta but results in no fetal abnormalities; can cause fetal tachycardia.
Sodium bicarbonate	Cardiac arrest unresponsive to other measures; documented preexisting metabolic acidosis	Category C. Studies to define risk of hypertonic sodium bicarbonate therapy in pregnancy have not been done.
Dopamine	Hemodynamically significant hypotension in the absence of hypovolemia	Category C. No teratogenic effects have been observed in laboratory animals but sufficient studies in humans are lacking. Use only when clearly indicated.
Dobutamine	Short term inotropic support of patients with depressed myocardial contractility	Category C. Not found to be teratogenic in animal studies but its effects in pregnant humans are unknown. Use only if clearly indicated.

*Tamari I, Eldar M, Rabinowitz B, Neufeld HN. Medical treatment of cardiovascular disorders during pregnancy. Am Heart J 104:1357, 1982
Gibler WB. Antiarrhythmics. In: Barsan WG, Jastremski MS, Syverud SA, eds. Emergency drug therapy. Philadelphia: WB Saunders, 1991:147
Saunders CE. Vasoactive agents. In: Barsan WG, Jastremski MS, Syverud SA, eds. Emergency drug therapy. Philadelphia: WB Saunders, 1991:281
Singal B. Acidifying and alkalizing agents. In: Barsan WG, Jastremski MS, Syverud SA, eds. Emergency drug therapy. Philadelphia: WB Saunders, 1991:281

may make the patient particularly susceptible to laceration of the liver; already compromised uteroplacental blood flow may be further jeopardized by decreased maternal perfusion pressures and vasopressor administration during resuscitation.[1]

Perimortem Cesarean Section

Since 1879 there have been less than 300 cases of perimortem cesarean section, with approximately half of the procedures yielding a live neonate.[20] Although a rare occurrence, the decision to perform postmortem cesarean section in the emergency department is a difficult one. Perinatal outcome is directly related to the gestational age of the fetus, the time from maternal death to delivery of the infant, the nature of the maternal insult, and to some extent, the availability of neonatal intensive-care facilities.[3,20–23]

Although the lower limit of fetal viability varies among institutions, in general, survival of the fetus is unlikely if gestational age is less than 28 weeks or fetal weight is less than 1000 g.[3,22,23] If the duration of gestation is unknown from the history, fetal maturity may be quickly estimated by measuring the height of the uterine fundus. At 28 weeks of gestation the fundus is approximately 28 cm above the symphysis pubis or halfway between the umbilicus and costal margin. In some institutions with advanced neonatal capabilities infant survival may be considered possible at 26 weeks of gestation or less.[23,24] Criteria for intervention should be established prospectively at each institution and should be in accordance with the institution's general neonatal policies.[16]

The frequency of infant survival decreases and the chance of neurologic damage increases as the time from maternal death to cesarean section rises. When cesarean section is performed within 5 minutes of maternal demise, outcome is generally considered excellent; within 5 to 10 minutes, good; within 10 to 15 minutes, fair; and within 15 to 20 minutes, poor. No cases of fetal survival have been reported when cesarean delivery was performed more than 25 minutes after maternal death.[3,22] Because even under optimal conditions cardiopulmonary resuscitation results in a cardiac output of 30% to 40% of normal and because placental perfusion may be severely compromised, every attempt should be made to begin cesarean delivery within 4 minutes of maternal cardiopulmonary arrest, completing the procedure within 5 minutes of arrest.[3,16] Fetal prognosis is generally better following the sudden death of a previously healthy mother than after death of a woman with a prolonged or debilitating illness.[3,23]

Perimortem cesarean section should be done by the most experienced personnel present, preferably an obstetrician; and when it is possible, a neonatologist should be in attendance. Cardiopulmonary resuscitation should, of course, be initiated on the mother at the time of cardiac arrest and continued until *after* delivery of the infant. A few seconds of sterile abdominal preparation are suggested but not necessary, and a Foley may be inserted to decompress the bladder. These preparations should not, however, delay delivery.

Rapid extraction of the infant while avoiding fetal injury is the goal of the procedure. A vertical incision extending from the level of the uterine fundus to the symphysis pubis is made through the abdominal wall to the peritoneal cavity (Fig. 5-1). Avoiding injury to the fetus, a small vertical incision is made in the lower uterine

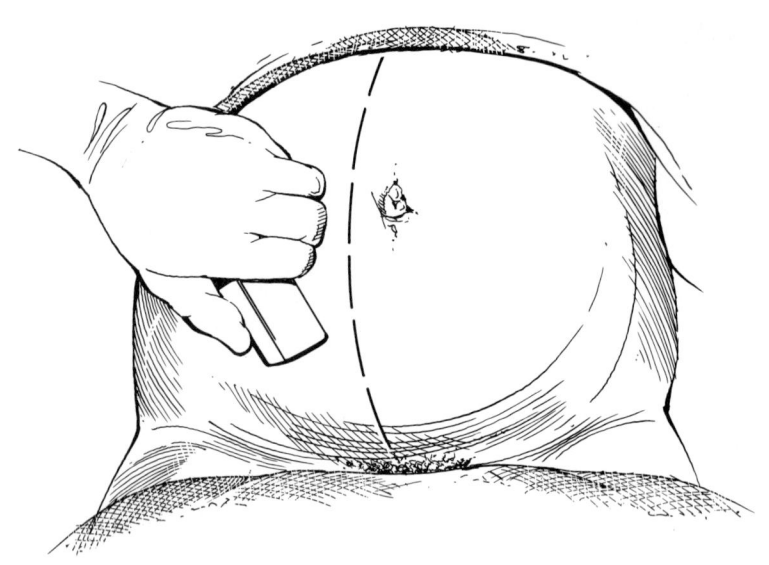

FIGURE 5-1
Site of incision for postmortem cesarean section.

segment just cephalad to the bladder until amniotic fluid is obtained or until the uterine cavity is clearly entered. Using scissors, this incision is extended cephalad to the uterine fundus while the physician's free hand is placed inside the uterus to lift the uterine wall away from the infant. If an anterior placenta is encountered, it is incised in order to reach the fetus. The infant is then gently delivered, the mouth and nares suctioned, and the cord clamped and cut.[20,25] Prompt resuscitation, conservation of the body heat, and transfer to a neonatal unit should be provided for the infant. Infrequently, relief of aortocaval compression by delivery of the infant will improve maternal hemodynamics enough for the mother to survive.[20,21,25]

No physician has ever been found liable for performing a perimortem cesarean section. Indeed, it is felt that the physician has the legal right and responsibility to provide the unborn fetus every possible chance of survival. Permission for operation should be obtained when possible but not at the expense of delaying the procedure. Failure to obtain permission should not preclude cesarean section.[3,22]

Summary

Although cardiopulmonary arrest during pregnancy occurs infrequently, its incidence is increasing in response to changing social and medical trends. With the exception of displacement of the gravid uterus during the latter part of pregnancy, most resuscitative procedures require little alteration. In the gravida of less than 24 weeks' gestation, resuscitative attempts should be directed primarily toward the mother, with the best chance of fetal survival being maternal survival. After the age of fetal viability, perimortem cesarean section should be considered in an attempt both to save the infant and to improve maternal hemodynamics.

REFERENCES

1. Lee RV, Rodgers BD, White LM, Harvey RC. Cardio-pulmonary resuscitation of pregnant women. Am J Med 81:311, 1986
2. Special resuscitation situations. In Textbook of Advanced Cardiac Life Support, p 227. Dallas: American Heart Association, 1987
3. Katz VL, Dotters DJ, Droegemueller W. Perimortem cesarean delivery. Obstet Gynecol 68:571, 1986
4. Arthur RK. Postmortem cesarean section. Am J Obstet Gynecol 132:175, 1978
5. Stokes IM, Evans J, Stone M. Myocardial infarction and cardiac arrest in the second trimester followed by assisted vaginal delivery under epidural analgesia at 38 weeks gestation. Case report. Br J Obstet Gynaecol 91:197, 1984
6. Curry JJ, Quintana FJ. Myocardial infarction with ventricular fibrillation during pregnancy treated by direct current defibrillation with fetal survival. Chest 58:82, 1970
7. McCubbin JH, Sibai BM, Abdella TN, Anderson GD. Cardiopulmonary arrest due to acute maternal hypermagnesaemia. Lancet 1:1058, 1981
8. Marx GF. Cardiopulmonary resuscitation of late-pregnant women. Anesthesiology 56:156, 1982
9. Sullivan JM, Ramanathan KB. Management of medical problems in pregnancy—severe cardiac disease. N Engl J Med 313:304, 1985
10. Lee W, Cotton DB. Cardiorespiratory changes during pregnancy. In Clark SL, Phelan JP, Cotton DB (eds): Critical Care Obstetrics, p 39. Oradell, NJ: Medical Economics Books, 1987
11. Kerr MG. The mechanical effects of the gravid uterus in late pregnancy. J Obstet Gynaecol Br Comm 72:513, 1965
12. Selden BS, Burke TJ. Complete maternal and fetal recovery after prolonged cardiac arrest. Ann Emerg Med 17:346, 1988
13. Bieniarz J, Crottogini JJ, Curuchet E, Romreo-Salinas G et al. Aortocaval compression by the uterus in late human pregnancy. Am J Obstet Gynecol 100:203, 1968
14. Archer GW, Marx GF. Arterial oxygen tension during apnoea in parturient women. Br J Anaesth 46:358, 1974
15. Sherman HF, Scott LM, Rosemurgy AS. Changes affecting the initial evaluation and care of the pregnant trauma victim. J Emerg Med 8:575, 1990
16. Phelan JP. Fetal considerations in the critically ill obstetric patient. In Clark SL, Phelan JP, Cotton DB (eds): Critical Care Obstetrics, p 436. Oradell: Medical Economics Books, 1987
17. Peeters LLH, Sheldon RE, Jones MD, Makowski EL, Meschia G. Blood flow to fetal organs as a function of arterial oxygen content. Am J Obstet Gynecol 135:637, 1979
18. Paneth N, Stark RI. Cerebral palsy and mental retardation in relation to indicators of perinatal asphyxia. Am J Obstet Gynecol 147:960, 1983
19. Adamsons K, Myers RE. Late decelerations and brain tolerance of fetal monkey to intrapartum asphyxia. Am J Obstet Gynecol 128:893, 1977
20. Strong TH, Lowe RA. Perimortem cesarean section. J Emerg Med 7:489, 1989
21. DePace NL, Betesh JS, Kotler MN. Postmortem cesarean section with recovery of both mother and offspring. JAMA 248:971, 1982
22. Weber CE. Postmortem cesarean section: review of the literature and case reports. Am J Obstet Gynecol 110:158, 1971
23. Dillon WP, Lee RV, Tronolone MJ, Buckwald S, Foote RJ. Life support during maternal brain death during pregnancy. JAMA 248:1089, 1982
24. Neufeld JDG, Moore EE, Marx JA, Rosen P. Trauma in pregnancy. Emerg Med Clin North Am 5:623, 1987
25. Doan-Wiggins L. Obstetric and gynecologic procedures. In Roberts JR, Hedges JR (eds): Clinical Procedures in Emergency Medicine, 2nd ed. Philadelphia: WB Saunders, 1991

CHAPTER 6

Perimortem Cesarean Section

Lance Sang

Cesarean section performed when survival of the mother is in doubt has been referred to as *perimortem cesarean section*.[1] This subject had previously been referred to in the literature as postmortem cesarean section, but relatively recent advances in both cardiopulmonary resuscitation and neonatal intensive care have combined to improve the potential for survival of both the mother and fetus after maternal cardiac arrest. Maternal death caused by chronic illness is now less commonplace than death from acute events, such as emboli, anesthetic complications, and cerebrovascular accidents. Furthermore, the fetus is more likely to survive in the absence of chronic maternal illness.

Cesarean section performed after the death of the mother is a procedure that has been reported since antiquity. Mythology holds that Apollo delivered Asklepios the physician from the dead Koronis, and Bacchus was delivered by postmortem cesarean section.[2,3] The *Lex Regia* of ancient Rome, which was later to become the *Lex Caesare* under the emperors, contained a decree dating from the eighth century BC that stated that no woman who died during late pregnancy could be buried until the child had been cut out of her abdomen. In 237 BC, Pliny the Elder recorded the earliest case of a postmortem cesarean section that was said to have resulted in a live-born infant; this was in reference to the birth of Scipio Africanus, who was later to become the general who conquered Hannibal.[2,3]

The operation was formally sanctioned by the Roman Catholic Church in 1280 AD, when the Council of Cologne decreed that postmortem cesarean section must be done so that the soul of the unborn child could be saved by baptism.

Changing Concepts Regarding Postmortem Cesarean Section

Older case reports in the literature, as well as reviews of the subject by Duer in 1879, Ritter in 1961, and Weber in 1971 were generally limited to the topics of fetal survival and to the examination of the changing causes of maternal mortality through the years.[2-4]

More recent studies have focused on acute maternal compromise and performance of the operation with not only improved chances for infant survival but also better maternal recovery.[5-7]

In 1879 Duer reported on 55 postmortem cesarean sections, with 36 infants surviving. In his series most maternal deaths were due to infections (cholera, dysentery, and tuberculosis) and eclampsia.[4] Ritter reviewed 120 cases of postmortem cesarean section, yielding live-born infants. The cause of maternal death was eclampsia (33%), tuberculosis (27%), trauma (7%), and cardiovascular disease (7%), including hypertension.[2] In 1961 Behney reported on the Michigan Maternal Mortality Study of 1950 to 1957; he detailed 72 cases of postmortem cesarean section among 987 maternal deaths. Thirty-eight (52.8%) of the infants were live-born, but only 11 (15%) were eventually discharged in good condition.[8] Behney noted that the causes of death among women undergoing postmortem section were changing. Polio and eclampsia were still the leading causes of death at that time, but embolic diseases, cerebral hemorrhage, and complications of spinal anesthesia were beginning to be reported in significant numbers.

Weber, who in 1971 reviewed the literature and added 33 cases of postmortem section with infant survival, was the first to analyze systematically the various factors associated with successful outcome. Weber's series included no deaths from poliomyelitis or tuberculosis, and only one case was related to infection.[3] Weber's conclusions follow:

1. Operation after 28 weeks offered the greatest chance for success, as defined by immediate survival of the fetus.
2. Promptness of operating was paramount; analysis of the elapsed time from maternal death to delivery revealed that delivery within 5 minutes offered excellent chances for survival; 5 to 10 minutes, good chances; 10 to 15 minutes, fair chances; 15 to 20 minute, poor chances. Within 20 to 25 minutes survival was unlikely. Delay of delivery for more than 15 minutes following maternal death would probably result in fetal death or severe cerebral damage. No cases of infant survival with delivery more than 25 minutes after the death of the mother could be documented.
3. Maternal resuscitative measures, ventilation, and cardiac massage should be continued throughout the cesarean section.
4. Intensive neonatal care should be readily available.
5. The impending maternal death should be anticipated whenever possible, and the operation should be prepared for.

In 1978 Arthur reported three cases of cesarean section being done immediately after the death of gravely ill mothers. (The diagnoses were pulmonary embolus, acute fatty liver of pregnancy, and amniotic fluid embolus.) Arthur commented that "postmortem cesarean section is done more frequently, but the results remain less than satisfying."[9] He noted that with the evolution of the disciplines of intensive medical care and perinatology, more aggressive management of critically ill mothers, along with surveillance of the fetus for its maturity and well-being, could likely result in an improvement of fetal survival and in the possible reversal of maternal disease.

Until 1980 all the series mentioned focused on the operation truly being done after the death of the mother. However, changing patterns of maternal mortality were noted within these series. Chronic illness became a less frequent cause of maternal death. Conversely, a trend toward acute events threatening maternal life was noted. For the first time there began to be suggestions that, in these cases, cesarean section might improve maternal salvage and might therefore become part of the resuscitative effort.

In the early 1980s sporadic case reports began to appear, reflecting two evolving concepts:

1. Increasing sophistication and success rate of maternal cardiopulmonary resuscitation led to the concept of cesarean section being performed as an integral part of the resuscitation procedure.
2. Antemortem cesarean section was reported to have been performed on brain-dead gravidas whose artificial life support continued until the fetus was deemed viable.

In 1982 DePace reported the case of a 27-year-old gravida who at 37 weeks of gestation sustained cardiopulmonary arrest as a result of massive hemoptysis.[10] After 25 minutes of intensive cardiopulmonary resuscitation, the patient had sinus tachycardia and absent femoral and carotid pulses. Fetal heart tones were not audible. Cesarean section was begun, all the while continuing cardiopulmonary resuscitation. The fetus had Apgar scores of 1 at 1 minute and of 2 at 5 minutes, with a cord pH of 6.9. Immediately after delivery of the fetus (30 minutes into the resuscitation), the mother regained femoral and carotid pulses and was found to have a systolic blood pressure of 80 mmHg. The mother's subsequent course included decerebrate rigidity and generalized seizures, but she was without focal neurologic signs on the first postpartum day. She went on to recover fully and ultimately became neurologically normal. The infant had no focal neurologic deficits at the time of discharge; she did have hypotonia and decreased sucking. The child was reported to be well at age 20 months and to be showing appropriate development. DePace commented that he believed that reversal of the supine hypotension syndrome by delivery of the fetus led to restoration of the patient's cardiac output and to the eventual success of the resuscitation.

In 1988 Oates reiterated the argument for prompt delivery as part of the overall management of cardiopulmonary resuscitation in late pregnancy.[11] She reported the case of a patient at 38 weeks' gestation who sustained cardiac arrest from an amniotic fluid embolism at home, 10 minutes before arrival at the hospital. Resuscitation was immediately begun but was found to be difficult with the patient in the left lateral position. Five minutes after hospital admission, cesarean section was performed, delivering a term infant with Apgar scores of 0, 4, and 5 at 1, 5, and 10 minutes, respectively. The infant had normal development at 6, 12, and 16 months of age. The mother's immediate cardiac status improved after delivery of the fetus and she survived, but not without significant neurologic impairment that reflected the hypoxia of long duration (15 minutes) during the cardiac arrest.

In a short report on cardiac arrest resulting from bupivacaine toxicity in five healthy women undergoing regional block for cesarean section, Marx noted the need for prolonged cardiac compression that is typically associated with such cases.[12] In addition, Marx commented on the prompt improvement of maternal circulation brought on by the relief of aortocaval compression resulting from delivery. Marx also noted that if immediate delivery could not be safely done, manual displacement of the uterus to the left and slightly cephalad was helpful in restoring maternal circulation. She also noted that the three patients who were "delivered with dispatch" all survived without sequelae; the other two patients, in whom delivery was delayed, suffered irreversible brain damage. She concluded that "prompt delivery of the infant should be considered part of the cardiopulmonary resuscitation of late-pregnant women."

In 1986 Katz commented on the changing causes of maternal death. He noted that in contrast to older data that showed that most maternal deaths occurred from infection, eclampsia, and hemorrhage, recent studies indicated that most maternal deaths occurred from acute causes, such as embolism, anesthesia, or cerebrovascular accidents. He noted that among the 60 cases of postmortem cesarean section that had been reported in the literature since the time of Weber's 1971 study, 20 were related to anesthesia or embolism and only two were related to infection. Katz believed that the importance of this shift in cause of maternal mortality in relation to postmortem cesarean delivery was that infants of mothers with chronic diseases have a poorer chance of survival than infants born of women who were previously healthy and died suddenly.[1] Therefore because of the possibility of a normal infant being delivered, cesarean section should be considered in any woman who has a cardiac arrest in the third trimester.

The diagnosis of maternal brain death in a patient with a previable fetus deserves consideration in reference to the performance of perimortem cesarean section. Sampson has reported comatose patients not requiring life support being capable of continuing pregnancy and delivering viable infants.[13]

Similarly, Dillon reported successful fetal outcome in cases of irreversible maternal coma in which life support was begun as early as 25 weeks. He commented that "considering the expense and futility of prolonging maternal life in the setting of brain death, at 28 weeks or beyond, the fetus should be delivered as soon as practical after confirming brain death" (i.e., when fetal maturity has been established).[14]

Heikkinen reported a patient at 21 weeks of pregnancy sustaining a massive intracerebral hemorrhage from a ruptured aneurysm. The patient was maintained on life support until 31 weeks of pregnancy, when cesarean section was performed because of maternal hypotension that was unresponsive to treatment.[15] Despite the initial insult having involved prolonged maternal hypoxia and hypotension, as well as repetitive periods of hypotension during the remainder of the pregnancy, development of the infant was normal, after a neonatal course consistent with prematurity.

Loewy has discussed the ethics of these clinical situations and has commented on the necessity of not prolonging the pregnancy beyond a point at which delivery would likely result in a normal infant.[16]

Special Considerations During Resuscitation

The following are some special areas to consider during resuscitation:

1. Analysis of successful cases in the literature by Katz has shown that the optimal timing of perimortem cesarean section that would allow fetal survival of good quality, as well as potential improvement of maternal circulation, is in the initiation of the procedure within 4 minutes of the start of the cardiac arrest, with delivery being accomplished within 1 minute more.[1] However, because of the many documented cases of infant survival well beyond the recommended 5 minutes, the procedure is justified for as long as the fetus is alive.
2. Since severe fetal bradycardia often accompanies the initial hypoxia of maternal cardiac arrest, simple auscultation for heart tones is not sufficient to assess the fetal condition. Sonography should be done whenever possible to confirm that the fetus is still alive.
3. Cardiopulmonary resuscitation should continue during the cesarean section, for increased fetal oxygenation, and for the possibility of a maternal response following delivery of the fetus.

Over the course of history the reasons for performing the operation, as well as the expected outcome, have dramatically changed. Postmortem cesarean section was initially performed to deliver a (usually) dead fetus from a dead mother "so as not to make the mother's body its coffin."[3] More recently, the goal changed to an attempt to salvage a living infant from a moribund or already dead mother.

With increasing knowledge of the physiology of cardiac arrest in pregnancy and with the advent of advanced techniques in cardiopulmonary resuscitation, perimortem cesarean section can now be done both to achieve delivery of a live-born infant and to improve the chances for maternal survival.

REFERENCES

1. Katz VL, Dotters DJ, Droegemueller W. Perimortem cesarean delivery. Obstet Gynecol 68:571, 1986
2. Ritter OW. Postmortem cesarean section. JAMA 175:715, 1961
3. Weber CE. Postmortem cesarean section: review of the literature and case reports. Am J Obstet Gynecol 110:158, 1971
4. Duer EL. Post-mortem delivery. Am J Obstet Gynecol 12:1, 1879
5. Strong TH, Lowe RA. Perimortem cesarean section. Am J Emerg Med 7(5):489, 1989
6. Selden BS, Burke TJ. Complete maternal and fetal recovery after prolonged cardiac arrest. Ann Emerg Med 17(4):346, 1988
7. Lopez-Zeno JA, Carlo WA, O'Grady JP, Fanaroff AA. Infant survival following delayed postmortem cesarean delivery. Obstet Gynecol 76:991, 1990
8. Behney CA. Cesarean delivery after death of the mother. JAMA 176:617, 1961
9. Arthur RK. Postmortem cesarean section. Am J Obstet Gynecol 132:175, 1978
10. DePace NL, Betesh JS, Kotler MN. "Postmortem" cesarean section with recovery of both mother and offspring. JAMA 248:971, 1982

11. Oates S, Williams GL, Rees GA. Cardiopulmonary resuscitation in late pregnancy. Br Med J 297:404, 1988
12. Marx GF: Cardiopulmonary resuscitation of the late pregnant woman. Anesthesiology 56:156, 1982
13. Sampson MB, Petersen LP. Posttraumatic coma during pregnancy. Obstet Gynecol 53:1, 1979
14. Dillon WP, Lee RV, Tronolone MJ, Buckwald S, Foote RJ. Life support and maternal brain death during pregnancy. JAMA 248:1089, 1982
15. Heikkinen JE, Rinne RI, Alahuhta SM et al. Life support for 10 weeks with successful fetal outcome after fatal maternal brain damage. Br Med J [Clin Res] 290:1237, 1985
16. Loewy EH. The pregnant brain dead and the fetus: Must we try to wrest life from death? Am J Obstet Gynecol 157:1097, 1987

CHAPTER 7

Hypertensive Disorders of Pregnancy: Preeclampsia/Eclampsia

Luis Sanchez-Ramos

Preeclampsia is a disorder that affects women exclusively during pregnancy. It is a disease of unknown etiology that presents in pregnant women at both extremes of reproductive age. Reported incidences range from 2 to 30%, depending on the diagnostic criteria used and the population studied.[1] Conditions associated with an increased incidence include previous preeclampsia, multifetal pregnancy, molar pregnancy, and triploidy. It is a clinical condition that comprises a wide spectrum of signs and symptoms that have been observed to develop alone or in combination. Complications resulting from preeclampsia are a leading cause of both maternal and perinatal morbidity and mortality.

The diagnosis of the disease is based on the presence of hypertension in association with proteinuria, edema, or both. Preeclampsia is usually classified clinically as mild or severe.[2] However, even in a seemingly stable patient with minimal signs and symptoms, this disease can rapidly progress to life-threatening eclampsia, with seizures and complications that may include pulmonary edema, intracerebral hemorrhage, acute renal failure, disseminated intravascular coagulation, and abruptio placentae. The criteria for severe preeclampsia are summarized in Table 7-1.

There appears to be an increased incidence of preeclampsia in patients with minimal or no prenatal care and in those of low socioeconomic status.[3] All these types of patients are frequently seen for the first time by physicians in the emergency department. Consequently, it is not unusual for such physicians to be the first in making the diagnosis and initiating appropriate management.

TABLE 7-1
Criteria for Severe Preeclampsia

Blood pressure ≥160 mmHg systolic or ≥110 mmHg diastolic, recorded on at least two occasions at least 6 hours apart with the patient at bed rest

Proteinuria ≥5 g in 24 hours (3+ or 4+ on qualitative examination)

Oliguria (≤400 mL in 24 hours)

Cerebral or visual disturbances

Epigastric pain

Pulmonary edema or cyanosis

Impaired liver function

Thrombocytopenia (<100,000)

Intrauterine growth retardation

Pathophysiology

The basic disorder underlying preeclampsia is vasospasm. Constriction of the arterioles causes resistance to blood flow and subsequent arterial hypertension. Vasospasm and damage to the vascular endothelium in combination with local hypoxia presumably lead to hemorrhage, necrosis, and other end-organ disturbances of severe preeclampsia.

Vascular reactivity to infused angiotensin II and other vasopressors is decreased in normotensive pregnancy.[4,5] The refractoriness to angiotensin II may be mediated by vascular endothelium synthesis of vasodilatory prostaglandins such as prostacyclin. There are data to suggest that preeclampsia may be associated with inappropriately increased production of prostaglandins with vasoconstrictor properties such as thromboxane. Several authors have shown increased vascular reactivity to pressor hormones in patients with early preeclampsia. The increased reactivity to vasopressors may be due to altered ratios of thromboxane and prostacyclin.[6]

Pregnancy normally increases blood volume by as much as 40%, but the expansion may not occur in a woman destined to develop preeclampsia. Vasospasm contracts the intravascular space and leaves her highly sensitive to fluid therapy or blood loss at delivery. The vascular contraction impairs uteroplacental blood flow, contributes to intrauterine growth retardation, and may lead to intrauterine fetal demise (Fig. 7-1). Circulatory impairment reduces renal perfusion and glomerular filtration, and swelling of intracapillary glomerular cells and glomerular endotheliosis may result. Edema probably occurs because of maldistribution of extracellular fluid, since plasma fluid is not increased.

Diagnosis

The diagnosis of preeclampsia is usually straightforward: The blood pressure is at least 140/90 mmHg, or there has been an increase of 30 mmHg systolic or 15 mmHg diastolic over baseline values on at least two occasions 6 or more hours apart. In

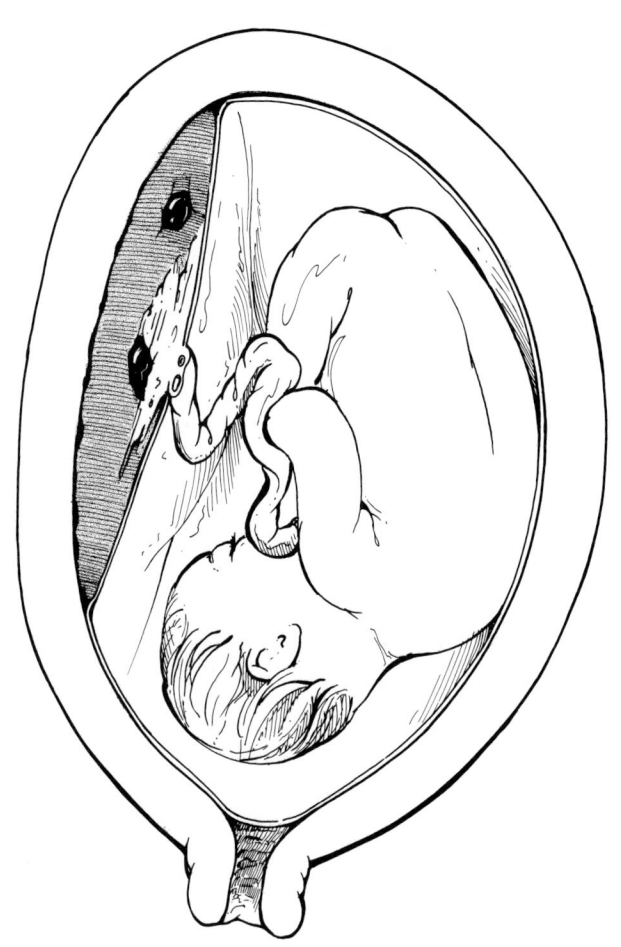

FIGURE 7-1
Placental with decreased placental flow.

addition to hypertension, the patient often presents with significant proteinuria, defined as the presence of at least 300 mg of protein in a 24-hour urine collection or 1+ or greater on dipstick on random samples. The degree of proteinuria often fluctuates widely over any 24-hour period. Therefore a single random sample may fail to detect significant proteinuria. Although edema is an accepted criterion for the diagnosis of preeclampsia, it is such a common finding in pregnant women that its presence should not validate the existence of preeclampsia any more than its absence should deny the diagnosis. However, significant edema of the hands and face associated with a sudden increase in weight may be a valuable diagnostic sign (Fig. 7-2). In addition to the classic triad of hypertension, proteinuria, and edema, other laboratory clues may be helpful in the diagnosis of preeclampsia. Thrombocytopenia may at times be an early warning in patients who subsequently will develop hypertensive disorders of pregnancy. Increased serum levels of uric acid may be of both prognostic and diagnostic value. It has been shown recently that patients with preeclampsia

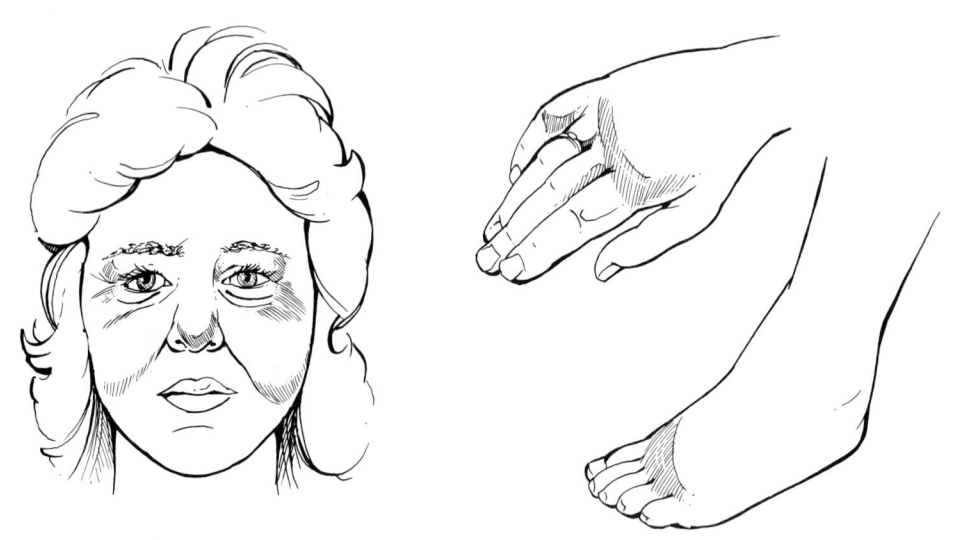

FIGURE 7–2
Preeclampsia—edema of hands, face, and feet.

have markedly decreased urinary excretion of calcium; in fact, hypocalciuria can be detected prior to the appearance of clinical signs and symptoms.

Hypertension and proteinuria, two important signs of preeclampsia, are usually not obvious. By the time the patient has developed symptoms, such as epigastric pain or severe headache, the disorder is far advanced. For this reason prenatal care for the early detection of this order is imperative (Fig. 7-3).

One of the earliest signs of preeclampsia may be a sudden increase in weight. Whenever weight gain exceeds more than 0.91 kg in any given week, or 2.73 kg in a month, early preeclampsia must be suspected. Sudden and excessive weight gain may be attributed to abnormal retention of fluid and is demonstrable before significant edema of the face or upper extremities.

The most dependable warning sign of preeclampsia is hypertension. The diastolic blood pressure is a more reliable prognostic sign than the systolic, and any persisting diastolic pressure of 90 mmHg is abnormal. Many patients have significant hypertension with diastolic blood pressures of less than 90 mmHg. It is therefore important to evaluate baseline blood pressures and look for an increase of 30 mmHg in systolic or 15 mmHg in diastolic pressures as early and important signs of preeclampsia.

Proteinuria varies greatly from case to case and, in the same patient, from hour to hour. This variability is likely due to intermittent renal vasospasm. Frequent urinary dipsticks or a 24-hour urinary collection is often necessary to diagnose proteinuria.

Other signs and symptoms of preeclampsia, such as severe headache, epigastric pain, blurry vision, shortness of breath, and decreased urinary output, are usually late in appearance and are seen in severe cases (see Table 7-1). However, hemolysis, elevated liver enzymes, and low platelets (HELLP syndrome) may be an early presentation of severe preeclampsia.[7–9]

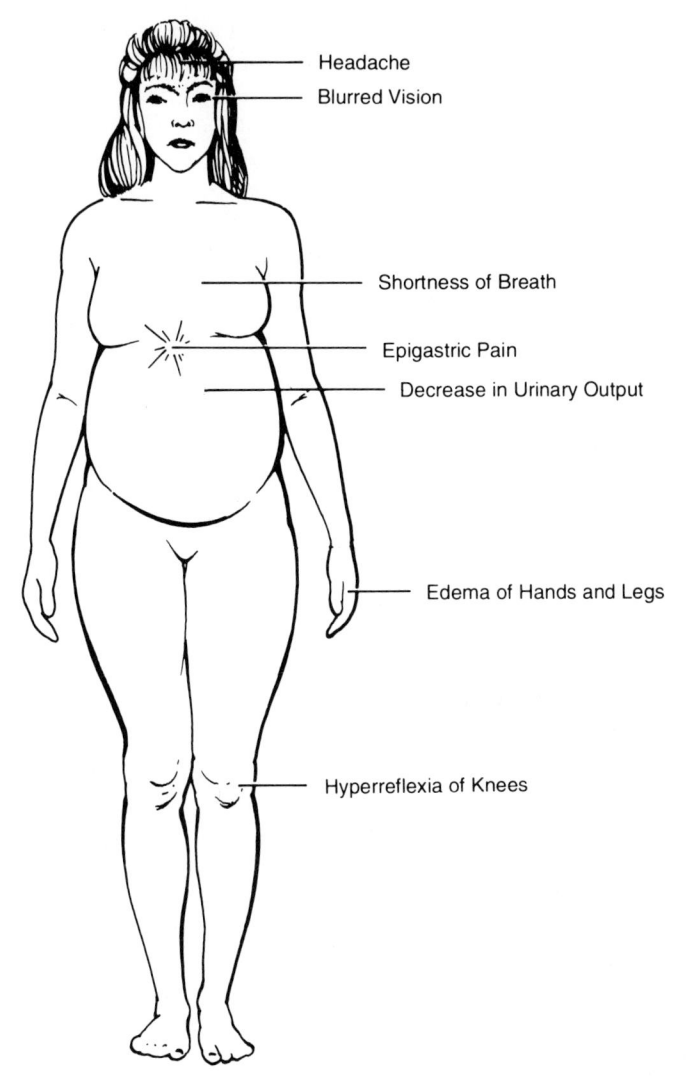

FIGURE 7–3
Signs and symptoms of preeclampsia.

Prepartum Management

The goal of therapy is to prevent eclampsia, as well as other severe complications of preeclampsia. The only definitive therapy for preeclampsia/eclampsia is delivery. Once this has been achieved in a form that assures maximum safety for both the mother and the newborn, the patient is usually on her way to full recovery. This decision is fairly simple in patients with mild preeclampsia at term or with severe preeclampsia at any time during gestation. However, the management of patients with mild preeclampsia remote from term is very controversial.[10] Some of the areas of controversy include the need for hospitalization of all patients, the use of antihypertensive agents, and the use of sedatives and anticonvulsants. Most obstetricians in this country usually advise bed rest in the hospital for the duration of the pregnancy. Ambulatory treatment may be appropriate for a minority of compliant private patients with very mild preeclampsia.

Preterm patients with mild preeclampsia are admitted to the hospital and placed on bed rest. Although this seems a reasonable form of therapy, its efficacy is not clearly established. Strict sodium restriction or diuretic therapy has no role in the prevention or treatment of preeclampsia. Patients are usually placed on a regular diet, although some authorities recommend a high-protein diet. Close monitoring of both mother and fetus is initiated. Daily monitoring should include hematocrit and platelet count, frequent blood pressure checks, maternal weight estimation, and search for clinical evidence of severe disease. Important clinical signs and symptoms of severe disease include headache, epigastric pain, blurred vision, and shortness of breath.

If deterioration is progressive, as determined by laboratory findings, symptoms, and clinical signs, the decision to continue the pregnancy must be reevaluated daily. Important clinical signs that need to be monitored include blood pressure, urinary output, and fluid retention as evidenced by daily weight increase. Laboratory studies (24-hour urinary collection for total protein and creatinine clearance, complete blood count, serum uric acid, BUN, and creatinine) should be performed at intervals of no more than 48 hours. Once it has been determined that the patient has developed severe preeclampsia, steps should be taken for prompt delivery.

Fetal size, determined by ultrasonic biometry, is an accurate guide to the functional status of the fetus. Lack of growth suggests insufficient blood flow, which places the fetus in danger because of lack of placental reserve. Another indirect measure of fetoplacental circulation is uterine artery Doppler velocimetry, which may serve as an early marker for preeclampsia (Fig. 7-4).

Every effort should be made to deliver the baby as close to term as possible. Regardless of fetal maturity, however, delivery is indicated whenever the fetoplacental unit is shown to be failing, as documented by a lack of fetal growth or lack of reassuring tests of fetal well-being. In severe preeclampsia, neonatal survival reportedly ranges from 10 to 37%, depending on gestational age at delivery and birth weight.

The most important test of maturity is the lecithin/sphingomyelin ratio, which can be used to determine the risk of severe respiratory distress syndrome. The risk is high when the ratio is less than 1.5 but insignificant when the ratio is 2 or greater.

Intrapartum Management

When labor commences, either naturally or by induction, the patient is transferred to the labor and delivery suite, where a magnesium sulfate infusion is begun. This agent has long been considered the anticonvulsant of choice. Magnesium sulfate therapy should be started with an intravenous loading dose of 4 g of 20% solution given slowly. The maintenance regimen is a continuous infusion of 1 to 3 g per hour, beginning immediately after the loading dose. Magnesium sulfate is maintained until at least 24 hours after delivery. Magnesium toxicity should be avoided: At plasma levels of 7 to 10 mEq/L the patellar reflex is lost, and severe respiratory

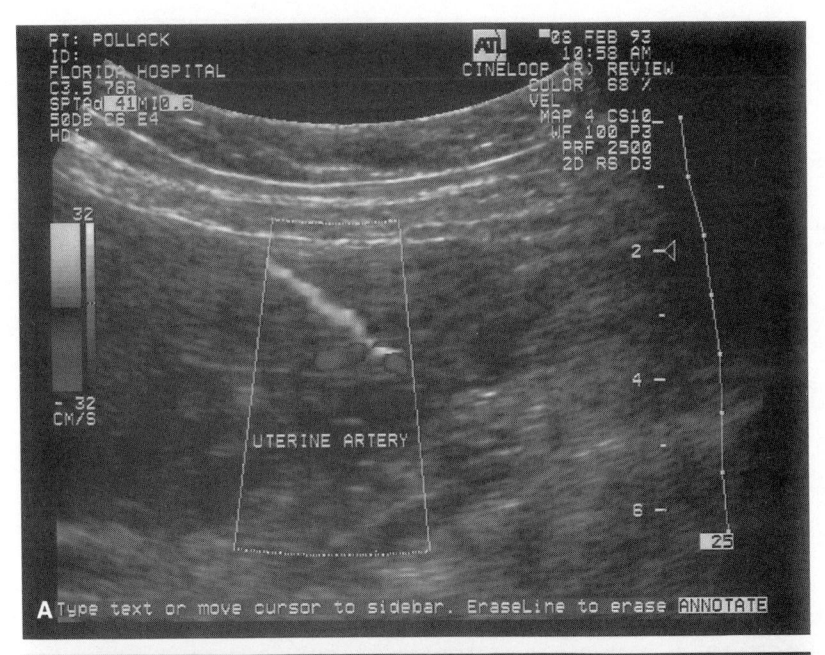

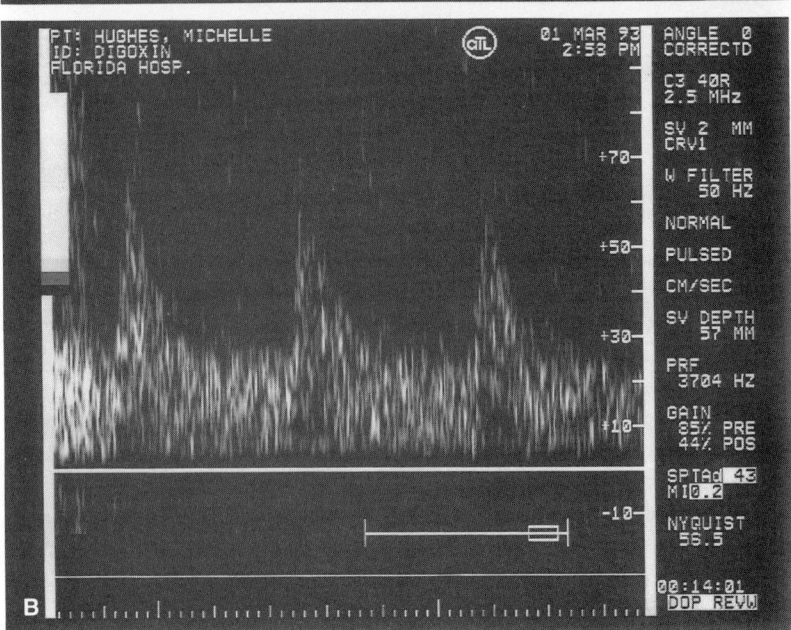

HYPERTENSIVE DISORDERS OF PREGNANCY: PREECLAMPSIA/ECLAMPSIA ♦ 99

FIGURE 7-4
(**A**) Identification of uterine artery with color Doppler. (**B**) Normal uterine artery velocimetry. (**C**) Abnormal velocimetry exhibiting notching. (continued)

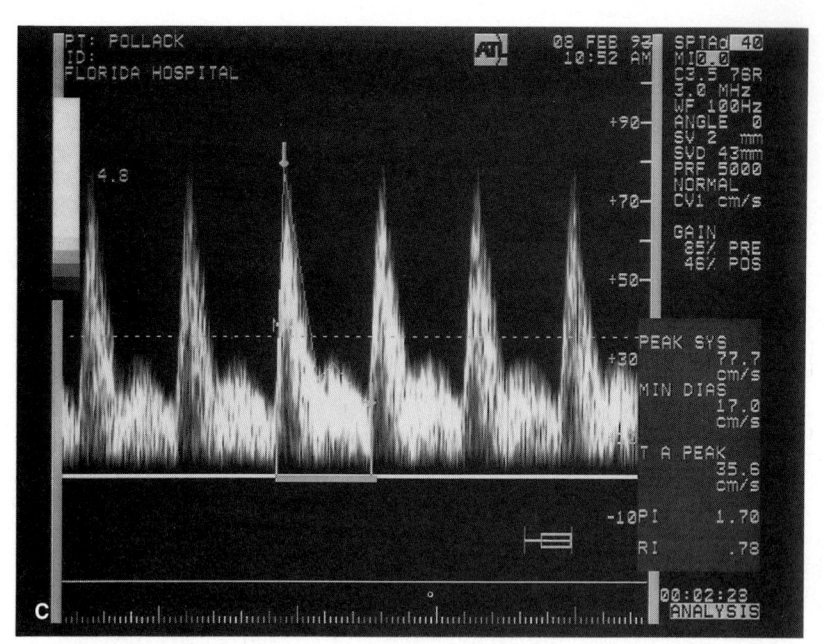

FIGURE 7–4
(Continued)

depression sets in at 12 mEq/L. Fortunately, the therapeutic level is 4 to 7 mEq/L. A 10% solution of calcium gluconate should be readily available to be utilized as an antidote for magnesium toxicity. In addition to checking serum magnesium levels and the patellar reflex, urinary output should be monitored, since magnesium is cleared almost entirely by the kidneys.

Patellar reflexes and respiratory rate should be checked regularly. A respiratory rate of less than 16 breaths per minute is an early sign of magnesium toxicity. Urinary output should be maintained at a minimum of 25 mL per hour to ensure adequate magnesium clearance. In cases of magnesium toxicity, especially respiratory depression, a slow intravenous injection of 10 to 20 mL of 10% calcium gluconate should be infused slowly.

One of the more frequent complications of preeclampsia is severe hypertension. Hydralazine has long been the agent of choice because it not only dilates arterioles but also increases cardiac output, renal blood flow, and placental blood flow. The goal is to lower diastolic pressure gradually to no less than 90 mmHg. This pressure should maintain adequate uteroplacental perfusion while avoiding the more serious complications of hypertension. The usual dosage of hydralazine is an initial intravenous dose of 5 mg followed by 5- to 10-mg doses at 20-minute intervals. The doses should be titrated to achieve the desired blood pressure level. Hydralazine may also be given in a continuous intravenous infusion of 80 mg in 500 mL of D5W beginning at a rate of 30 mL per hour (5 mg) and increased every 15 minutes as needed. Most patients will respond to 5 to 20 mg of hydralazine; an alternative agent should be considered if there is no response to a total dose of 30 mg of hydralazine.

Alternative, rapid-acting antihypertensive agents are diazoxide and nitroprusside, but their use in pregnancy is controversial and they should be reserved for emergencies that do not respond to hydralazine. Diazoxide given in a standard 300-mL bolus may cause maternal hypotension, fetal hypoxia, and maternal and fetal hyperglycemia. Therefore it should be administered in small doses of either 30 mg every 1 to 2 minutes or as a continuous infusion of 15 mg a minute to a total dose of 5 mg/kg.

Nitroprusside is a less desirable choice for the treatment of pregnancy-induced hypertension because it crosses the placenta and may cause cyanide toxicity in the fetus. It may be used, however, when hypertension is refractory to other agents. In short-term use, cyanide toxicity may be avoided. Infusion is started at a rate of 0.25 μg/kg a minute and increased by 0.25 μg/kg a minute every 5 minutes until the desired blood pressure is achieved.

Eclampsia occurs most frequently in a hospitalized patient being treated for preeclampsia. However, anyone who presents initially with eclampsia must be hospitalized and treated at once.[11,12] The first priorities are to clear the patient's airway, aspirate mucus, give oxygen, and start anticonvulsant therapy with magnesium sulfate. The patient should be placed in the left lateral decubitus position. An indwelling catheter should be inserted to collect 24-hour urine specimens for protein and urinary estriol measurements until delivery.

Seizures usually stop minutes after the loading dose of magnesium sulfate, and within 2 hours a comatose patient should regain consciousness and be oriented to place and time. Patients whose seizures persist may be given a quick-acting barbiturate, such as sodium amobarbital, 250 to 500 mg in a slow intravenous injection.

Postpartum Management

Hypertension that persists after delivery may be reduced by intramuscular administration of hydralazine, 10 mg every 4 to 6 hours. A woman may be discharged while still hypertensive as long as her blood pressure appears to be falling and she is otherwise well. The patient must be reexamined within 2 weeks, by which time the pregnancy-induced hypertension should be gone. If hypertension persists after 8 weeks, essential hypertension is the likely cause.

Prevention

Several clinical trials have suggested that administration of low-dose aspirin (50 to 150 mg) in high-risk pregnant women can reduce the incidence and severity of preeclampsia.[13-15] These studies provide promising evidence that low-dose aspirin reduces the risks of hypertension, preeclampsia, and cesarean delivery. But the effects of low-dose aspirin on more substantive outcomes, such as perinatal death or serious neonatal morbidity, still remain unclear. To date, the old standbys of early prenatal care and good nutrition are still the most effective means of decreasing the incidence of this disease.

REFERENCES

1. MacGillivray I. Some observations on the incidence of preeclampsia. J Obstet Gynaecol Br Empire 65:536, 1958
2. Hughes EC, ed. Obstetric-Gynecologic Terminology. Philadelphia: Davis, 1972:422
3. Gant NF, Daley GL, Chand S, Whalley PJ, MacDonald PC. A study of angiotensin II pressor response throughout primigravid pregnancy. J Clin Invest 52:2682, 1973
4. Talledo OE, Chesley LC, Zuspan FP. Renin-angiotensin system in normal and toxemic pregnancies. III. Differential sensitivity to angiotensin II and norepinephrine in toxemia of pregnancy. Am J Obstet Gynecol 100:218, 1968
5. Sibai BM. The HELLP syndrome (hemolysis, elevated liver enzymes, and low platelets): much ado about nothing? Am J Obstet Gynecol 162:311, 1990
6. Sibai BM, Taslimi MM, El-Nazer A et al: Maternal perinatal outcome associated with the syndrome of hemolysis, elevated liver enzymes, and low platelets in severe preeclampsia-eclampsia. Am J Obstet Gynecol 155:501, 1986
7. Cunningham FG, Leveno KJ. Management of pregnancy-induced hypertension. In Rubin PC (ed): Handbook of Hypertension, vol 10, p 290. Hypertension in Pregnancy. Amsterdam: Elsevier, 1988
8. Sibai BM, McCubbin JH, Anderson GD, Lipshitz J, Dilts PV Jr. Eclampsia. I. Observations from sixty-seven recent cases. Obstet Gynecol 58:609, 1981
9. Adams EM, MacGillivray I. Long-term effect of preeclampsia on blood pressure. Lancet 2:1373, 1961
10. Fisher KA, Luger A, Spargo BH, Lindheimer MD. Hypertension in pregnancy: clinical-pathological correlations and remote prognosis. Medicine 60:267, 1981
11. Aarnoudse JG, Houthoff HJ, Weits J, Vellenga E, Huisjes HJ. A syndrome of liver damage and intravascular coagulation in the last trimester of normotensive pregnancy: a clinical and histopathological study. Br J Obstet Gynaecol 93:145, 1986
12. Hinselmann H. Allgemeine Krankheitslehre. In Hinselmann H (ed): Die Eklampsie, p 1. Bonn: Cohen, 1924
13. Beaufils M, Uzan S, Donsimoni R, Colau JC. Prevention of pre-eclampsia by early antiplatelet therapy. Lancet 1:840, 1985
14. Wallenburg HC, Dekker GA, Makovitz JW, Rotmans P. Low-dose aspirin prevents pregnancy-induced hypertension and pre-eclampsia in angiotensin-sensitive primigravidae. Lancet 1:1, 1986
15. Schiff E, Peleg E, Goldenberg M et al. The use of aspirin to prevent pregnancy-induced hypertension and lower the ratio of thromboxane A_2 to prostacyclin in relatively high-risk pregnancies. N Engl J Med 321:351, 1989
16. Benigni A, Gregorini G, Frusca T et al. Effect of low dose aspirin on fetal and maternal generation of thromboxane by platelets in women at risk for pregnancy-induced hypertension. N Engl J Med 321:357, 1989

CHAPTER 8

Infections in Pregnancy

Joseph G. Pastorek II

Physicians should be aware of the possibility, even the probability, that they will ultimately encounter, in the course of the "routine" labor and delivery of an apparently "normal" patient, some life-threatening catastrophe that seems to arise at the most inopportune minute, in the most untimely and inconvenient circumstances. Historically, the most deadly triad of illnesses befalling the obstetric patient has consisted of hemorrhage, hypertensive disease, and infection. Recently, with adequate medical technology, blood banking, and antibiotics, the really frightening cases may seem few and far between. This only lulls the doctor into a false sense of security.

There are still a number of infectious complications of pregnancy that may develop at different points in gestation (including postpartum) and that raise the specter of the emergent and the life-threatening. Those that will be covered in this chapter include chorioamnionitis, pyelonephritis, septic shock, primary varicella, and primary herpes. Though these entities may seem to have appropriate and efficacious therapies, their abrupt occurrence and diverse sequelae are still cause for concern.

Chorioamnionitis

Infection of the uterus and the intrauterine contents is variably termed *intra-amniotic infection*, *chorioamnionitis*, *amnionitis*, *amniotic fluid infection*, and *intrapartum infection*. Each term has its utility and proponents; *intra-amniotic infection* is perhaps the most correct, but *chorioamnionitis* may be more common in general usage. Whatever the term, the clinical disease is common in obstetric practice, with an incidence of between 0.5% and 1.0% quoted by many authors.[1]

Diagnosis

Clinical chorioamnionitis is characterized by fever, maternal and/or fetal tachycardia, uterine tenderness, foul amniotic fluid odor, and leukocytosis.[2] However, none of these parameters are invariably present in all patients with chorioamnionitis. Leukocytosis and fever, the most common signs, are present in roughly 85% of cases.[1] Therefore many patients will present with subtle signs that may easily be overlooked by the practitioner. If histologic evidence of chorioamnionitis is sought—namely, polymorphonuclear leukocytic infiltration of the chorioamnion—then 15% of term placentas and up to 75% of premature placentas may be so diagnosed.[3] Most of these patients do not meet the criteria for clinical disease, which suggests that the disease represents a spectrum extending from an asymptomatic inflammatory cell invasion to an overt, febrile illness.

Unfortunately, there are no definitive laboratory tests to identify patients with chorioamnionitis reliably. Although the presence of microorganisms in amniotic fluid as detected by Gram stain is of value, it is not exclusive to symptomatic patients, nor is it universally present in symptomatic women.[4] Similarly, the presence of white blood cells—or alternatively, leukocyte esterase—is not foolproof.[5] The physician must therefore be quite alert to the possibility of chorioamnionitis in the laboring patient, the patient with premature rupture of the membranes, and the gravida with unexplained fever.

Pathophysiology

Clinical parameters independently associated with the development of chorioamnionitis include duration of ruptured membranes and duration of internal monitoring.[4] This type of association leads researchers to conclude that most cases of chorioamnionitis result from ascension of bacteria from the cervicovaginal microbial flora, through the cervix and point of membrane rupture, into the amniotic cavity. Alternatively, occasional cases may be due to hematogenous seeding by particular bacteria. *Listeria monocytogenes* chorioamnionitis is a classic result of this route of spread. Finally, although it is rare, invasive procedures (eg, amniocentesis) may lead to clinical infection.[6]

Patients with clinical evidence of intra-amniotic infection have been shown to have higher rates of recovery of bacteria from the amniotic cavity, particularly so-called high-virulence bacteria.[4] Gram-negative isolates, such as *Escherichia coli;* gram-positive organisms, such as group B streptococci and enterococci; and such anaerobes as the *Bacteroides* and *Peptococcus* species are all much more commonly encountered in women with symptoms of chorioamnionitis than in asymptomatic patients.

E. coli, group B streptococci, and other high-virulence organisms are commonly associated with significant illness in mothers and their infants, including postpartal or postcesarean endometritis, urinary tract infection, septic shock, and neonatal sepsis and pneumonia. Histologically, the inflammatory reaction extends from the chorioamnion and endometrium into the myometrium,[7] indicating that the uterine muscle is often involved.

Outcome and Sequelae

One consequence of chorioamnionitis commonly encountered is endometritis, especially if the patient is delivered by cesarean section. Less frequently, sepsis and maternal death may follow intra-amniotic infection.[1,8] Rates of perinatal sepsis and death are also significantly increased in pregnancies complicated by chorioamnionitis. Mortality may be increased by as much as 400%.[9]

Neonatal outcome is not always determined by infection, however. Because of the strong relationship of chorioamnionitis with preterm labor and delivery,[3,6] many newborns are premature, suffering the usual respiratory distress syndrome, intracranial hemorrhage, or other effects of prematurity.[9,10] Even so, babies delivered in the face of chorioamnionitis seem to have a poorer prognosis even from noninfectious illnesses.[9,11]

Noninfectious sequelae of intra-amniotic infection in the mother revolve about dysfunction of infected uterine musculature. Apparently, the effects of the inflammatory process interfere with normal myometrial activity, leading to dystocia and failure to progress (and resultant higher cesarean delivery rates). Cesarean section is also commonly performed for ominous fetal heart rate patterns, though Apgar scores do not indicate a serious problem with fetal asphyxia in most cases.[12] An extremely serious result of myometrial dysfunction frequently encountered in women with amnionitis is uterine atony, presumably caused by biochemical imbalances within the myometrial cells incited by infection or the inflammatory response. Whether delivered vaginally or abdominally, women with intra-amniotic infection are prone to develop severe uterine relaxation and postpartum hemorrhage. Chorioamnionitis tends to make the myometrial cell refractory to the usual pharmacologic therapies for uterine atony. Potent agents such as prostaglandin preparations have cases of uterine atony associated with chorioamnionitis among their few failures.[13]

Management

The patient with suspected chorioamnionitis must undergo thorough physical examination, both for evidence of uterine involvement and for signs of other, distant sources of infection. If the patient is having uterine contractions, the diagnosis is one of exclusion, as uterine irritability and tenderness are often impossible to differentiate in the patient in labor. Fetal evaluation includes external fetal heart rate monitoring or direct fetal electrocardiography if membranes are ruptured (Table 8-1).

Bacteriologic evaluation should include cultures of urine, blood, and amniotic fluid. If feasible, amniotic fluid may be aspirated through an internal uterine pressure catheter. Otherwise, amniotic fluid may be collected directly as it flows from the cervix (assuming the membranes are ruptured). Whether membranes are ruptured

TABLE 8-1
Protocol for Management in Cases of Chorioamnionitis

Diagnosis
  Physical examination (including vital signs)
  Maternal WBC count and differential
  Amniotic fluid culture/Gram stain
  Vaginal culture
  Blood culture
  Catheterized urine for culture and analysis
  Fetal monitoring

Management
  Antibiotic therapy (after cultures taken)
  Fetal monitoring
  Blood type and screened
  Induction of labor (if membranes are ruptured and labor has not ensued spontaneously)
  Oxytocics as needed for laboring patient
  Close maternal observation during labor
  Cesarean delivery for usual obstetric indications
  Appropriate neonatal resuscitation and care (ie, septic "work-up" ± antibiotics)
  Careful observation during the immediate puerperium for evidence of uterine atony

or not, a vaginal swab should be obtained for culture for group B streptococcus. This organism has neonatal implications, and microbial inoculum is generally heavier in the vaginal barrel than at the level of the cervix.

As soon as cultures have been taken, appropriate antibiotics should be initiated. Retrospective comparisons of women receiving antimicrobial therapy before delivery with those treated after delivery indicate that both the mother and the baby benefit from timely therapy.[14,15] This has been confirmed in a prospective, randomized study, which demonstrated higher neonatal sepsis rates in patients from whom antenatal antibiotics were withheld.[16] It is considered proper current medical practice therefore to initiate antibiotic therapy as soon as the diagnosis of chorioamnionitis is made, once cultures are obtained. Since chorioamnionitis is usually a polymicrobial infection, a drug regimen that covers the usual aerobic and anaerobic bacteria resident in the cervicovaginal environment is indicated. Many physicians, because of recommendations concerning group B streptococcus, often use ampicillin. This is reasonable for sensitive microorganisms, since ampicillin has been shown to cross the placenta in therapeutic amounts.[17] However, most single agents and combination antibiotics commonly used by obstetricians—including cefoxitin, mezlocillin, clindamycin, and gentamicin—penetrate into fetal membranes and cord blood in amounts that would be sufficient to inhibit most vaginal flora participating in the usual case of chorioamnionitis.[18]

After antibiotics are initiated, the patient in labor should be followed in a manner consistent with standard obstetric care. In particular, careful electronic fetal monitoring and uterine tocodynamometry are essential, with the increased rate of fetal heart rate abnormalities and myometrial dysfunction noted earlier. Oxytocin is used in the usual fashion. Cesarean section should be performed only for the usual obstetric indications. Though the cesarean section rate in these patients will be relatively high, because of failure to progress and fetal (monitor) distress, if the procedure can be avoided, the maternal outcome would be better.

Finally, at delivery, there should be appropriate facilities and personnel to evaluate adequately and resuscitate a possibly septic newborn. In addition, the obstetrician should be prepared for the possibility of severe uterine atony, even in apparently mild cases of chorioamnionitis. The graduated sequence of maneuvers addressing a case of massive postpartum hemorrhage, from uterine massage and uterotonics through emergency operative intervention, should be available immediately.

Pyelonephritis

Acute bacterial infection of the renal parenchyma, pyelonephritis has long been known to be a serious complication of gestation, complicating 1% to 2% of pregnancies.[19] Rates can be lowered by screening and eradication of bacteriuria and close urine culture follow-up.[20] Routine urine culture and appropriate therapy of asymptomatic bacteriuria during pregnancy, however, have not prevented acute pyelonephritis from remaining one of the most common serious infections in the gravid patient.

Diagnosis

The pregnant patient with acute pyelonephritis presents with the triad of fever, costovertebral angle or flank tenderness (most commonly of the right), and pyuria (Table 8-2).[19,21] Nonspecific symptoms may include nausea, vomiting, chills, and various lower-urinary-tract manifestations of coincident cystitis (eg, frequency, dysuria, urgency). In modest to severe cases, the patient's temperature may be high, on the order of 40°C (104°F), with intermittent spikes. If vomiting and insensate water loss have caused significant dehydration, the patient may be weak and appear debilitated. Clinical hypotension may ensue and rarely progress to overt septic shock.

A voided urine specimen resulting in the growth of ≥ 10^5 colonies per milliliter is

TABLE 8–2
Protocol for Management in Cases of Pyelonephritis in Pregnancy

Diagnosis
  Physical examination (including vital signs, urinalysis)
  Complete blood count, WBC differential, platelet count
  Baseline chemistry profile (including liver and renal evaluation)
  Urine culture
  Blood culture
  Uterine contraction monitoring

Management
  Intravenous access and fluid resuscitation, as needed
  Antibiotic therapy (after cultures taken)
  Close monitoring of maternal vital signs
  Observation for premature uterine contractions, with tocolysis as necessary
  Antipyretics for temperature in excess of 39°C
  Symptomatic treatment of nausea and/or vomiting
  Appropriate outpatient follow-up (ie, serial urine cultures ± suppressive antibiotics)

generally accepted as diagnostic of infection in any symptomatic individual. However, if a pregnant patient exhibits fever, flank tenderness, and pyuria, smaller colony counts are sufficient for diagnosis. Additionally, any growth in a catheterized specimen is reasonable evidence of infection. With significant disease, leukocytosis with left shift is present. Occasionally, though rarely of clinical significance, there is evidence of hemolysis, moderate anemia, and possibly thrombocytopenia.[22] Nearly a quarter of gravidas with pyelonephritis may be shown to have transient diminution of renal function. This may be demonstrated as a decreased creatinine clearance as low as 80 mL per minute or less, indicating a decreased glomerular filtration rate.[23]

Pathophysiology

The development of pyelonephritis during pregnancy is usually due to lower-urinary-tract colonization by potentially pathogenic bacteria. It is estimated that asymptomatic bacteriuria, present in up to 10% of pregnant women, will develop into acute pyelonephritis in 20% to 40% of cases.[24] Presumably, microbes present in the urethra and bladder ascend the ureters into the renal collecting systems, ultimately invading susceptible tissue and inciting an inflammatory response. Subsequently, either the patient's own immunomodulators, both humoral and cellular, or various bacterial toxins mediate the systemic symptoms and laboratory derangements characteristic of the disease. As noted earlier, effective screening and therapy of such bacteriuria significantly decrease the incidence of pyelonephritis.

The bacteria responsible for most cases of pyelonephritis are primarily the aerobic inhabitants of the lower female genital tract. Members of the Enterobacteriaceae, such as *Escherichia coli*, *Klebsiella pneumoniae*, and *Proteus mirabilis*, are most commonly recovered, along with other gram negatives (eg, *Enterobacter, Citrobacter*) and the occasional gram-positive organism (eg, group B streptococcus).[25] Lower-genital-tract bacteria colonize the lower urinary tract through various mechanisms, including adhesion to uroepithelium mediated by fimbria on the bacterial cell wall.[26] Access to the upper tract is facilitated during pregnancy by urinary stasis and upper-urinary-tract dilation as a result of mechanical obstruction by the enlarging uterus and engorged pelvic vasculature, as well as the smooth-muscle relaxation effects of progesterone. This upper-tract dilation is more pronounced in women with pyelonephritis during pregnancy.[27]

Outcome and Sequelae

The effects of antepartum pyelonephritis may be serious for both mother and baby. Maternal complications indicative of acute end-organ dysfunction occur in roughly 25% of women with the infection, mediated in part by lipopolysaccharide endotoxin released from the cell wall of the various gram-negative bacteria involved, or occasionally exotoxin produced by gram positives, and caused by the patient's own immunologic responses. Transient renal dysfunction[23] has been mentioned, as have hematologic aberrations.[22] Although up to 15% of pyelonephritis patients are bacteremic, overt septic shock is rare. Most incidents of hypotension are due to dehydration from fever and vomiting rather than to the vascular dilatory effects found in true septic shock.

One recently described end-organ repercussion of pyelonephritis during pregnancy is a respiratory insufficiency syndrome, occurring in about 1 to 2% of gravid women with clinically apparent pyelonephritis.[28-33] This entity is characterized by dyspnea, tachypnea, hypoxemia, pulmonary infiltrates, and the occasional effusion (Fig. 8-1). Pulmonary damage is presumably initiated by gram-negative bacterial endotoxin or immunologic mediators (or both), which alter alveolar-capillary membrane permeability, leading to a type of adult respiratory distress syndrome or noncardiogenic pulmonary edema.

Fetal effects of maternal pyelonephritis are controversial. There is a concern, not completely supported by the literature, that maternal urinary tract infection and pyelonephritis predispose to low birth weight and small-for-gestational-age infants.[24] Many studies antedate the era of modern antibiotics and support technology. More modern reports show no such association of pyelonephritis and fetal growth disturbances.[25] However, both immunologic modulators mobilized during an acute, febrile illness and bacterial endotoxin are capable of inciting uterine activity.[34] It is not

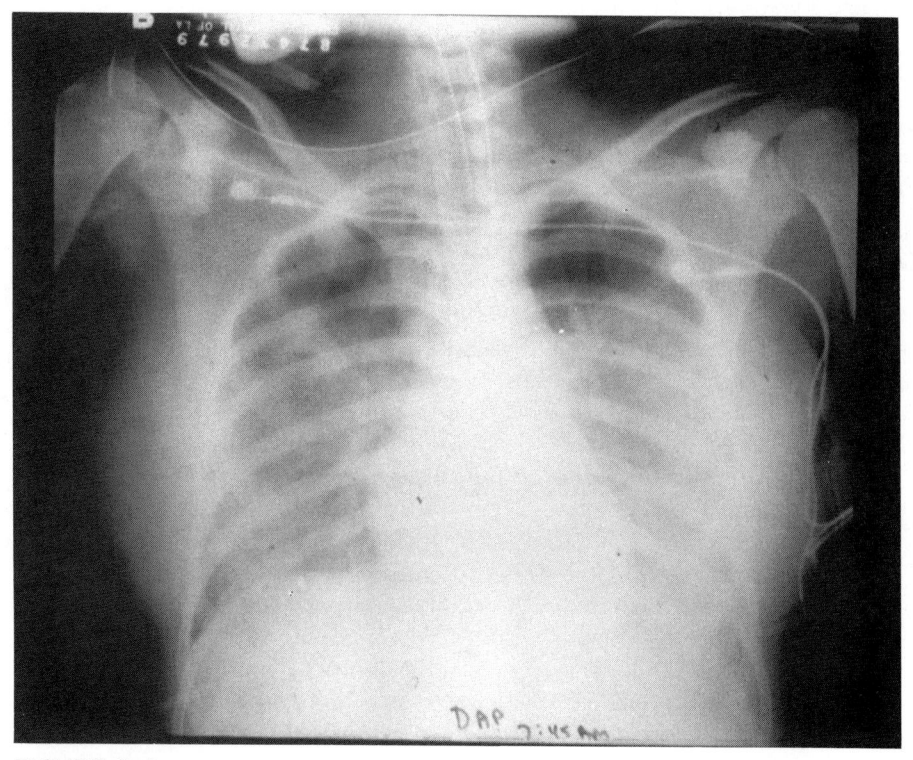

FIGURE 8–1
Bilateral fluffy infiltrates in the chest roentgenograph of a 23-year-old secunda gravida admitted with a temperature of 39°C and pyelonephritis at 26 weeks of gestation. The patient developed tachypnea after approximately 24 hours of hydration and antibiotic administration. Her condition responded to diuretic administration and positive end expiratory pressure respiratory therapy.

surprising, then, that premature uterine contractions accompany pyelonephritis and may lead to premature delivery. Of course, significant maternal illness (eg, septic shock) will have the expected untoward effects upon the unborn child.

Management

Pregnant women presenting with complaints of fever and side pain may depict a straightforward case of pyelonephritis. The obstetrician must not be cavalier in making this diagnosis, however. A number of other infectious conditions might manifest as right-sided pain and obvious infection, including appendicitis, hepatitis, cholecystitis, and perhaps Meckel's diverticulitis. Noninfectious conditions, such as preeclampsia/HELLP syndrome, may also mimic right-sided renal infection. Of course, basilar pneumonia may exist on either the right or the left. For these reasons the physician evaluating a patient with pyelonephritis must thoroughly question and examine the patient and consider appropriate laboratory data before reaching the final diagnosis (see Table 8-2).

The initial approach to the management of a gravida with pyelonephritis, once the diagnosis has been made, includes urine and blood culture, followed by the administration of intravenous fluids and parenteral antibiotics. Hydration is achieved with normal saline, lactated Ringer's solution, or some other balanced salt solution, which is infused at a rate to ensure a urine output of 30 to 50 mL per hour. Care must be taken not to overhydrate a patient, remembering the possibility of the development of pulmonary insufficiency. A complete blood count and baseline chemistries should also be performed for evaluation of the patient's status with respect to the pyelonephritis as well as for use in excluding other similar maladies. It is also wise, in the initial acute phase of the disease, to monitor the patient for any uterine activity that may become organized into overt premature labor.

Antibiotic therapy is directed primarily at the community gram-negative flora, including *E. coli, K. pneumoniae,* and *P. mirabilis,* as well as the occasional group B streptococcus and *Staphylococcus saprophyticus.* While ampicillin has previously been the antibiotic of choice, in recent years ampicillin resistance has been so widespread among these organisms[35,36] that first-generation cephalosporins (eg, cephalothin, cephapirin, cefazolin) have become the workhorse drugs utilized for this purpose. Unfortunately, resistance to these drugs is approaching 10% in some centers,[25,36] though clinical failures do not seem to be as frequent. Other drugs that have been used and that may be increasingly useful in the future (if first-generation cephalosporins must be abandoned) include the newer semisynthetic penicillins[37] and higher-generation cephalosporins (eg, cefuroxime).[38]

Parenteral antibiotic therapy is the rule in the treatment of pyelonephritis of pregnancy. Inpatient observation is necessary in the usual case, because of the threat of premature labor, pulmonary insufficiency, dehydration, and other complications. However, in the case of patients without bacteremia, oral therapy has been shown, at least in one study, to be efficacious.[39] After the patient has been initially treated with antibiotics and fluid resuscitation, she should be observed for evidence of septic shock, pulmonary dysfunction, and response to antibiotics. Temperatures in excess of 39°C should be lowered with acetaminophen to prevent any untoward fetal effects of prolonged hyperthermia. The physician should be aware that the first 24 to 36 hours of therapy may involve higher temperatures than initially, since the killing of gram-negative organisms releases pyrogenic lipopolysaccharides associated with the cell wall. Therefore the patient may look worse after a day or so of appropriate therapy, as did two patients in the oral antibiotic study mentioned earlier.[39] During this time most patients destined to experience premature labor develop uterine contraction and may require short-term tocolytic therapy.

After 24 to 48 hours of appropriate drug therapy, most patients with pyelonephritis defervesce and become symptomatically improved. Parenteral therapy should be continued until the patient is afebrile for 48 hours and bacterial antibiotic sensitivities are known. The patient may then be switched to an oral drug that fits the organism's sensitivities, usually an oral first-generation cephalosporin (eg, cephalexin, cephradine) if that was the parenteral class of drugs used at the outset. She may be discharged with the prescription to complete a total of 10 to 14 days of antibiotics. Upon follow-up in an outpatient setting, the patient should be tested for cure with a repeat urine culture after completion of her medication. In addition, urine cultures should be repeated monthly during gestation to detect recurrence or new infection. Use of suppressive antibiotics is recommended by some to decrease the recurrence rates.[36] This is not a foolproof strategy and does not excuse the need for monthly urine cultures.

Finally, patients who are not clinically responding to what appears to be appropriate antibiotics, who have significant hematuria, and who have frequently recurrent disease may benefit from ultrasonographic evaluation of the urinary tract for evidence of obstruction or stone. A limited intravenous pyelogram may be of value in this instance. Alternative antibiotic therapy, such as with an aminoglycoside, aztreonam, or imipenem/cilastatin, is predicated upon persistence of symptoms, persistent bacteriuria, demonstration of in vitro antibiotic resistance, and perhaps frequent recurrence in spite of seemingly appropriate therapy.

Septic Shock

Hypotension and decreased tissue perfusion resulting from the body's response to various byproducts of infection is termed *septic shock*. In obstetrics and gynecology, septic shock is one of the more frightening, but thankfully rare, sequelae of the various infectious complications of pregnancy, gynecologic surgery, or pelvic inflammatory disease. Perhaps 8 to 10% of infected ob-gyn patients are bacteremic, and at most 12% of these experience shock. The relative youth and health of these patients result in a fatality rate of at most 3%, compared to upward of 81% in some populations of nonobstetric patients.[40]

Diagnosis

By definition septic shock entails a sepsis-mediated decrease in tissue perfusion, leading to deficient oxygen and nutrition supply to tissues. If left unchecked, shock ultimately causes serious impairment of cellular function and death.[41] Even though a decrease in blood pressure is usually perceived as fairly essential for the condition, in the earliest stage, so-called warm shock, hypotension may be subtle or absent. The patient will have an elevated temperature with warm extremities, low systemic vascular resistance, tachycardia, and leukocytosis and may otherwise appear to be obviously infected, often precipitating a "fever work-up" and initiation of antibiotics. Ancillary laboratory findings, including transient hyperglycemia, thrombocytopenia, and other evidence of coagulopathy, may be present if investigated. However, the physician may overlook low blood pressure, merely assuming that the patient's condition represents a "normal" infection. Therefore misdiagnosis in the warm shock stage may be quite dangerous.

Subsequently, endogenous catecholamine release produces marked vasoconstriction, which reduces peripheral tissue perfusion, and cellular hypoxia, resulting in cool extremities, high systemic resistance, cyanosis, and oliguria, the so-called cold shock. Hypoxia at the cellular level leads to lactic acidosis from anaerobic metabolism. If significant myocardial depression leads to cardiovascular collapse, in the face of hypotension and hypoxia, the stage of *irreversible shock* is diagnosed.[40,41]

The diagnosis of septic shock is therefore based upon the demonstration of infection of some source, coupled with clinical hypotension or other findings noted earlier. Besides clinical examination, including vital signs, diagnostic evaluation should include bacterial cultures of appropriate sources as well as complete blood count (including platelets and WBC differential), clotting studies, general chemistries, and urinalysis. If pulmonary infection (or pulmonary decompensation) is suspected, chest roentgenography is in order. The clinician must be aware of other disorders that may give similar clinical symptomatology, including hemorrhagic (hypovolemic) shock, pulmonary embolus, amniotic fluid embolus, diabetic ketoacidosis, cardiac tamponade, and such rarities in the ob-gyn patient as acute aortic dissection.[42]

Pathophysiology

Septic shock is the most common form of distributive shock, wherein aberrant blood flow distribution is the initial physiologic defect (the other two types of shock being cardiogenic and hypovolemic). It should be noted that in general, after an hour or more of clinical shock, a patient will exhibit all three types of shock, because of the interaction of reflex vasoconstriction, vascular permeability, and hypoxic cardiac dysfunction that result no matter what the initial type of insult was.[41]

Septic shock is commonly caused by gram-negative bacilli, though infection by gram positives, fungi, rickettsiae, and viruses may precipitate shock as well. Bacterial products, including endotoxin and exotoxin, provoke activation of macrophages, the intrinsic and extrinsic coagulation pathways, the fibrinolytic pathway, and the direct and properdin complement pathways. The subsequent release of diverse mediators of these various and complex pathways (eg, histamine, bradykinin, kallikrein, hydrogen peroxide, and superoxide free radicals) causes increased capillary permeability, vasodilation (initially), and endothelial damage. Intravascular volume is lost to the extracellular space, which, coupled with vasodilation, results in hypotension. Decreased blood pressure, in turn, causes a reflex increase in cardiac output and heart rate. If this hypotension is unrelieved, the sympathetic nervous system becomes activated, causing marked and generalized vasoconstriction and ultimately tissue hypoperfusion (which may be made worse by the local effects of epithelial damage). Finally, lengthy tissue hypoxia has long been recognized to cause a shift to anaerobic metabolism and subsequent lactic (metabolic) acidosis.[43]

The sequelae of metabolic acidosis include relaxation of arteriolar smooth muscle and constriction of venule walls, leading to pooling of blood in the capillary beds. This causes more loss of fluid into the extravascular space and further decrease in circulating volume, and hence continued hypotension and decreased cardiac output. Added to this cycle of decreasing perfusion is the impairment of myocardial function by endogenous opioids (ie, endorphins) and by myocardial depressant factor. Ultimately, failure of tissue oxygenation and nutrition leads to generalized tissue death, as the patient succumbs.[44]

Septic shock in the pregnant patient appears to be more severe than in the nonpregnant individual. Studies in animal models indicate that less endotoxin, in cases of induced gram-negative shock, is required to induce shock and organ necrosis in gravid animals.[45] Effects are much more pronounced near term, and metabolic acidosis is much worse in pregnant animals compared to nonpregnant controls. Surprisingly, the fetus is more resistant than the mother, at least to the effects of endotoxin. It appears that adverse effects on the baby are predicated upon the mother's condition, rather than on any direct effects of the offending toxins.[46]

Outcome and Sequelae

It may seem superfluous to speak of sequelae of septic shock, which is itself considered a sequel to serious infectious conditions. However, aside from the possibility of death due to prolonged hypotension and acidosis, the patient in various stages of septic shock runs the risk of end-organ damage and dysfunction. As tissue hypoxia and physiologic failure affect the various systems, individual organ function may continue to be suboptimal, even if the shock itself resolves. In particular, shock may incite acute renal failure, adult respiratory distress syndrome, disseminated intravascular coagulation, myocardial ischemia/infarction, and gastrointestinal hemorrhage. Perhaps the most troublesome of these is adult respiratory distress syndrome, which is a common cause of death in septic shock patients.[47] Finally, it must be remembered that patients who do not expire from sepsis itself are at risk of complications of therapy, such as anesthetic effects, pulmonary collapse or hemorrhage from invasive monitoring, infectious sequelae of blood component transfusion, and the like.

Fetal sequelae of septic shock will be more indirect, since, as noted earlier, the fetus seems more resistant to the effects of endotoxin. However, maternal hypotension and vasoconstriction will cause detrimental changes to uterine perfusion, resulting in both decreased oxygen transfer to the fetus and increased uterine activity. Therefore while she is aggressively managed for hypotension and other manifestations of shock, the pregnant woman with sepsis must be observed judiciously for signs both of premature labor, to ensure that prematurity does not complicate the situation, and of fetal distress brought on by maternal hemodynamic instability.

Management

The treatment of septic shock consists of four basic components: hemodynamic stabilization, with improvement of functional intravascular volume; maintenance of an adequate airway, including endotracheal intubation, if necessary; identification of

114 ♦ OBSTETRIC AND GYNECOLOGIC EMERGENCIES

the specific focus of infection and its extirpation, if possible; and initiation of appropriate antibiotics.[43,46] It should be appreciated that the urgency of the situation compels the physician to perform the specific tasks necessary for these four goals simultaneously, in concert with support personnel such as nursing, anesthesia, laboratory, blood bank, and others (Table 8-3). Volume replacement is the first and most important therapeutic strategy in the treatment of septic shock. Patients will have either absolute or relative hypovolemia, depending upon the degree of vasodilation and third-spacing of fluid. With judicious use of the Swan-Ganz[48] or other pulmonary artery catheter, isotonic crystalloid (eg, normal saline, lactated Ringer's solution) may be given freely as pulmonary capillary wedge pressures (PCWP) are monitored. If the PCWP increases by more than 7 mmHg, fluid administration may be curtailed to avoid pulmonary edema; if it does not rise by at least 3 mmHg, then more volume is administered (the so-called 7–3 rule).[49] It is important to emphasize the utility of the PCWP, especially in the obstetric patient. Use of the traditional central venous pressure has been demonstrated to be inadequate in the estimation of pulmonary pressure dynamics.[50]

Especially in cases of warm shock, fluid administration (along with appropriate antibiotic therapy or removal of the infected focus) may be all that is necessary for resuscitation of the patient. However, if the patient is refractory, especially if significant sympathetic-mediated vasoconstriction is thought to be present, dopamine hydrochloride may be used to improve cardiovascular parameters.[51] Dopamine has dose-dependent alpha- and beta-adrenergic activity, such that at low doses it in-

TABLE 8–3
Protocol for Management in Cases of Septic Shock

Diagnosis
 Physical examination (including vital signs)
 Insertion of triple lumen pulmonary artery flotation catheter
 Maternal complete blood count and coagulation profile
 General chemistry panel
 Amniotic fluid or endometrial culture, if available
 Blood culture
 Catheterized urine for culture and analysis
 Culture of other operative site, if available
 Fetal monitoring, if appropriate

Management
 Large-bore venous access and arterial catheter
 Indwelling urinary bladder catheter
 Fluid replacement (crystalloid)
 Serial blood gas and central pressure monitoring
 Antibiotic therapy (after cultures taken)
 Pressor agents, as necessary (dopamine)
 Electrolyte replacement
 Acidosis correction (with sodium bicarbonate)
 Correction of clinically significant coagulopathy or anemia with appropriate blood component replacement
 Surgical removal of infected focus, as soon as the patient is adequately resuscitated (including evacuation of uterus in cases of septic abortion or retained products of conception)
 Fetal monitoring, if appropriate
 Narcotic antagonists (naloxone)?

creases myocardial contractility and heart rate and causes vasodilation of renal, coronary, cerebral, and splanchnic vessels by its beta-adrenergic effects. There is also vasoconstriction in skeletal muscle, in effect shunting blood to more important organs. Initial doses of 2 to 5 µg/kg per minute are titrated upward until blood pressure, cardiac output, and other hemodynamic parameters are stabilized. Administration should not exceed 15 to 20 µg/kg per minute, as this allows alpha-adrenergic predominance and vasoconstrictive reduction in tissue perfusion. It should be noted that dopamine administration during pregnancy decreases uterine blood flow, at least in the animal model.[52]

Oxygen supplementation should be initiated immediately. Nasal prongs or mask may be utilized initially, including the continuous positive airway pressure mask. At the first sign of respiratory decompensation, however, intubation and mechanical ventilation should be instituted. Serial arterial blood gas measurements should document the patient's oxygenation status, as well as evidence of carbon dioxide retention and acidosis. As mentioned earlier, attention to the PCWP will aid in the prevention of pulmonary edema due to overhydration.

Treatment of the infection itself is centered about the administration of antibiotics and the removal, if possible, of the focus of infection. Initial antibiotic therapy should consist of a combination of antibiotics that covers most bacteria anticipated in the infectious process. Combinations that include a penicillin (penicillin G, ampicillin), an aminoglycoside (gentamicin, tobramycin), and a specifically anti-anaerobic antibiotic (clindamycin, metronidazole) are appropriate as empiric therapy in cases of septic shock. If *Staphylococcus aureus* is suspected, as in the case of purulent wound infection, vancomycin may be substituted for the penicillin if methicillin resistance is significantly prevalent in the community. However, although antibiotics are absolutely essential in the management of these patients, removal of the septic focus is extremely desirable, if at all possible. This may entail evacuation of the uterus in cases of septic abortion, delivery in cases of chorioamnionitis, hysterectomy in cases of abscess after cesarean section, "total pelvic sweep" in instances of ruptured tubo-ovarian abscess, debridement of necrotic tissue resulting from necrotizing fasciitis, or drainage of pus in cases of postoperative wound abscess.[42,43] Occasionally, the practitioner will balk at such an undertaking in the severely ill patient, with the protest, "She's too sick to take to surgery!" Often, however, the patient's condition will only deteriorate until surgery is accomplished, leading to the sagacious reply, "She's too sick not to take to surgery!"

Another measure historically utilized in the therapy of septic shock is the use of corticosteroids, which presumably enhance cardiac function by several mechanisms, dilate cerebral and visceral vasculature, and prevent third-spacing of fluid by various actions.[53] However, clinical studies have not convincingly proven any positive effect of steroids on survival in severe, late shock, though they may be helpful in some patients early in the illness.[54] There has also been some interest in the use of opiate antagonists in shock patients. Compounds such as naloxone are thought to exert some benefit through the blockade of naturally occurring endorphins, which mediate some of the deleterious effects of the condition. However, even though positive results have been achieved in animal models, insufficient work has been done in humans to make opiate antagonists a standard of therapy in the treatment of septic shock.[41]

Primary Varicella

Varicella zoster virus, a member of the family of herpesviruses, is known to cause two separate clinical syndromes: acute or primary varicella, the (usually childhood) illness commonly known as chickenpox, and recurrent herpes zoster, also known as shingles. Although the recurrent form of the disease may occasionally disseminate and cause severe disease, especially in the immunocompromised patient, it is primarily acute chickenpox that is responsible for significant morbidity and mortality from this virus. In the decade of the 1980s, chickenpox occurred at an annual rate of 0.15 to 0.22 cases per 10,000 population in the United States, resulting in about 50 to 90 deaths per year.[55]

Diagnosis

Acute chickenpox in the otherwise normal, nonimmune individual is heralded by a viral syndrome of fever, headache, myalgia, and malaise that is not particularly distinct from other viral illnesses. However, when crops of characteristic pruritic maculopapular lesions appear on the face, head, and trunk, progressing through a vesicular phase to pustules that scab over, the clinical diagnosis is straightforward. If there is any reason to doubt the diagnosis, seroconversion may be documented with a variety of antibody assays, including fluorescent-antibody-membrane-antigen and enzyme-linked immunoassay. Of course, acute and convalescent serum specimens need to be drawn and tested simultaneously.[56]

The differential diagnosis of acute chickenpox includes generalized herpes simplex infection, disseminated zoster (most commonly in an immunocompromised host), generalized vaccinia and eczema vaccinatum, rickettsial pox, and hand-foot-and-mouth disease. Chickenpox typically occurs in yearly outbreaks in late winter, thus making the diagnosis of a characteristic disease in an otherwise healthy patient quite easy.

Pathophysiology

Varicella zoster virus is generally contracted through the respiratory tract. This is followed by local multiplication and an asymptomatic viremia, with seeding of the reticuloendothelial system. There is a secondary wave of viremia 10 to 21 days later, with dissemination to the skin and viscera. This results in the characteristic skin lesions and any other end-organ effects within 2 days of the second viremia.[57] Patients may be contagious therefore from 2 days before the onset of the rash.

Two to 5 days after the onset of the rash, antibody to varicella virus appears in the blood, peaking in 2 to 3 weeks. Antibody is somewhat protective, since modified disease (ie, disease with reduced symptoms) occurs in patients given varicella zoster immune globulin (VZIG) or in young infants with residual maternal antibody. Interestingly, after a modified case of chickenpox, the patient may still be susceptible to reinfection, followed by either overtly symptomatic or mild to asymptomatic illness. On the other hand, cell-mediated immunity is depressed and modified during an acute primary infection, apparently allowing the virus to escape immunologic recognition and establish latency in the sensory ganglia.[57]

Outcome and Sequelae

Most children with primary varicella (ie, chickenpox) develop the appropriate immunologic response and clear themselves of the acute infection with little damage beyond a few cutaneous pock marks. Latent virus may reappear months or years later as a case of zoster. However, adults who contract the disease may develop clinical varicella pneumonia in up to 50% of cases, often with severe morbidity and mortality. The pregnant patient seems to be two or three times as susceptible to mortality from this complication as the nonpregnant woman.[58,59] In recent reports the benefits of antiviral chemotherapy do not completely eliminate maternal mortality.[60,61]

Fetal effects of maternal varicella take three forms: fetal wastage from maternal disease; intrauterine infection, resulting in the congenital varicella syndrome; and neonatal infection at delivery, allowing disseminated neonatal varicella. Severe maternal disease is apt to incite premature uterine activity and possible preterm delivery. Maternal viremia during the first trimester is associated with a syndrome of limb hypoplasia, cutaneous scarring, microcephaly, cortical atrophy, chorioretinitis, cataracts, and other teratogenic effects in the infant. This appears to occur in up to 5% of such cases, though infants infected in the second and third trimesters do not appear to suffer any ill effects directly.[62] Finally, infants born to mothers who have developed symptomatic varicella within 5 days of delivery are at risk of contracting neonatal disease without the benefit of passively acquired maternal antibody. Infection in this instance may be severe, with dissemination and neurologic damage in 30% of cases.[63]

Management

Varicella, like viral diseases in general, is not curable. Prevention is the only sure way to avert any potential adverse sequelae. Research in this area is promising,[64] and as of this writing active immunization will soon be clinically available. One strategy that is effective is the administration of VZIG to prevent or ameliorate the course of disease in susceptible persons exposed to the virus.[65] Identification of susceptible pregnant individuals is somewhat problematic, since antibody assays are not yet widely available for routine screening purposes. On the other hand, a positive history of chickenpox is almost a guarantee of immunity, while patients with a negative history may be demonstrated to have antibody nearly 80% of the time. Still, a negative history gives the obstetrician enough evidence to warrant screening and administration of VZIG in the exposed gravida near term to prevent severe neonatal varicella. Unfortunately, maternal VZIG has not been shown to prevent congenital varicella syndrome. In addition, VZIG, though currently readily available, is too expensive to use merely to modify maternal disease.[66]

Pregnant women who actually develop acute primary varicella should be carefully monitored for evidence of dissemination and visceral involvement (eg, pneumonia) (Table 8-4). At the same time, uterine activity should be monitored so

TABLE 8-4
Protocol for Management in Cases of Primary Varicella in Pregnancy

Diagnosis
  Physical examination (including chest auscultation and respiratory rate determination)
  Acute and convalescent serology, if necessary
  Serial ultrasonography for fetal effects of intrauterine infection

Management
  Symptomatic relief (eg, for itching)
  Fetal and uterine activity monitoring
  Liberal hospitalization
  Close observation of respiratory status
  Chest roentgenography, if indicated
  Baseline and serial arterial blood gas measurements, as indicated by pulmonary status
  Oxygen administration, if indicated by blood gas measurements
  Intubation and ventilatory support, as necessary
  Parenteral acyclovir, as indicated

---

that tocolysis may be instituted if organized uterine contractions or cervical change is documented. If delivery is unavoidable in the face of acute maternal disease, the neonate is given VZIG shortly after birth to prevent or modify neonatal infection.

The pulmonary status of the infected gravida should be carefully monitored, including frequent determination of respiratory rate and auscultation of the chest. If suggestive findings arise, chest x-ray and arterial blood gases should be obtained, at least as baseline comparisons. If symptoms worsen and the diagnosis of varicella pneumonia is made, oxygen supplementation should be initiated and consideration should be given to the administration of high-dose intravenous acyclovir, given at a dose of 10 to 15 mg/kg, or 500 mg/m^2 three times a day for a week.[61] If clinical deterioration occurs, endotracheal intubation should be instituted, and mechanical ventilation with positive end expiratory pressure or continuous positive airway pressure should be started at appropriate levels. Transient maternal side-effects that may be anticipated include elevated hepatic studies, central nervous system toxicity, and renal dysfunction. Although significant levels of acyclovir cross the placenta, there appear to be no adverse fetal effects.[67]

Primary Herpes

Genital herpes, which may be caused by either of the human herpes viruses, herpes simplex virus type 1 (HSV-1) and HSV-2, is a viral disease that may become chronic and recurrent. Since the 1960s the number of physician consultations for symptomatic disease has increased by a factor of more than 15. In addition, neonatal disease, the most common serious consequence of genital herpes infection, has increased in a parallel fashion.[68] Since men and women in their 20s are most likely to seek medical care for this disease, it is not unexpected that genital herpes commonly complicates pregnancy.

Diagnosis

Primary infection with either HSV-1 or HSV-2, in particular genital infections, usually is more severe than recurrent disease. Thus clinical presentation is often diagnostic. Multiple, painful small vesicles in the vulvar area, coupled with systemic signs such as malaise, fever, photophobia, and myalgia, can be dramatic. However, a manifestation this severe occurs in only about 40% of primary infections. Therefore a less dramatic presentation may compel the practitioner to depend upon laboratory testing for definitive diagnosis. Although scraping of suspect lesions and performance of Tzanck preparations or Papanicolaou smear may give persuasive evidence of viral infection (eg, giant cells) if positive, their sensitivities are at most 50%. Therefore viral isolation in cell culture is considered the gold standard of diagnosis for HSV infection.[69]

Viral culture takes a week or more when performed in the traditional manner. Therefore the addition of indirect and direct staining of clinical material with fluorescent antibody, including monoclonal antibody, has been used to produce immediate results in many cases.[70,71]

Of great concern is the diagnosis of HSV infection complicating pregnancy. Though recurrent infections and asymptomatic viral shedders are most troublesome from the standpoint of diagnosis, even mild first infections are difficult to identify. The strategy of making the diagnosis of HSV in pregnancy by searching for clinical findings and then applying viral culture techniques only has a sensitivity of 77% in first infections, and this is much worse in asymptomatic shedding. Therefore measuring serum antibodies is perhaps the only way to identify patients adequately with mild or subclinical infection.[72] Of course, positive serology does not necessarily mean viral shedding or infectivity. Thus these strategies must be clarified further.

Pathophysiology

HSV enters the body through mucosal surfaces or abrasions in skin, replicating in the local epidermal and dermal cell layers. At this point clinical lesions may or may not develop. The exact cause of severe disease in some patients, versus mild to nonexistent illness in others, is not clear. Patients with significant immunocompromise, especially individuals with depressed cell-mediated immunity, may have much more severe outbreaks, even of recurrent HSV. However, the exact mechanisms are not clear. In any event, if virus reaches sensory or autonomic nerve endings, it is transferred intra-axonally to the dorsal nerve root ganglia, where a chronic source of virus may cause variably intermittent recurrent outbreaks along the route of the nerve. The exact mechanism by which the virus remains latent in the nerve roots and sallies forth to cause recurrent outbreaks is still unknown.[73] Depending upon the status of the host, HSV may disseminate and affect nearly all organ types. Cutaneous and mucosal lesions are common, but dissemination to central nervous system, liver, lungs, and other sites is not unusual. Generally speaking, HSV-2 tends to be more virulent and disseminates more often than HSV-1. In addition, HSV-2 infection is more often recurrent; HSV-1 primary infection is followed less often by recurrent outbreaks.

Outcome and Sequelae

In pregnant women, as well as in adults generally, primary HSV infection (and recurrent infection in patients with immunocompromise) has been documented to result in pneumonia,[74] meningitis and encephalitis,[75,76] hepatitis,[77] and general dissemination.[78] All these manifestations may be extremely severe, or fatal. Pregnant women with severe HSV infection are also at risk for premature uterine activity and preterm delivery, much as with any systemic febrile illness.

Of particular concern, however, is the syndrome of neonatal herpes infection,[79] which occurs in newborns exposed to maternal virus at or after delivery. Disseminated HSV infection is extremely serious in the neonate, fatal even with appropriate antiviral therapy. Survivors have been neurologically damaged. This syndrome is rare in babies of women with recurrent disease,[80] making the recognition of primary HSV infection in pregnancy that much more important.

Management

Primary HSV infection can be treated with acyclovir to shorten the duration of symptoms, decrease viral shedding, and lessen symptoms of the disease.[81] However, this therapy is not recommended during pregnancy unless evidence of dissemination, hepatitis, or the like is present. Therefore the pregnant woman with primary herpes is treated symptomatically with attention to documentation of visceral or central nervous system involvement (Table 8-5). Hospitalization should be liberally employed. Hepatic transaminases, mental status, and pulmonary condition are all observed closely during the acute phase of the disease. Unfortunately, women with unapparent disease (eg, herpetic cervicitis) may occasionally present a diagnostic dilemma and appear to "go down the tubes" without demonstrable infection unless closely scrutinized.[82] This underscores the importance of accurate diagnosis and gives a high index of suspicion in pregnant women with unexplained fever and apparent systemic infection.

If the patient is deemed ill enough for parenteral acyclovir therapy, the drug is administered at a dose of 5 mg/kg every 8 hours for 5 to 7 days or until symptoms

TABLE 8–5
Protocol for Management in Cases of Primary Herpes Simplex in Pregnancy

Diagnosis
  Physical examination
  Acute and convalescent serology, if necessary
Management
  Symptomatic relief (eg, for pain)
  Fetal and uterine activity monitoring
  Liberal hospitalization
  Vigilance for signs of visceral damage (eg, central nervous system signs, evidence of hepatic involvement)
  Serial observation of hepatic enzymes
  Tocolysis, if necessary
  Parenteral acyclovir, as indicated
  Cesarean section if delivery of an otherwise viable infant is imminent
  Parenteral acyclovir for neonate if delivery occurs during the acute illness

resolve.[81] As mentioned earlier, acyclovir seems to have no adverse effects upon the fetus. Indeed, if the baby is delivered during the mother's acute infection, it should doubtless be treated similarly, either empirically or at the onset of suspicious symptoms. On the other hand, delivery is best delayed in the face of acute maternal HSV infection. Tocolysis has been used successfully in such a circumstance.[78]

Because of the severity of the effects of first-episode HSV infection on the neonate, various strategies to prevent vertical transmission have been employed.[83] In recent decades weekly viral cultures in the third trimester were felt to be advantageous in identifying women with a previous history of genital herpes whose infants would benefit by cesarean delivery.[84] However, more recent studies indicated that this strategy failed to select most infants at risk.[85,86] Therefore in concert with the Infectious Disease Society for Obstetrics-Gynecology, the American College of Obstetricians and Gynecologists forwarded the recommendation that weekly viral cultures were not indicated in women with a previous history of genital herpes and that only those women demonstrating lesions (or prodrome) at the onset of labor should be considered for cesarean delivery. In addition, the patient must be counseled that cesarean delivery does not totally exclude the possibility of neonatal herpes infection.[87]

Conclusion

Certain infections that complicate pregnancy may lead, quite rapidly in many cases, to severe manifestations and even death for the mother, infant, or both. Some of the maladies mentioned have less than foolproof therapies, though even those that do respond may not always do so completely. In the final analysis, it is the physician who is responsible for the possession of the knowledge and the skill to handle the emergency at hand appropriately. This should be a stimulus for the practitioner to persevere in his education with the knowledge that this skill and expertise may be called upon at a moment's notice, often in the dark of night or at some other inopportune moment.

REFERENCES

1. Gibbs RS, Castillo MS, Rodgers PJ. Management of acute chorioamnionitis. Am J Obstet Gynecol 136:7009, 1980
2. Gibbs RS. Diagnosis of intra-amniotic infection. Semin Perinatal 1:71, 1977
3. Meuller-Heuback E, Rubinstein DN, Schwarz SS. Histologic chorioamnionitis and preterm delivery in different patient populations. Obstet Gynecol 75:622, 1990
4. Gibbs RS, Blanco JD, St. Clair PJ, Castaneda YS. Quantitative bacteriology of amniotic fluid from women with clinical intraamniotic infection at term. J Infect Dis 145:18, 1982
5. Hoskins IA, Johnson TRB, Winkel CA. Leukocyte esterase activity in human amniotic fluid for rapid detection of chorioamnionitis. Am J Obstet Gynecol 157:730, 1987
6. Gibbs RS, Duff P. Progress in pathogenesis and management of clinical intraamniotic infection. Am J Obstet Gynecol 164:1317, 1991
7. Azziz R, Cumming J, Naeye R. Acute myometritis and chorioamnionitis during cesarean section of asymptomatic women. Am J Obstet Gynecol 159:1137, 1988

8. Koh KS, Chan FH, Monfared AH, Ledger WJ, Paul RH. The changing perinatal and maternal outcome of chorioamnionitis. Obstet Gynecol 53:730, 1979
9. Morales WJ. The effect of chorioamnionitis on the development outcome of preterm infants at one year. Obstet Gynecol 70:183, 1987
10. Naeye RL, Peters EC. Amniotic fluid infections with intact membranes leading to perinatal death: a prospective study. Pediatrics 61:171, 1978
11. Garite TJ, Freeman RK. Chorioamnionitis in the preterm gestation. Obstet Gynecol 59:539, 1982
12. Duff P, Sanders R, Gibbs RS. The course of labor in term patients with chorioamnionitis. Am J Obstet Gynecol 147:391, 1983
13. Hayashi RH, Castillo MS, Noah ML. Management of severe postpartum hemorrhage with a prostaglandin F2α analogue. Obstet Gynecol 63:806, 1984
14. Sperling RS, Ramamurthy RS, Gibbs RS. A comparison of intrapartum versus immediate postpartum treatment of intra-amniotic infection. Obstet Gynecol 70:861, 1987
15. Gilstrap LC, Leveno KJ, Cox SM, et al. Intrapartum treatment of acute chorioamnionitis: impact on neonatal sepsis. Am J Obstet Gynecol 159:579, 1988
16. Gibbs RS, Dinsmoor MJ, Newton ER, Ramamurthy RS. A randomized trial of intrapartum versus immediate postpartum treatment of women with intra-amniotic infection. Obstet Gynecol 72:823, 1988
17. Adamkin DH, Marshall E, Weiner LB. The placental transfer of ampicillin. Am J Perinatol 1:310, 1984
18. Gilstrap LC, Bawdon RE, Burris J. Antibiotic concentration in maternal blood, cord blood, and placental membranes in chorioamnionitis. Obstet Gynecol 72:124, 1988
19. Cunningham FG, Morris GB, Mickal A. Acute pyelonephritis of pregnancy: a clinical review. Obstet Gynecol 42:112, 1973
20. Harris RE, Gilstrap LC. Prevention of recurrent pyelonephritis during pregnancy. Obstet Gynecol 44:637, 1974
21. Hibbard L, Thrupp L, Summeril S, et al. Treatment of pyelonephritis in pregnancy. Am J Obstet Gynecol 98:609, 1967
22. Cox SM, Shelburne P, Mason R et al. Mechanisms of hemolysis and anemia associated with acute antepartum pyelonephritis. Am J Obstet Gynecol 164:587, 1990
23. Whalley PJ, Cunningham FG, Martin FG. Transient renal dysfunction associated with acute pyelonephritis of pregnancy. Obstet Gynecol 46:174, 1975
24. Sweet RL. Bacteriuria and pyelonephritis during pregnancy. Semin Perinatol 1(1):25, 1977
25. Fan Y-D, Pastorek JG, Miller JM, Mulvey J. Acute pyelonephritis in pregnancy. Am J Perinatol 4:324, 1987
26. Lomberg H, Hanson LA, Jacobsson B, Jodal U, Leffler H, Eden CV. Correlation of P blood group, vesicoureteral reflux, and bacterial attachment in patients with recurrent pyelonephritis. N Engl J Med 308:1189, 1983
27. Twickler D, Little BB, Satin AJ, Brown CEL. Renal pelvicalyceal dilation in antepartum pyelonephritis: ultrasonographic findings. Am J Obstet Gynecol 165:1115, 1991
28. Cunningham FG, Leveno KJ, Hankins GDV, Whalley PJ. Respiratory insufficiency associated with pyelonephritis during pregnancy. Obstet Gynecol 63:121, 1984
29. Elkington KW, Greb LC. Adult respiratory distress syndrome as a complication of acute pyelonephritis during pregnancy: case report and discussion. Obstet Gynecol 67:18S, 1986
30. Soisson AP, Eldridge E, Kopelman JN, Duff P. Acute pyelonephritis complicated by respiratory insufficiency. A case report. J Reprod Med 36:525, 1986
31. Pruett K, Faro S. Pyelonephritis associated with respiratory distress. Obstet Gynecol 69:444, 1987
32. Cunningham FG, Lucas MJ, Hankins GDV. Pulmonary injury complicating antepartum pyelonephritis. Am J Obstet Gynecol 156:797, 1987

33. Yazigi R, Lerner S, Tejani N. Association of acute pyelonephritis with pulmonary complications in pregnancy. A report of two cases. J Reprod Med 35:563, 1990
34. Miller JM, Pastorek JG. The microbiology of premature rupture of the membranes. Clin Obstet Gynecol 29(4):739, 1986
35. Duff P. Pyelonephritis in pregnancy. Clin Obstet Gynecol 27:17, 1984
36. Van Dorsten JP, Lenke RR, Shifrin BS. Pyelonephritis in pregnancy: the role of in-hospital management and nitrofurantoin suppression. J Reprod Med 32:895, 1987
37. Cox SM, Cunningham FG. Ureidopenicillin therapy for acute antepartum pyelonephritis. Curr Ther Res 44:1029, 1988
38. Faro S, Pastorek JG, Plauché W, Korndorffer F, Aldridge K. Short-course parenteral antibiotic therapy for pyelonephritis in pregnancy. South Med J 7:455, 1984
39. Angel JL, O'Brien WF, Finan MA et al. Acute pyelonephritis in pregnancy: a prospective study of oral versus intravenous antibiotic therapy. Obstet Gynecol 76:28, 1990
40. Gonik B. Bacteremia and septic shock. Chapter 67. In Mead PB, Hager WD (eds): Infection Protocols for Obstetrics and Gynecology, p 324. Montvale, NJ: Medical Economics, 1992
41. Houston MC, Thompson WL, Robertson D. Shock. Diagnosis and management. Arch Intern Med 144:1433, 1984
42. Duff WP. Management of septic shock in the pelvic surgery patient. Infect Surg 4(2):101, 1985
43. Motsay GJ, Dietzman RH, Ersek RA et al. Hemodynamic alterations and results of treatment in patients with gram-negative shock. Surgery 67:577, 1970
44. Rackow EC, Astiz ME. Pathophysiology and treatment of septic shock. JAMA 266:548, 1991
45. Morishima HO, Niemann WH, James LS. Effects of endotoxin on the pregnant baboon and fetus. Am J Obstet Gynecol 131:899, 1978
46. Gonik B. Considerations in managing septic shock in the obstetric patient. Infect Med 5:191, 1988
47. Kaplan RL, Sahn SA, Petty TL. Incidence and outcome of the respiratory distress syndrome in gram-negative sepsis. Arch Intern Med 139:867, 1979
48. Swan HJ, Ganz W, Forrester J et al. Catheterization of the heart in man with use of a flow-directed balloon-tipped catheter. N Engl J Med 283:447, 1970
49. Shubin H, Weil MH, Carlson RW. Bacterial shock. Am Heart J 94:112, 1977
50. Cotton DB, Gonik B, Dorman K et al. Cardiovascular alterations in severe pregnancy-induced hypertension: relationship of central venous pressure to pulmonary capillary wedge pressure. Am J Obstet Gynecol 151:762, 1985
51. Goldberg LI. Dopamine: clinical uses of an endogenous catecholamine. N Engl J Med 291:707, 1974
52. Rolbin SH, Levinson G, Shnider DM et al. Dopamine treatment of spinal hypotension decreases uterine blood flow in the pregnant ewe. Anesthesiology 51:36, 1979
53. Sladen A. Methylprednisolone: pharmacologic doses in shock lung syndrome. J Thorac Cardiovasc Surg 74:800, 1976
54. Sprung CL, Caralis PV, Marcial EH et al. The effects of high-dose corticosteroids in patients with septic shock. N Engl J Med 311:1137, 1984
55. Centers for Disease Control. Summary of notifiable diseases, United States, 1991. MMWR 40(53):57, 1991
56. McGregor JA, Madinger NE. Varicella-zoster infection in pregnancy. Chapter 20. In Mead PB, Hager WD (eds): Infection Protocols for Obstetrics and Gynecology, p 94. Montvale, NJ: Medical Economics Books, 1992
57. Weller TH. Varicella and herpes zoster. Changing concepts of the natural history, control, and importance of a not-so-benign virus. N Engl J Med 309:1362, 1983
58. Harris RE, Rhoades ER. Varicella pneumonia complicating pregnancy: report of a case and review of the literature. Obstet Gynecol 25:734, 1965

59. Pickard RE. Varicella in pregnancy. Am J Obstet Gynecol 104:504, 1968
60. Hockberger RS, Rothstein RJ. Varicella pneumonia in adults: a spectrum of disease. Ann Intern Med 15:931, 1986
61. Smego RA, Asperilla MO. Use of acyclovir for varicella pneumonia during pregnancy. Obstet Gynecol 78:1112, 1991
62. Paryani SG, Arvin AM. Intrauterine infection with varicella-zoster virus after maternal varicella. N Engl J Med 314:1542, 1986
63. Fuccillo DA. Congenital varicella. Teratology 15:329, 1977
64. Hardy I, Gershon AA, Steinberg SP, LaRussa P. The incidence of zoster after immunization with live attenuated varicella vaccine. N Engl J Med 325:1545, 1991
65. Immunization Practices Advisory Committee. Varicella-zoster immune globulin for the prevention of chickenpox. MMWR 33:84, 1984
66. McGregor JA, Mark S, Crawford GP, Levin MJ. Varicella zoster antibody testing in the care of pregnant women exposed to varicella. Am J Obstet Gynecol 157:281, 1987
67. Andrews EB, Yankaskas BC, Cordero JF, Schoeffler K, Hampp S. Acyclovir in pregnancy registry: six years' experience. Obstet Gynecol 79:7, 1992
68. Becker TM, Stone KM, Cates W. Epidemiology of genital herpes infections in the United States: the current situation. J Reprod Med 31:359, 1986
69. Corey L. The diagnosis and treatment of genital herpes. JAMA 248:1041, 1982
70. Nerurkar LS, Namba M, Sever JL. Comparison of standard tissue culture, tissue culture plus staining, and direct staining for detection of genital herpes simplex virus infection. J Clin Microbiol 19:631, 1984
71. Volpi A, Lakeman AD, Pereira L, Stagno S. Monoclonal antibodies for rapid diagnosis and typing of genital herpes infections during pregnancy. Am J Obstet Gynecol 146:813, 1983
72. Koutsky LA, Stevens CE, Holmes KK et al. Underdiagnosis of genital herpes by current clinical and viral-isolation procedures. N Engl J Med 326:1533, 1992
73. Corey L, Spear PG. Infections with herpes simplex viruses. N Engl J Med 314:686, 1986
74. Ramsey PG, Fife KH, Hackman RC, Meyers JD, Corey L. Herpes simplex virus pneumonia: clinical, virologic, and pathologic features in 20 patients. Ann Intern Med 97:813, 1982
75. Soper JT, Warenski JC. Culture-proven herpes simplex type 2 meningitis associated with genital herpes. A case report. J Reprod Med 28:607, 1983
76. Whitley RJ, Alford CA, Hirsch MS et al. Vidarabine versus acyclovir therapy in herpes simplex encephalitis. N Engl J Med 314:144, 1986
77. Goyert GL, Bottoms SF, Sokol RJ. Anicteric presentation of fatal herpetic hepatitis in pregnancy. Obstet Gynecol 65:585, 1985
78. Cox SM, Phillips LE, DePaolo HD, Faro S. Treatment of disseminated herpes simplex virus in pregnancy with parenteral acyclovir. A case report. J Reprod Med 31:1005, 1986
79. Stone KM, Brooks CA, Guinan ME, Alexander ER. National surveillance for neonatal herpes simplex virus infections. Sex Transm Dis 16:152, 1989
80. Prober CG, Sullender WM, Yasukawa LL, Au DS, Yeager AS, Arvin AM. Low risk of herpes simplex virus infections in neonates exposed to the virus at the time of vaginal delivery to mothers with recurrent genital herpes simplex virus infections. N Engl J Med 316:240, 1987
81. Centers for Disease Control. 1989 Sexually transmitted diseases treatment guidelines. MMWR 38(No. S-8):16, 1989
82. Wertheim RA, Brooks BJ, Rodriguez FH et al. Fatal herpetic hepatitis in pregnancy. Obstet Gynecol 62:38S, 1983
83. Brown ZA, Vontver LA, Benedetti J et al. Effects on infants of a first episode of genital herpes during pregnancy. N Engl J Med 317:1246, 1987
84. Boehm FH, Estes W, Wright PF, Growdon JF. Management of genital herpes simplex virus infection occurring during pregnancy. Am J Obstet Gynecol 141:735, 1981

85. Arvin AM, Hensleigh PA, Prober CG et al. Failure of antepartum maternal cultures to predict the infant's risk of exposure to herpes simplex virus at delivery. N Engl J Med 315:796, 1986
86. Prober CG, Hensleigh PA, Boucher FD, Yasukawa LL, Au DS, Arvin AM. Use of routine viral cultures at delivery to identify neonates exposed to herpes simplex virus. N Engl J Med 318:887, 1988
87. American College of Obstetricians and Gynecologists. Perinatal herpes simplex virus infection. ACOG Tech Bull 122. Washington, DC: ACOG, 1988

CHAPTER 9

Bleeding in Pregnancy

Donald Willis

Other than slight bleeding that can occur with the onset of labor at term, vaginal bleeding during pregnancy is abnormal. The health care professional treating a woman with bleeding during pregnancy should remember that this can be an extremely emotional period. Mother/infant bonding occurs early in pregnancy, and bleeding is often perceived as an early sign of pregnancy loss. Patients are best managed in a professional, caring atmosphere. Appropriate laboratory tests, including ultrasound evaluation, or consultation with an obstetrician/gynecologist will be helpful to alleviate maternal anxiety. Discussions with the patient should be honest but not unduly pessimistic. Patient education in the emergency department is important. However, this can be easily overlooked or rendered quickly without a detailed explanation. Staff members may find it easier to say nothing than to risk saying the wrong thing to an already worried patient. In an effort to improve patient education, information handouts have been developed.[1] This may be especially helpful in busy emergency department settings.

Bleeding in The First 20 Weeks of Pregnancy

Vaginal bleeding occurs in about 20% to 30% of pregnancies during the first 20 weeks. Half of these pregnancies will end with a spontaneous abortion. Therefore about 15% of all human pregnancies end in clinically recognized abortion. The actual abortion rate is much higher, probably 30% to 40% of all pregnancies.[2,3] This difference in actual versus recognized pregnancy loss is because over half of all early pregnancy losses occur at about the same time as expected menses and are not clinically recognized. Several studies monitoring serial human chorionic gonadotropin (HCG) levels have confirmed this high rate of subclinical early-pregnancy loss.[3,4]

There are many known causes for spontaneous abortion. The most common is chromosomal abnormality, which accounts for approximately 50% of all miscarriages.[5] A list of the possible causes for miscarriage is shown in Table 9-1. Whatever the etiology, it has been suggested that bleeding in early pregnancy without other symptoms is almost always the result of marginal separation of the placenta.[6] It is apparent that once bleeding occurs, with few exceptions, little can be done to prevent pregnancy loss among those pregnancies destined to end in abortion. The physician's primary role is to establish whether a pregnancy is viable or not and to limit maternal morbidity and anxiety.

Abortion

Abortion is defined as pregnancy loss before 20 weeks of gestation from last menstrual period (LMP) or loss of a fetus weighing less than 500 g.[2] There are basically four types of spontaneous abortion (Table 9-2). Speculum examination of the cervix and, when indicated, ultrasound evaluation will allow the correct differential diagnosis.

Threatened Abortion

Threatened abortion represents the most common type of abortion seen in the emergency department or physician's office. The patient presents in early pregnancy (less than 20 weeks) with vaginal bleeding. Physical examination reveals the cervix to be closed with no evidence of fetal tissue protruding through the cervical os. Essentially, the examination is normal, other than the presence of vaginal bleeding. As mentioned previously, almost half of these pregnancies will end in miscarriage. Pregnancies that are destined to end in miscarriage are more likely to have associated uterine cramps and pain.[2] Ultrasound findings will be normal for the appropriate gestational age. If fetal cardiac activity is present in normal pregnancies that have reached 8 weeks, the subsequent abortion rate is decreased to only 3.2%,

TABLE 9-1
Etiology of Spontaneous Abortion

1. Chromosome abnormalities
2. Congenital uterine malformations
3. Incompetent cervix
4. Luteal phase defect
5. Fibroid uterus
6. Diabetes—poor control
7. Asherman's syndrome
8. Unknown

TABLE 9–2
Differential Diagnosis: Bleeding in Early Pregnancy

1. Abortion
   a. Threatened
   b. Inevitable
   c. Missed
   d. Incomplete
2. Ectopic pregnancy
3. Cervical/vaginal infection or lesions
4. Hydatiform mole
5. Incompetent cervix

whereas when vaginal bleeding is present, the abortion rate is increased to about 12%.[7,8] This is still considerably less than the 50% overall expected miscarriage rate quoted for women with threatened abortions.

There is no known medical treatment that will prevent pregnancy loss among most women with threatened abortions. Though not substantiated by scientific data, recommendations include avoidance of strenuous activity and sexual intercourse (pelvic rest) until the bleeding has stopped for approximately 7 days. When pregnancy does not end in miscarriage, bleeding in early pregnancy is an important predictor of adverse fetal outcome during the remainder of pregnancy. A two- to three-fold increase in preterm birth, low birth weight, and neonatal death has been reported.

Threatened abortion carries some risk of fetal/maternal bleed.[9] Therefore sensitization of an Rh-negative woman is possible. The Rh antigens have been demonstrated to be present on fetal blood cells by 6 to 7 weeks of gestation by LMP. Since a woman can become sensitized by as little as 0.1 mL of Rh-positive blood, the possibility of a fetal/maternal bleed large enough to cause sensitization is possible by the seventh week from LMP.[10] At present there is no standard recommendation concerning the administration of D immunoglobulin in the clinical setting of a threatened abortion. The American College of Obstetricians and Gynecologists simply states that the risk of isoimmunization among women with antepartum bleeding has not been established.[11] Other investigators recommend the administration of D immunoglobulin (300 µg) for Rh-negative women with threatened abortion.[9,12]

In summary, it appears that a fetal/maternal bleed of enough quantity to cause sensitization is possible with threatened abortion as early as 7 weeks of gestation. However, no information is available to quantify what this risk is. Not administering D immunoglobulin to a woman with threatened abortion is acceptable.[11] The author's institution is not routinely administering D immunoglobulin to such patients. If the attending physician elects to administer D immunoglobulin to Rh-negative women with threatened abortion, it seems reasonable to do so for patients at least 7 weeks in gestation with ultrasound evidence of a viable fetus.

Inevitable Abortion

An abortion is considered inevitable when the cervix has dilated, the amniotic membranes have ruptured, or the bleeding is severe and potentially life-threatening. These pregnancies will not continue and termination is generally advised. When rupture of the membranes occurs between 16 and 24 weeks (previable gestational age), expectant management should be discussed. With improved neonatal care, continuation of pregnancy is an alternative in selected cases. Overall perinatal survival remains poor at only 13 to 15%.[13,14] However, for some patients this may be sufficient to warrant continuation of the pregnancy. Before this decision is made the patient should be aware that of the 13 to 15% of survivors, less than half can be expected to be developmentally normal. Serious neurologic sequelae, such as cerebral palsy, occur in 20% of survivors.[13] Maternal death due to sepsis has been reported.[13] When rupture of the membranes occurs after 24 weeks, perinatal survival improves considerably to over 50%.[13] Referral or consultation with a qualified perinatologist or obstetrician/gynecologist is advised.

Incomplete Abortion

Once products of conception have been passed or can be seen protruding through the cervical os, the pregnancy is obviously lost (Fig. 9-1). Termination is recommended. This is generally done with suction curettage to remove the remaining fetal

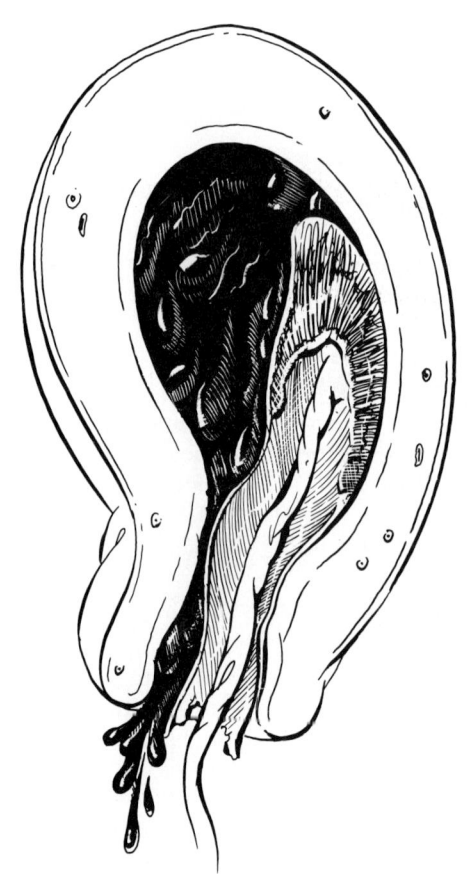

FIGURE 9-1
Incomplete abortion.

and placental tissue. Suction curettage is preferable to sharp curettage, since the latter can result in more blood loss and possible uterine damage. Overzealous curettage, especially with a sharp curette, can result in the development of Asherman's syndrome.[2] Generally, miscarriages that occur between 6 and 14 weeks of gestation are considered incomplete and curettage is recommended.

Rh sensitization can occur after both induced and spontaneous abortions. The risk is 2 to 4%.[11] All unsensitized Rh-negative women should receive D immunoglobulin following abortion, unless the father of the baby is known to be Rh negative.[11] For pregnancies of less than 12 weeks of gestation, a dose of 50 μg is sufficient. Abortions occurring after 12 weeks should receive the standard 300-μg dose.

Complete Abortion

Very early pregnancy loss occurring by 6 weeks from last menstrual period may result in the complete expulsion of the products of conception. The cervix will be closed and bleeding will be minimal after the tissue is passed. In this situation curettage may not be necessary. However, during the remainder of the first trimester, until about 12 to 14 weeks, spontaneous abortions are not usually complete. Failure to perform a suction curettage may lead to persistent or profuse bleeding, anemia, or infection.

Missed Abortion

In the preultrasound era the lack of diagnosis of missed abortion frequently resulted in retention of a dead fetus for several weeks. The diagnosis of missed abortion can be made when a pregnancy is determined to be nonviable by ultrasound. After the fetus dies, disseminated intravascular coagulation (DIC) can develop. Generally, this will not occur until 3 to 4 weeks after fetal demise. Blood-clotting studies (platelet count and fibrinogen) should be obtained before dilatation and suction curettage. Once the diagnosis of missed abortion is made, there is no reason to delay treatment.

Ultrasound Use in the Diagnosis of Abortion

With the introduction of high-resolution ultrasound and especially vaginal probe technology, fetal structures can be identified at earlier gestational ages than previously possible. Vaginal probe ultrasound places a transducer in close proximity to the uterus and fetus, allowing better resolution.

A gestational sac can be seen at about 5 weeks of gestation based on last menstrual period.[15,16] This structure grows approximately 1 mm per day.[17] When the gestational sac measures 15 mm in mean diameter, a fetal pole is consistently seen. The finding of a mean gestational sac diameter of more than 25 mm without a fetal pole identified is definitely abnormal and strongly suggests a nonviable pregnancy.[18] Fetal cardiac activity can be identified by 6 to 7 weeks of gestation with vaginal probe ultrasound.[19] Early identification of fetal cardiac activity before 7 weeks may be associated with a slower than expected fetal heart rate of about 90 beats per minute (bpm). By about 7 weeks the fetal heart rate has increased to 120 to 140 bpm, probably related to a change from idioventricular to an atrial initiated rhythm.[20] By the eighth week of pregnancy, fetal movement is consistently seen even with transabdominal scanning.

Subchorionic hematoma, resulting from a concealed hemorrhage, can be detected by ultrasound in about 20% of women with bleeding in the first half of pregnancy.[21,22] Before 9 weeks of gestation the incidence of detectable hematoma is less. In some cases the hematoma may actually increase in size, then gradually diminish. Subchorionic hematomas are reported to resolve by 24 weeks of gestation. Initial reports suggested that either the presence of subchorionic hematoma or large hematoma (>40 mL) was associated with significantly increased abortion rates and preterm deliveries.[23] However, more recent studies have shown that neither the presence nor the size of a subchorionic hematoma is associated with an increased abortion rate.[22] Therefore it appears that subchorionic hematomas are common and probably an insignificant finding among women with threatened abortion.

Laboratory Test

The need for a laboratory test should be based on clinical presentation. Laboratory evaluation may not be necessary in the emergency department for patients in whom ectopic pregnancy is not suspected and who have only spotting or light vaginal bleeding. Those with more bleeding should have a complete blood count (CBC). Women who are hemodynamically unstable or who have profuse bleeding sufficient to require immediate hospital admission or suction curettage should be typed and matched for packed red blood cells. Rh blood type should be obtained if it is the policy of the individual physician or department to give D immunoglobulin to Rh-negative women with threatened abortion. Unless indicated by clinical presentation, additional laboratory tests are generally unnecessary and only serve to increase the cost of medical care.

With the introduction of vaginal probe ultrasound, maternal serum β-HCG levels are of little value in the diagnosis or management of threatened abortion. The primary role for β-HCG is in the diagnosis of ectopic pregnancy. In a normal pregnancy β-HCG levels should double every 2.4 days. However, one third of ectopic pregnancies may also show a normal increase in β-HCG levels.[24] In these pregnancies a gestational sac should be identified by transabdominal ultrasound when the level is more than 6500 mIU/mL (International Reference Preparation) or about 1500 mIU/mL (IRP) using transvaginal ultrasound.[24] Failure to identify a gestational sac under these circumstances should indicate the possibility of an ectopic pregnancy rather than of a threatened abortion.

Cervical Incompetence

For all practical purposes, cervical incompetence does not present until the second trimester of pregnancy (more than 14 weeks). This condition accounts for 15 to 20% of all second-trimester abortions.[25] It is usually due to prior trauma to the cervix, which could include childbirth, cervical laceration or dilation, and curettage. Patients may have a history of short labors with delivery at progressively earlier gestational ages in successive pregnancies. The clinical presentation is that of gradual, relatively painless, and progressive dilation of the cervix resulting in pregnancy loss, often with delivery of a live fetus. The amniotic membranes may be seen bulging from the cervical os, commonly resulting in spontaneous rupture. The clinical presentation may include vaginal bleeding resulting from cervical dilation. Although the standard diagnosis is based on cervical effacement and dilation in the absence of preterm labor, some uterine activity may be present. Ultrasound can be helpful in demonstrating a shortened and dilated cervix, but more diagnostic is the finding of the amniotic sac protruding into the cervical canal. Caution must be used in making the diagnosis based solely on cervical dilation, since almost 30% of women may have cervical dilation of more than 2 cm by the end of the second trimester.[26,27]

If the diagnosis of cervical incompetence is suspected, the patient should be placed at bed rest in a slight Trendelenburg position, have continuous electronic monitoring for uterine contractions to rule out preterm labor, and consult with an obstetrician or perinatologist.

Hydatidiform Mole

Hydatidiform moles result from abnormal fertilization of an ovum. Usually both sets of chromosomes are of paternal origin.[28] This results in abnormal placental development with typical grapelike vesicles. The diagnosis can be made by gross and microscopic evaluation of placental tissue. The finding of characteristic "snowstorm pattern" on ultrasound is diagnostic.[28] Ovarian thecalutein cysts, which are often very large, are common ultrasound findings.

Patients present as a threatened or incomplete abortion. The uterus may be larger than expected for gestational age. Easily palpable ovarian cyst may be found on bimanual examination. No fetal cardiac activity will be detected. Hydatidiform mole has been associated with the development of early-onset preeclampsia, occurring before the 20th week of pregnancy. Consultation with an obstetrician is indicated when hydatidiform mole is suspected. Tissue that is passed spontaneously or at time of suction curettage should be sent to pathology to confirm the diagnosis. Since 10% of hydatidiform moles will undergo malignant transformation, proper diagnosis and management are important.[29] Unlike true hydatidiform moles, partial moles may have a fetus present. The fetal karyotype is triploidy.[29] Fetal malformations are also common. Since fetal demise generally occurs during pregnancy, a partial mole will usually present as a missed abortion. Ultrasound will show some normal placental tissue as well as areas that resemble the "snowstorm pattern" seen with a true hydatidiform mole. Partial moles only rarely result in persistent trophoblastic disease.[20]

Cervical and Vaginal Infections or Lesions

Although cervicitis and vaginitis are listed in the differential diagnosis of spotting or light vaginal bleeding during pregnancy, these are relatively uncommon causes. Attributing bleeding in pregnancy to these diagnoses should be done with caution. Cervical polyps, ulceration, or gross malignancy should be ruled out by speculum examination. Any vaginal or cervical lesion warrants evaluation for biopsy to establish a definitive diagnosis.

Bleeding After 20 Weeks in Pregnancy

The differential diagnosis for bleeding that occurs after the 20th week in pregnancy is listed in Table 9-3. Cervical/vaginal lesions or infection as well as incompetent cervix were discussed in the prior section and will not be repeated. For all practical purposes, bleeding after 20 weeks is usually due to preterm labor, abruptio placenta, or placenta previa, all of which require hospitalization once the diagnosis is made. A helpful approach to proper diagnosis and management follows.

Stabilization of the Patient

Patients with significant blood loss show evidence of hypovolemia. When clinically indicated, these patients require one or more large-bore intravenous catheters for fluid resuscitation and appropriate blood replacement when clinically indicated.

Assessment of Fetal Well-being

Pregnancies that are at or beyond 24 to 25 weeks of gestation are potentially viable. Continuous electronic fetal monitoring of fetal heart rate and uterine activity is indicated to determine if immediate delivery is necessary for fetal distress. Abnormal fetal heart rate patterns such as bradycardia (less than 120 bpm), decelerations, or lack of normal fetal heart rate variability require immediate transfer to the labor and delivery suite for obstetric care. Other than for ultrasound or other diagnostic procedures, fetal monitoring should be uninterrupted until a diagnosis and/or disposition is made. In the event that continuous fetal monitoring is not available, the patient should be transferred to a hospital with an obstetric service.

Rule Out Placenta Previa

Among patients with significant vaginal bleeding, ultrasound should be performed to rule out placenta previa (Fig. 9-2). Digital examination in a patient with a placenta previa can result in life-threatening hemorrhage and possible fetal loss. Ultrasound, especially vaginal probe, will effectively diagnose placenta previa. If ultrasound is not available, gentle speculum examination can be performed to determine cervical dilation to rule out advanced labor. However, speculum exami-

TABLE 9–3
Differential Diagnosis: Bleeding After 20 Weeks in Pregnancy

1. Preterm labor
2. Abruptio placenta
3. Placenta previa
4. Incompetent cervix
5. Cervical or vaginal lesions

BLEEDING IN PREGNANCY ♦ 135

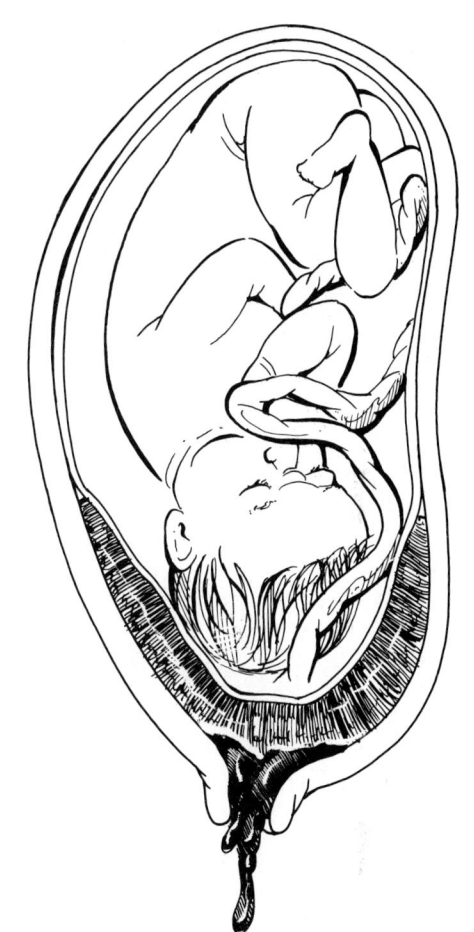

FIGURE 9–2
Placenta previa.

nation cannot be used to exclude placenta previa. Ultrasound can also detect abruptio placenta in some cases (Fig. 9-3). Since the detection rate has been reported to be as low as only 2%, normal findings do not exclude the diagnosis of abruptio placenta.

Rule Out Labor

After placenta previa is excluded, digital examination can be performed to determine cervical dilation and effacement. Patients in labor are transferred directly to the labor and delivery suite. Emergency departments that do not have access to a labor and delivery unit should arrange patient transfer as soon as the patient is determined to be hemodynamically stable. This assumes that the patient is not in advanced labor and that delivery is not anticipated before transfer is completed.

Laboratory Test

Patients in labor with minimal bleeding and stable vital signs do not require laboratory evaluation in the emergency department. Appropriate studies including CBC, type and screen, urinalysis, and VDRL are best obtained in the labor and delivery

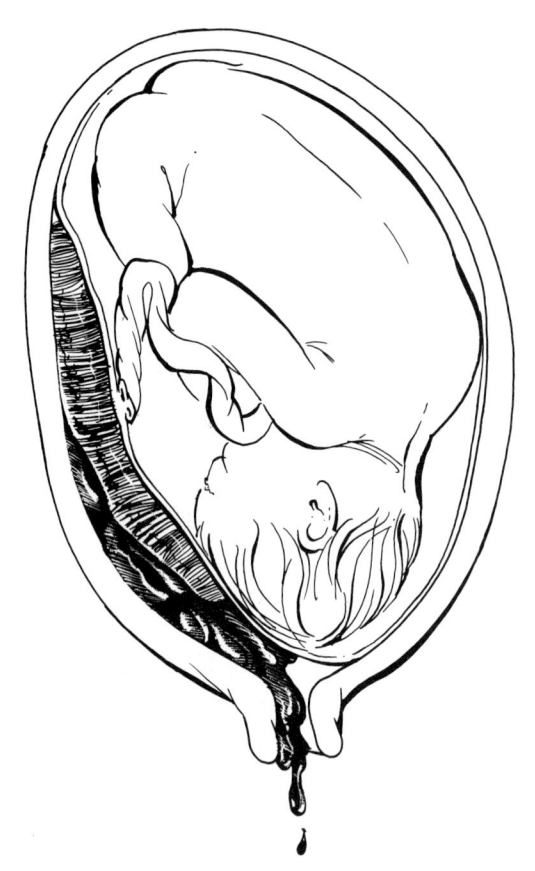

FIGURE 9-3
Abruptio placenta with visible vaginal bleeding.

suite. Patients that present in acute distress with vaginal bleeding, severe pain, or clinical evidence of hypovolemia require hospital admission and immediate consultation with an obstetrician or perinatologist. Laboratory tests should be ordered on a stat basis and should include a CBC, type and match for two or more units of blood, and clotting studies (platelet count, fibrinogen, PT, PTT). For patients that are not in acute distress, initial evaluation with ultrasound is most helpful. After obtaining the ultrasound results, more appropriate laboratory tests can be ordered. It should also be noted that maternal cocaine use is associated with preterm labor and abruptio placenta.[30,31] A urine toxicology screen is becoming a standard laboratory test in the evaluation of patients with pain and bleeding during pregnancy.

Patients with ultrasound diagnosis of placenta previa and vaginal bleeding require hospital admission. Appropriate laboratory tests in the emergency department include a CBC and type and match for two or more units of packed red blood cells. Placenta previa is not associated with disseminated intravascular coagulation (DIC), unless this results from excessive blood loss. Therefore blood-clotting studies are not necessary for these patients. If placenta previa and labor are excluded, the diagnosis of abruptio placenta should be suspected unless another etiology is obvious. It should be remembered that approximately 20% of patients with abruptio placenta have concealed hemorrhage and that therefore no visible bleeding is seen (Fig. 9-4). However, blood loss may still be significant, and therefore the lack of vaginal bleeding should not limit the resuscitation efforts. Abruptio placenta is often associated

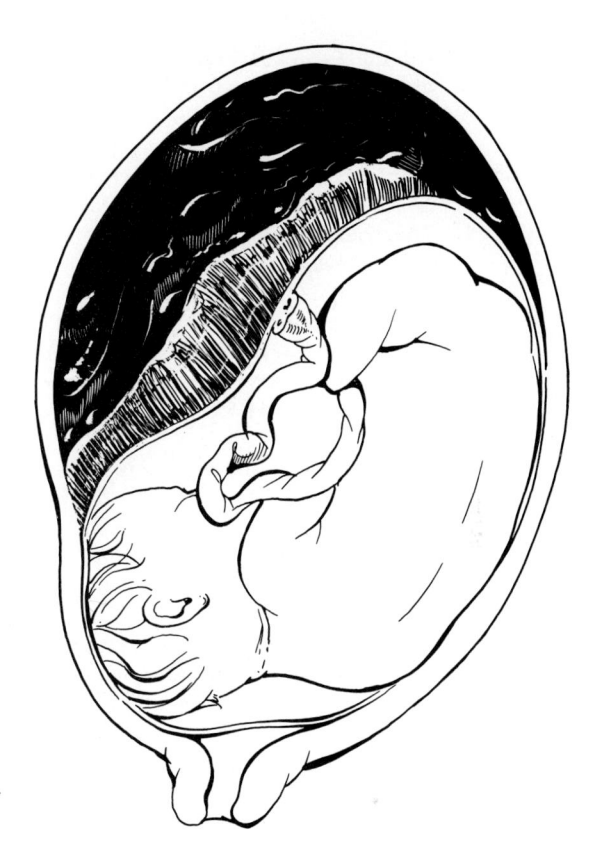

FIGURE 9–4
Abruptio placenta with concealed bleeding.

with fetal distress, renal failure secondary to hypovolemia, and DIC. When abruptio placenta is suspected, appropriate laboratory studies include a CBC, platelet count, fibrinogen, PT, PTT, serum BUN and creatinine, type and match for four or more units of blood, and a urine toxicology screen. Immediate consultation with the obstetric service is indicated.

REFERENCES

1. Stockman M. Nurse educator, patient teaching in the emergency department: vaginal bleeding during early pregnancy. J Emerg Nursing 17:424, 1991
2. Mishell DR. Abortion. In Herbst AL, Mishell DR, Stenchever MA, Droegemueller W (eds): Comprehensive Gynecology, 2nd ed, p 425. St Louis: CV Mosby, 1992
3. Wilcox AJ, Weinberg CR, O'Connor JF et al. Incidence of early pregnancy loss. N Engl J Med 319:189, 1988
4. Miller JF, Williamson E, Glue J. Fetal loss after implantation: a prospective study. Lancet 2:554, 1980
5. Simpson JL. Fetal wastage. In Gabbe SG, Niebyl JR, Simpson JL (eds): Obstetrics: Normal and problem pregnancies, 2nd ed, p 786. New York: Churchill Livingstone, 1991
6. William MA, Mittendorf R, Lieberman E, Monson RR. Adverse infant outcomes associated with first-trimester vaginal bleeding. Obstet Gynecol 78:14, 1991
7. Simpson JL, Mills JL, Holmes LB et al. Low fetal loss rates after demonstration of a live fetus in the first trimester. JAMA 258:2555, 1987

8. Hill LM, Guzick D, Fries J, Hixson J. Fetal loss rate after ultrasonically documented cardiac activity between 6 and 14 weeks, menstrual age. J Clin Ultrasound 19:221, 1991
9. Dayton VD, Anderson DS, Crosson JT, Cruikshank SH. A case of Rh isoimmunization: should threatened first-trimester abortions be an indication for Rh immune globulin prophylaxis? Am J Obstet Gynecol 163:63, 1990
10. Ascari WQ. Abortion and maternal Rh immunization. Clin Obstet Gynecol 14:625, 1971
11. American College of Obstetricians and Gynecologist. Prevention of D isoimmunization. ACOG Technical Bulletin 147. Washington, DC: ACOG, 1990
12. Bowman JM. Controversies in Rh prophylaxis: who needs Rh immune globulin and when should it be given? Am J Obstet Gynecol 151:289, 1985
13. Moretti M, Sibai B. Maternal and perinatal outcome of expected management of premature rupture of the membranes. Am J Obstet Gynecol 159:390, 1988
14. Taylor J, Garite TJ. Premature rupture of the membranes before fetal viability. Obstet Gynecol 64:615, 1984
15. DeCherny AH, Romero R, Polan ML. Ultrasound in reproductive endocrinology. Fertil Steril 37:323, 1982
16. Fossum GT, Davajon V, Kletzky OH. Early detection of pregnancy with transvaginal ultrasound. Fertil Steril 49:788, 1988
17. Goldstein SR. Early detection of pathologic pregnancy by transvaginal sonography. J Clin Ultrasound 18:262, 1990
18. Nyberg DA, Filly RA, Filho DLD et al. Abnormal pregnancy: early diagnosis by ultrasound and serum chorionic gonadotropin levels. Radiology 158:393, 1986
19. Levi CS, Lyons EA, Zheng XH et al. Endovaginal us: demonstration of cardiac activity in embryos of less than 5.0 mm in crown rump length. Radiology 176:71, 1990
20. Walton D, Ludlow D. Abrupt rise in the fetal heart rate at the end of the sixth gestational week. Am J Obstet Gynecol 164:265, 1991
21. Goldstein SR, Subramanyam BR, Raghavendvra BN et al. Subchorionic bleeding in threatened abortion: sonographic findings and significance. AJR 141:975, 1983
22. Pedersen JF, Mantoni M. Prevalence and significance of subchorionic hemorrhage in threatened abortion: a sonographic study. AJR 154:535, 1990
23. Pedersen JF, Mantoni M. Large intrauterine haematomata in threatened miscarriage: frequency and clinical consequences. Br J Obstet Gynaecol 97:75, 1990
24. Decherney AH, Seifer DB. Ectopic pregnancy. In Gabbe SG, Niebyl JR, Simpson JL (eds): Obstetrics, normal and problem pregnancies, 2nd ed, p 816. New York: Churchill Livingstone, 1991
25. Main DM, Main EK. Preterm birth. In Gabbe SG, Niebyl JR, Simpson JL (eds): Obstetrics, normal and problem pregnancies, 2nd ed, p 858. New York: Churchill Livingstone, 1991
26. Leveno KJ, Cox K, Roark ML. Cervical dilatation and prematurity revisited. Obstet Gynecol 68:434, 1986
27. Schaffner F, Schanger SN. Cervical dilatation in the early third trimester. Obstet Gynecol 27:130, 1966
28. Parmley TH. The placenta. In Gabbe SG, Niebyl JR, Simpson JL (eds): Obstetrics: Normal and problem pregnancies, 2nd ed, p 52. New York: Churchill Livingstone, 1991
29. Vejerslev LO, Fisher RA, Surti U et al. Cytogenetically unusual cases and their implications for the present classification. Am J Obstet Gynecol 157:180, 1987
30. Dombrowski MP, Wolf HM, Welch RA et al. Cocaine abuse is associated with abruptio placentae and decreased birth weight, but not shorter labor. Obstet Gynecol 77:139, 1991
31. Handler A, Kistin N, Davis F et al. Cocaine use during pregnancy: perinatal outcomes. Am J Epidemiol 133:818, 1991

CHAPTER 10

Delivery in the Emergency Department

Isaac Delke

In the first half of this century most births occurred at home. In response to concerns about maternal deaths due to hemorrhage, infection, and eclampsia, the hospital replaced the home as the site for labor and delivery. This change in the place of birth resulted in a welcomed decrease in maternal mortality. Furthermore, as maternal mortality decreased, fetal well-being during labor was increasingly emphasized. By 1980 over 95% of births in the United States occurred in hospitals; the rest were in birthing centers and at home.[1,2] In several localities the emergency department (ED) is the site of entry of obstetric patients to the hospital. These patients are subsequently sent to the labor and delivery suite if the hospital has an obstetrics service. Sometimes, however, the ED staff is faced with a gravida ready to deliver and must be ready to handle such a situation.

This chapter presents basic steps in the management of imminent delivery. It focuses on the management of (1) normal spontaneous vaginal delivery of infant and placenta (including episiotomy) and (2) abnormal delivery of infant (shoulder dystocia, breech) and perineal lacerations. Knowledge of the management of conditions that commonly confront the ED staff will maximize the potential for effective intervention and optimal outcome.

Spontaneous Vaginal Delivery

Delivery of the Head

If delivery is already well on its way, the operator should proceed with a vaginal delivery after a stat call to an obstetrician and pediatrician. Ideally, the patient should be on a delivery table in the lithotomy position. If the patient is on a bed or stretcher, her legs should be supported. If the fetus is dead, there is no risk of further fetal trauma, and concern is totally maternal.

As the head becomes increasingly visible, the vaginal outlet and vulva are stretched until they ultimately encircle the largest diameter of the baby's head (Fig. 10-1). This is termed *crowning*. Unless an episiotomy has been made, the perineum is extremely thin and, particularly in the case of the nulliparous woman, is almost at the point of tear.

Ritgen Maneuver

Once the head distends the vulva and perineum sufficiently to open the vaginal introitus to a diameter of 5 cm or so, a towel should be draped over one gloved hand to protect it from the anus. Forward pressure should be extended on the chin of the fetus through the perineum just in front of the coccyx while the other hand exerts pressure superiorly against the occiput (Fig. 10-2). This allows the physician to control the delivery of the head and prevents "popping." It also favors extension, so that the head is delivered with its smallest diameters passing through the introitus and over the perineum. The head is delivered slowly with the base of the occiput rotating around the lower margin of the symphysis pubis as a fulcrum, while the bregma (anterior fontanel), brow, and face pass successively over the perineum.[1]

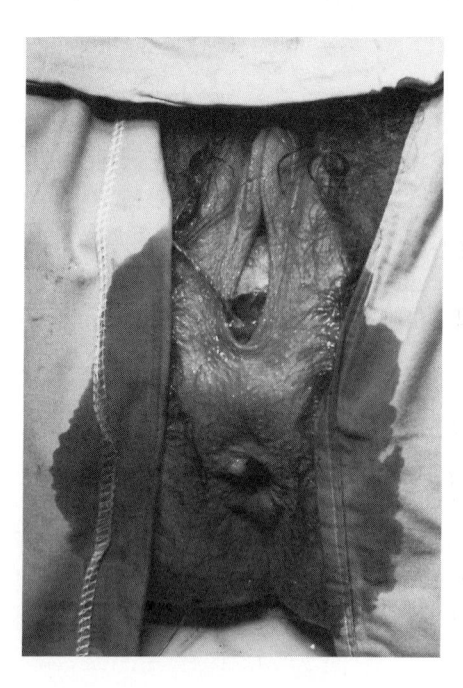

FIGURE 10-1
Crowning.

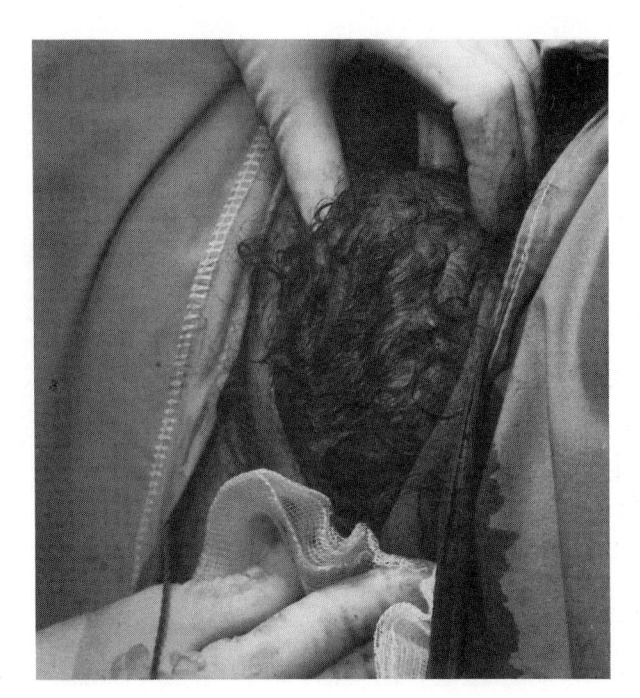

FIGURE 10-2
Ritgen maneuver.

Clearing the Nasopharynx

To minimize the likelihood of aspiration of amniotic fluid debris and blood that might occur once the thorax is delivered and the infant can inspire, the face is quickly wiped and the nares and mouth are aspirated (Fig. 10-3). A soft rubber ear syringe or its equivalent inserted with care is suitable for this. If the amniotic fluid is meconium stained, a wall suction system is necessary.

Nuchal Cord

Once the head is delivered, a finger should be passed to the neck of the fetus to ascertain whether is it encircled by one or more coils of the umbilical cord (Fig. 10-4). A nuchal cord occurs in about 25% of cases and ordinarily does no harm. If a coil is felt, it should be drawn down between the fingers and, if loose enough, slipped over the infant's head. If it is applied too tightly to the neck to be slipped over the head, it should be cut between two clamps and the infant should be delivered promptly.

Delivery of Shoulders

After delivery, the head falls posteriorly, bringing the face almost into contact with the anus. The occiput promptly turns toward one of the maternal thighs so that the head assumes a transverse position. The successive movements of restitution and external rotation indicate that the bisacromial diameter (transverse diameter of the thorax) has rotated into the anteroposterior diameter of the pelvis.

In most cases the shoulders appear at the vulva just after external rotation and

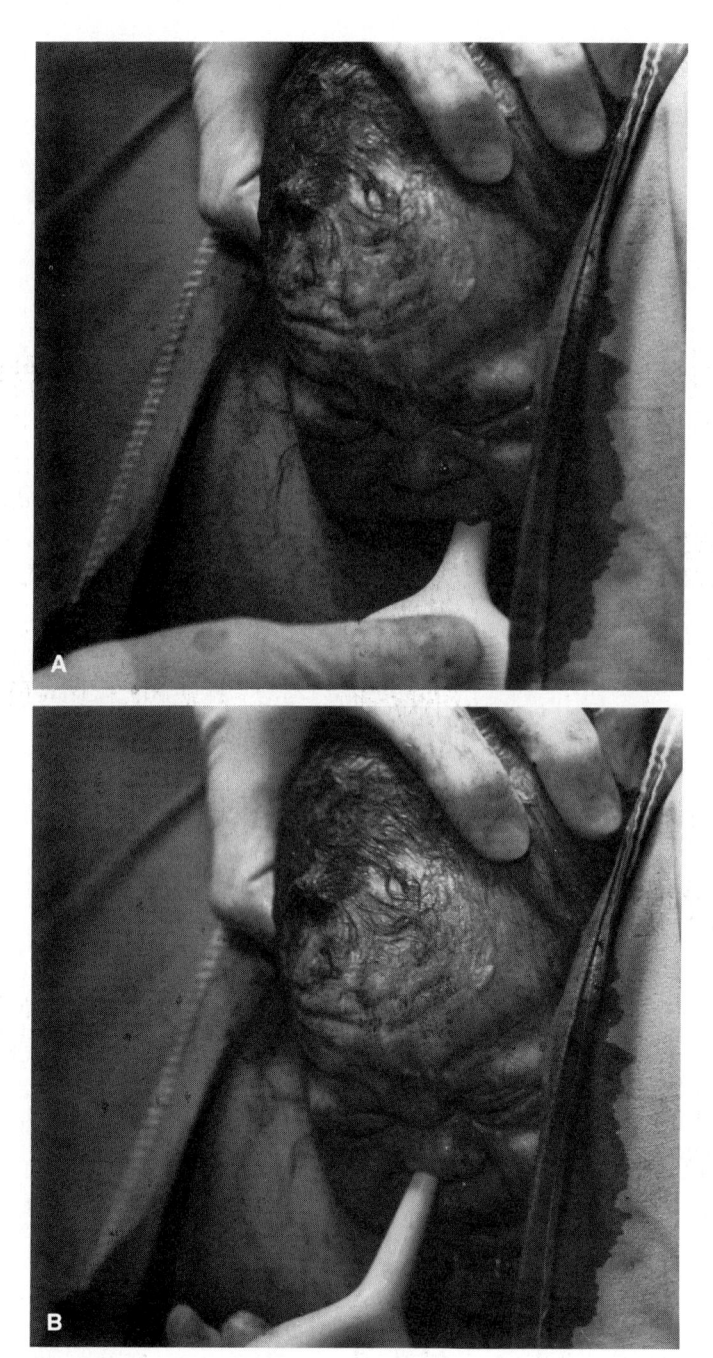

FIGURE 10-3
(**A**) Aspiration of mouth. (**B**) Aspiration of nose.

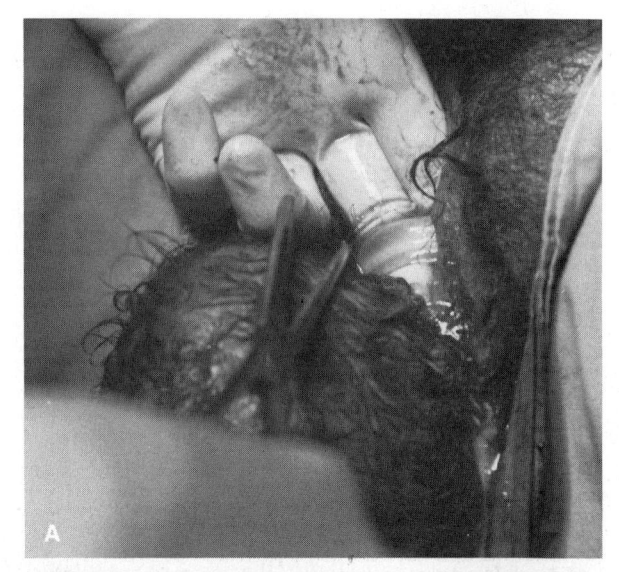

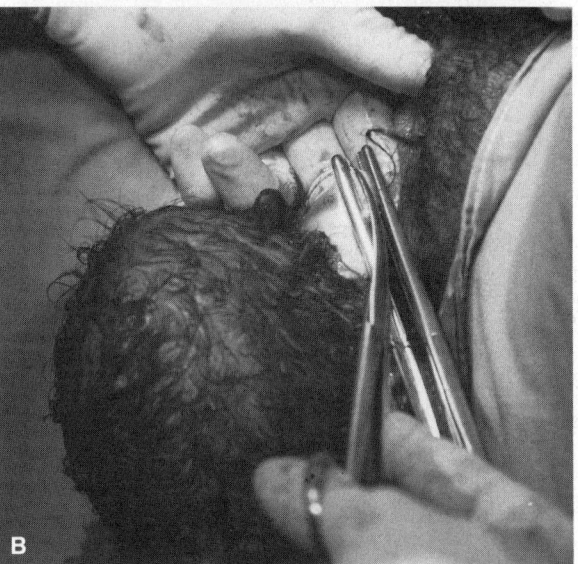

FIGURE 10–4
(A) Nuchal cord. **(B)** Nuchal cord—clamped.

are born spontaneously. Occasionally, a delay occurs and immediate extraction may appear advisable. In that event, the sides of the head are grasped with the two hands and *gentle* downward traction is applied until the anterior shoulder appears under the pubic arch. Then, by an upward movement, the posterior shoulder is delivered and the anterior shoulder usually drops down from beneath the symphysis. An equally effective method entails completion of delivery of the anterior shoulder before that of the posterior (Fig. 10-5).[1,2]

The rest of the body almost always follows the shoulders without difficulty, but in case of prolonged delay its birth may be hastened by *moderate* traction on the head and moderate pressure on the uterine fundus. Hooking the fingers in the axillae

144 ♦ OBSTETRIC AND GYNECOLOGIC EMERGENCIES

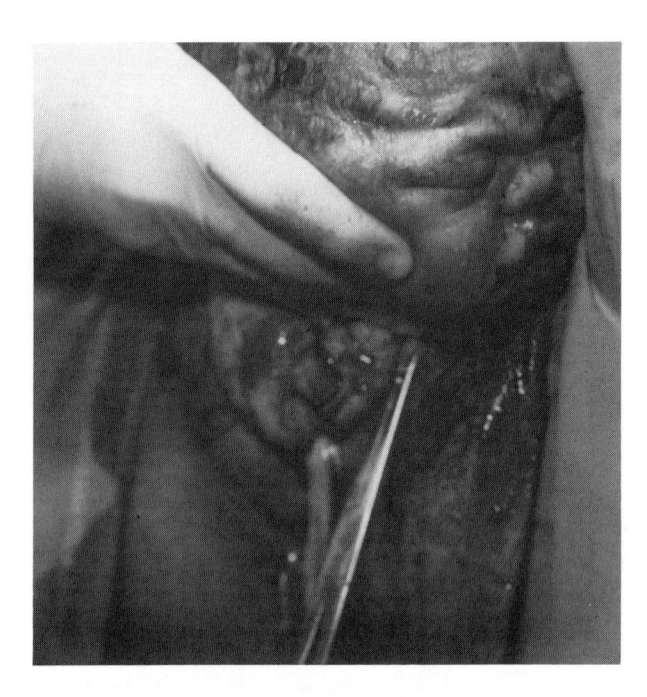

FIGURE 10-5
Delivery of posterior shoulder.

should be avoided, however, since this may injure the nerves of the upper extremity, producing a transient or possibly permanent paralysis. Furthermore, traction should be exerted only in the direction of the long axis of the infant, for if applied obliquely it causes bending of the neck and excessive stretching of the brachial plexus.

Clamping of the Cord

The cord is clamped after thoroughly clearing the infant's airway, which usually takes about 30 seconds. The infant is not elevated above the introitus at vaginal delivery. The umbilical cord is cut between two clamps placed 4 or 5 cm from the fetal abdomen. Later, an umbilical cord clamp is applied 2 or 3 cm from the fetal abdomen. A segment of the umbilical cord is saved for blood gas analysis.

Once the cord has been divided, the infant is immediately placed supine with the head lowered and turned to the side in a heated unit that has appropriate thermal regulation. If such a unit is unavailable, the infant should be wiped dry, wrapped, and have its head covered, to minimize heat loss.

Delivery of the Placenta

Some bleeding is inevitable during the third stage of every labor as the result of transient partial separation of the placenta. As the placenta separates, the blood from the implantation site may escape into the vagina immediately ("Duncan mechanism"), or it may be concealed behind the placenta and membranes ("Schultze mechanism") until the placenta is delivered.[1]

In the presence of any external hemorrhage during the third stage, the uterus should be massaged if it is not firmly contracted. If the signs of placental separation have appeared, expression of the placenta should be attempted by manual pressure on the fundus of the uterus. Descent of the placenta is indicated by the cord becoming slack. If bleeding continues, manual removal of the placenta is mandatory.

Immediately after delivery of the infant, the height of the uterine fundus and its consistency are ascertained. As long as the uterus remains firm and there is no unusual bleeding, the usual practice is to watch carefully for any of the following signs of placental separation:

1. The uterus becomes globular and, as a rule, firmer. This sign is the earliest to appear.
2. There is often a sudden gush of blood.
3. The uterus rises in the abdomen because the placenta, having separated, passes into the lower uterine segment and vagina, where its bulk pushes the uterus upward.
4. The umbilical cord protrudes farther out of the vagina, indicating that the placenta has descended.

These signs sometimes appear within about a minute after delivery of the infant and usually within 5 minutes. The mother may be asked to bear down, and the intra-abdominal pressure so produced may be adequate to expel the placenta. If these efforts fail, the physician, again having made certain that the uterus is contracted firmly, lifts the fundus cephalad with the abdominal hand, keeping the umbilical cord slightly taut. This maneuver is repeated until the placenta reaches the introitus. Traction on the cord, however, must not be used to pull the placenta out of the uterus. Placental expression should never be forced before placental separation, lest the uterus be turned inside out. *Inversion of the uterus* is one of the grave accidents associated with delivery.[1,2]

As the placenta passes through the introitus, pressure on the uterus is stopped. The placenta is then gently lifted away from the introitus. Care is taken to prevent the membranes from being torn off and left behind. If the membranes start to tear, they are grasped with a ring forceps and removed by gentle traction. The placenta, membranes, and umbilical cord should be examined for completeness and anomalies.

The hour immediately following delivery of the placenta is critical. Even though oxytocics are administered, postpartum hemorrhage as the result of uterine relaxation is most likely to occur at this time. It is mandatory that the uterus be evaluated very frequently throughout this period by a competent attendant, who places a hand frequently on the fundus and massages it at the slightest sign of relaxation. At the same time, the vaginal and perineal regions are also inspected frequently to allow prompt identification of any excessive bleeding.

Oxytocin Agents

After the uterus has been emptied and the placenta has been delivered, the primary mechanism by which hemostasis is achieved at the placental site is by a well-contracted myometrium. Oxytocin (Pitocin, Syntocinon), ergonovine maleate

(Ergotrate), and methylergonovine maleate (Methergine) are employed in various ways in the conduct of the third stage of labor, principally to stimulate myometrial contractions and thereby reduce the blood loss.

Oxytocin, ergonovine, and methylergonovine are all employed widely in the conduct of the normal third stage of labor, but the timing of their administration differs in various institutions. Oxytocin, and especially ergonovine, given before delivery of the placenta will decrease blood loss somewhat. However, the use of oxytocin, and especially ergonovine or methylergonovine, before delivery of the placenta may entrap an undiagnosed and therefore undelivered second twin. This may prove injurious, if not fatal, to the entrapped fetus. In most cases following uncomplicated vaginal delivery, the third stage of labor can be conducted with reasonably small blood loss without using alkaloids of ergot.

If an intravenous infusion is in place, a common practice is to add 20 units (2 mL) of oxytocin per liter, which is administered after delivery of the placenta at a rate of 10 mL per minute for a few minutes until the uterus remains firmly contracted and the bleeding is controlled. Then the infusion rate is reduced to 1 to 2 mL per minute until the mother is ready for transfer from the recovery suite to the postpartum unit, when the infusion is usually discontinued.

Episiotomy and Repair

Episiotomy (perineotomy) is incision of the perineum. The incision may be made in the midline (median), or it may begin in the midline but be directed laterally and downward away from the rectum (mediolateral).

Except for cutting the umbilical cord, episiotomy is the most common operation in obstetrics. The reasons for its popularity among obstetricians include the substitution of a straight, neat, surgical incision for the ragged laceration that otherwise frequently results; ease of repair; ease of healing. With mediolateral episiotomy, the likelihood of lacerations into the rectum is reduced.[3,4]

Most obstetricians in the United States have abandoned the routine use of mediolateral episiotomy. The disadvantages of mediolateral episiotomy include increased blood loss from incision of the bulbocavernosus and pubococcygeus muscles, and severe postpartum discomfort. Despite the increased risk of sphincter injury with midline episiotomy, satisfactory repair and healing can be expected in nearly all cases.

Extensions or lacerations complicating midline episiotomies are classified as first degree (involving only vaginal mucosa), second degree (involving vaginal mucosa and perineal body without sphincter injury), third degree (rectal sphincter injury), and fourth degree (injury to rectal mucosa).

Timing of Episiotomy

In most vertex vaginal deliveries it is common to allow distention of the perineum prior to episiotomy incision. As the head crowns, the operator's index and second fingers are placed inside the introitus to expose the mucosa, posterior fourchette, and perineal body (see Fig. 10-5). Mayo scissors are placed in the midline at the fourchette, and a 3-cm incision is made either directly posteriorly (midline) or posterolaterally at a 45° angle to the midline (mediolateral) (Fig. 10-6). Under visu-

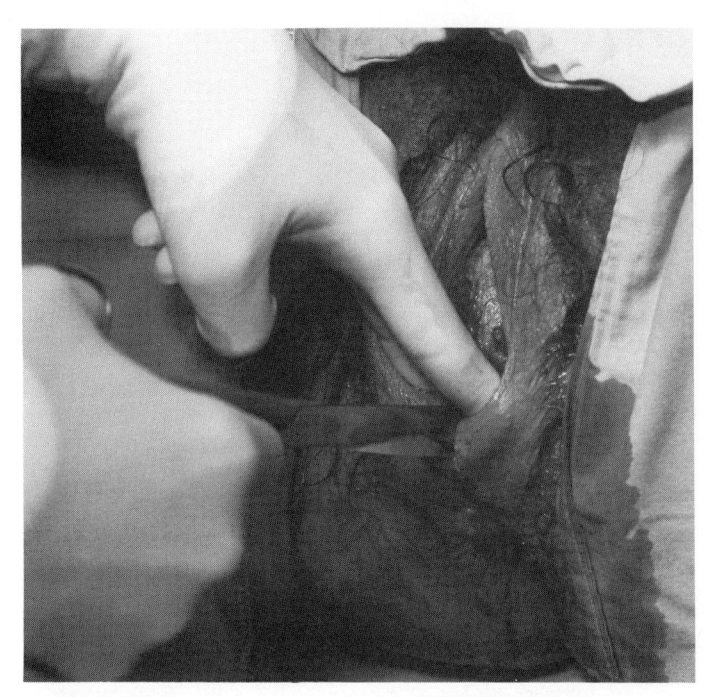

FIGURE 10-6
Episiotomy incision.

alization the incision is extended approximately 6 cm into the vaginal mucosa. The anatomic structures incised during midline episiotomy include the posterior vaginal fourchette, the vaginal mucosa and submucosa, the interdigitating fibers of the superficial and deep transverse perinei and pubococcygeus muscle group, and the inferior fascia of the urogenital diaphragm. During mediolateral episiotomy, in addition to the preceding, the medial portions of the bulbocavernosus and pubococcygeus muscles also may be incised.[3,4]

Timing of the Repair of Episiotomy

The most common practice is to defer repair of the episiotomy until after the placenta has been delivered. This permits the obstetrician to give undivided attention to the signs of placental separation and to deliver the organ just as soon as it has separated. Early delivery of the placenta is believed to decrease the loss of blood from the implantation site, since it prevents the development of extensive retroplacental bleeding. A further advantage of this practice is that the episiotomy repair is not interrupted or disrupted by the obvious necessity of delivering the placenta, especially if manual removal must be performed.

Technique. There are many ways to close the episiotomy incision, but hemostasis and anatomic restoration without excessive suturing are essential for success with any method. A technique that is commonly employed in episiotomy repair is shown in Figure 10-7. The suture material ordinarily used is 000 chromic catgut.

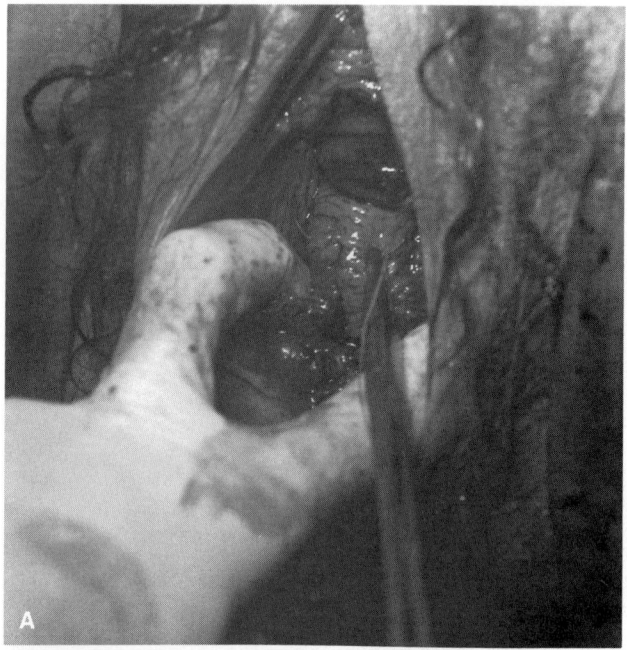

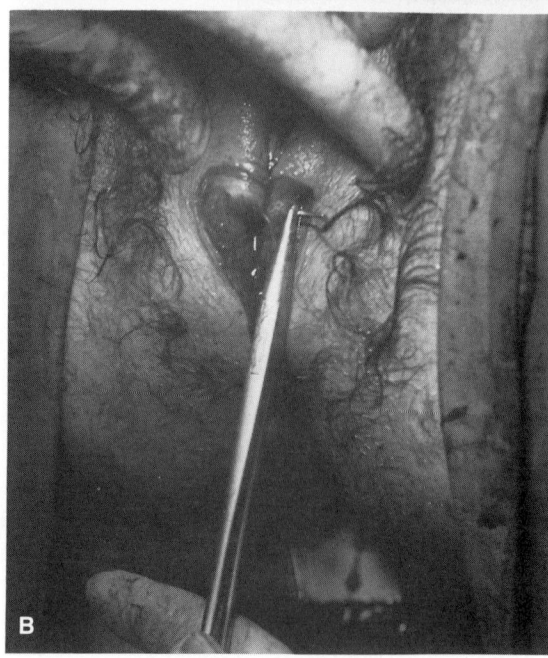

FIGURE 10-7
Episiotomy repair. (**A**) Suturing of vaginal mucosa. (**B**) Perineal body repair.

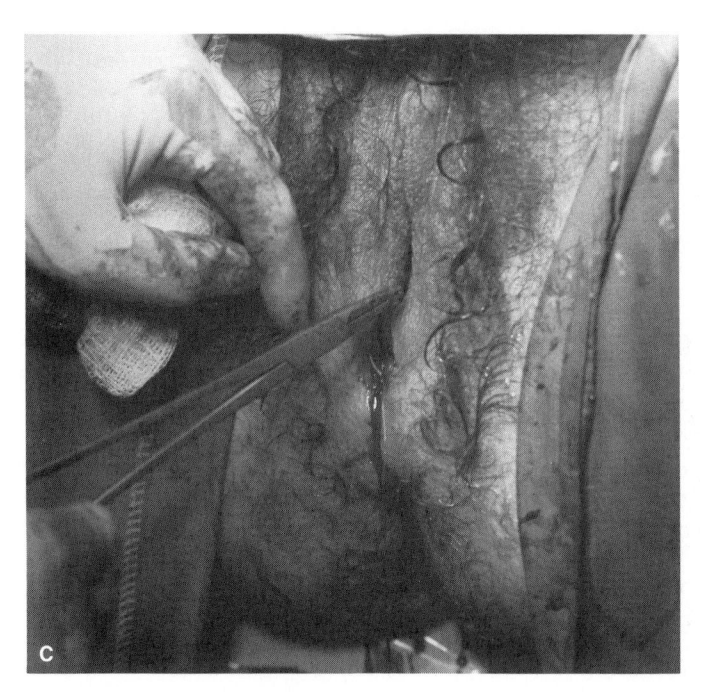

Figure 10-7 (Continued)
(**C**) Subcuticular skin closure.

Repair of the midline episiotomy begins with a careful survey of the region to rule out rectal mucosa or rectal sphincter injury. Suture repair proceeds by reapproximation of tissues in layers. Repair of an uncomplicated episiotomy begins with suturing of the vaginal mucosa with a continuous suture of 2–0 or 3–0 chromic catgut. When the level of the hymenal ring is reached, the bulbocavernosus muscles are reapproximated at the midline ("crown stitch"). The needle is then passed through the vaginal tissues, to exit on the perineal side of the episiotomy incision. The continuous suture is held at that point, and interrupted sutures of 2–0 chromic catgut are used to approximate the muscles and fascia of the perineal body. The remainder of the continuous suture is then used to close the subcutaneous layer of muscle and fascia. When the inferior margin of the incision has been reached, the suture is carried upward as a subcuticular suture to close the skin.

1. The apex of the vaginal incision is identified and, beginning at this point, the mucosa and submucosa are reapproximated with a continuous interlocking suture. Deep to the hymenal ring, the suture is directed under the posterior fourchette and into the anterior portion of the perineal body and laid aside untied.
2. Reapproximation of the superficial transverse perinei is critical in the repair of the midline episiotomy. Interrupted deep horizontal sutures are placed, reapproximating the perineal muscle and fascia from the subvaginal vestibule posteriorly to the rectal sphincter. After thus reconstructing the perineal body, the continuous vaginal mucosal suture is continued posteriorly, to ap-

proximate the subcutaneous tissue overlying the perineal body. The suture is brought out subcuticularly at the posterior apex of the cutaneous incision. It is then used to reapproximate the skin as a subcuticular continuous suture. Upon arrival at the posterior fourchette, the suture is again directed beneath the fourchette and hymenal ring and tied inside the vaginal introitus, thus burying all knots. Reabsorbable sutures should be used in episiotomy repair. The synthetic sutures are reabsorbed by hydrolysis rather than by polymorphonuclear phagocytosis and are associated with less postpartum discomfort.

As with most surgical procedures, episiotomy carries risks of anesthesia, bleeding, and infection. Additional risks include extension of the incision with rectal and anal sphincter involvement and postpartum pain and dyspareunia. Infiltration of the perineal body with a local anesthetic may be used for episiotomy. Measures to avoid intravascular injection of local anesthetic and proper aseptic techniques minimize risks. Although third-degree extension of median episiotomy occurs in approximately 4% of cases, repair is successful and without sequelae 99% of the time. Postpartum discomfort and dyspareunia associated with episiotomy may be minimized by use of fine-gauge absorbable suture material and by avoidance of knots near the hymenal ring or on the perineal skin.[4]

Shoulder Dystocia

Shoulder dystocia is the failure of the shoulders to traverse the pelvis spontaneously after delivery of the fetal head. Shoulder dystocia is a serious complication of delivery. The problem is that the head is delivered, causing the cord to be drawn into the pelvis and compressed before it is realized that there is an arrest to the delivery of the shoulders. The incidence of shoulder dystocia is 0.15% for all fetus-infants weighing more than 2500 g and 1.7% for those weighing more than 4000 g. The contributing factors include maternal obesity, diabetes mellitus, postterm pregnancy, prolonged second stage of labor, oxytocin induction or augmentation of labor, and use of midforceps or a vacuum extraction during delivery. Unfortunately, *shoulder dystocia cannot be predicted from clinical characteristics or labor abnormalities.*[5,6]

Shoulder dystocia also occurs with an extremely rapid delivery of the head, as can occur with vacuum extraction or forceps. It could also result from overzealous external rotation of the fetal head by the operator. Deliveries in bed increase the difficulty of reducing a shoulder dystocia, because the bedding precludes fullest use of the posterior pelvis and outlet.

Once a vaginal delivery has begun, the operator must resist the temptation to rotate the head to a transverse axis. *Aggressive fundal pressure often worsens the impaction.* The specific method used is probably not as critical as a careful, methodical approach to the problem and the avoidance of desperate, potentially traumatic traction.

If it is not appropriately managed, shoulder dystocia may be associated with significant neonatal morbidity (fractured humerus or clavicle, Erb's palsy) and mortality (severe asphyxia).

The major maternal consequence of shoulder dystocia is postpartum hemorrhage, usually from uterine atony but also from vaginal and cervical lacerations.

Management

Because shoulder dystocia cannot be predicted, there always will be the unexpected case. Therefore the attendant *must* be prepared to manage this occasionally devastating complication.[5,6]

Reduction in the interval of time from delivery of the head to delivery of the body is of great importance to survival, but overly vigorous traction on the head or neck, or excessive rotation of the body may seriously damage the infant.

Various methods or techniques have been described to free the anterior shoulder from its impacted position beneath the maternal symphysis pubis. The most popular techniques include the following:

1. *Suprapubic pressure.* This involves moderate suprapubic pressure applied obliquely by an assistant while downward traction is applied to the fetal head.
2. *The McRobert's maneuver.* The maneuver consists of sharply flexing the woman's legs upon her own abdomen (Fig. 10-8). This supposedly results in a straightening of the sacrum relative to the lumbar vertebrae with accompanying rotation of the symphysis pubis toward the patient's head and a decrease in the angle of pelvic inclination. This maneuver does not increase the dimensions of the pelvis, but the cephalic rotation of the pelvis frees the impacted anterior shoulder.
3. *Woods corkscrew maneuver.* The impacted anterior shoulder is released by progressively rotating the posterior shoulder 180° in a corkscrew fashion.
4. *Delivery of the posterior shoulder.* This consists of carefully sweeping the posterior arm of the fetus across the chest, followed by delivery of the arm. The shoulder girdle then is rotated into one of the oblique diameters of the pelvis with subsequent delivery of the anterior shoulder.
5. *Deliberate fracture of the clavicle.* The anterior clavicle is deliberately fractured by pressing against the ramus of the pubis so that the shoulder is freed of impaction. The fracture will heal rapidly and is not nearly as serious as a brachial nerve injury, asphyxia, or death.
6. *Zavanelli maneuver* (cephalic replacement). The first part of the maneuver consists of returning the head to the occipitoanterior or occipitoposterior po-

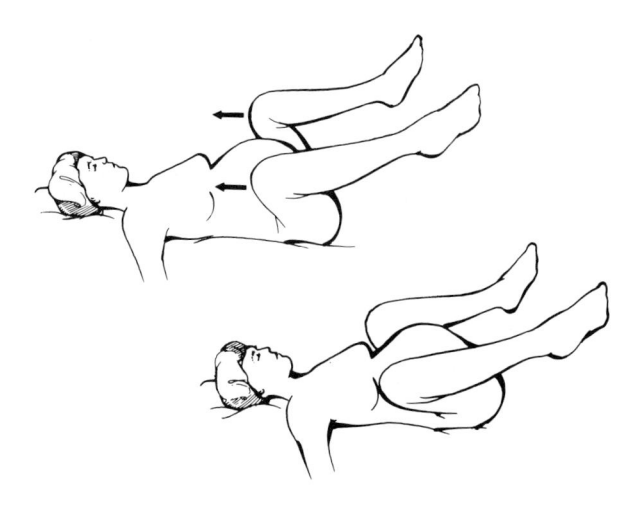

FIGURE 10-8
McRobert's maneuver.

sition if the head has rotated from either position. The second step is to flex the head and slowly push it back into the vagina, following which a cesarean delivery is performed.

Documentation

It is essential that there be clear documentation in the chart of the exact events that have taken place during delivery of an infant after shoulder dystocia. If the infant is unfortunate enough to suffer permanent brachial plexus injury, there is a high likelihood of malpractice litigation. The best defense can be mounted if there is a clearly documented description of the efforts made to deliver the fetus.[5-7]

Breech

A major current dilemma is that of obtaining sufficient experience at breech delivery. Little or minimal experience is gained in many training programs. Thus many recently trained obstetricians may have great difficulty when faced with imminent delivery of a breech fetus in a facility unable to perform an emergency cesarean section (CS). About 12% of breeches deliver vaginally before CS can be performed.[8] Paradoxically, some ED physicians may be more experienced than obstetricians with breech birth.

The patient who enters the ED with a breech baby about to deliver (ie, buttocks crowning or legs through the introitus) requires rapid mobilization of forces for delivery. If available, anesthesia personnel, an obstetrician, a nurse assistant, and a pediatrician should be called. Where possible, a quick sonogram to determine the presence of a head, its attitude, and possible hydrocephaly is ideal because it would help in managing the delivery.

If delivery is already well on its way (ie, the buttocks are born), the operator should proceed with a vaginal delivery. Ideally, the patient should be on a delivery table in lithotomy position. If the fetus is dead, there is no risk of further fetal trauma, and concern is totally for the mother.

No traction should be exerted until the buttocks are delivered. The infant's body should be supported. The head is delivered by flexion (Fig. 10-9). If a labor suite is available, subcutaneous terbutaline 0.25 mg may be given to inhibit uterine activity until the patient can be transferred to the labor and delivery unit.

If a leg is showing it should not be pulled down because the patient may not be ready to deliver. This may be a footling presentation through a cervix that is not fully dilated. There is time to transfer the patient to labor and delivery, preferably in knee/chest position to avoid possible cord compression. Generally, unless the infant has been delivered to the umbilicus, there is time for transfer to labor and delivery.

Lacerations of the Birth Canal

Lacerations of the vagina and perineum are classified as first, second, or third degree. Such lacerations most often are preventable with an appropriate episiotomy.[9,10]

DELIVERY IN THE EMERGENCY DEPARTMENT ♦ 153

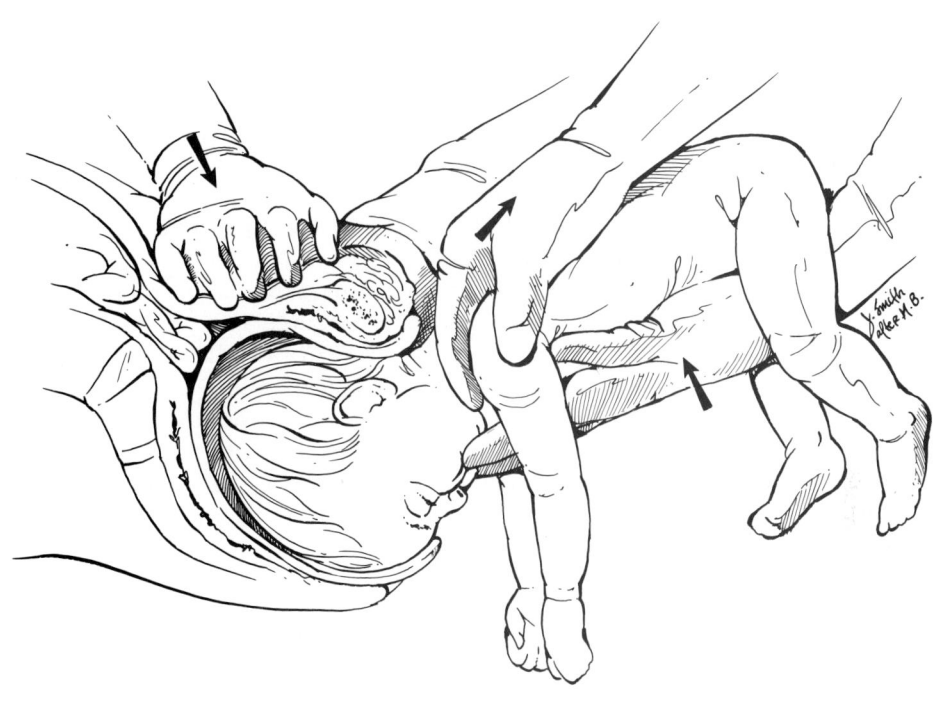

FIGURE 10–9
Delivery of head by flexion.

First-degree lacerations involve the fourchette, the perineal skin, and vaginal mucous membrane but not the underlying fascia and muscle. Tears in the region of the urethra are also likely to occur unless an adequate episiotomy is performed, and they may bleed profusely.

Second-degree lacerations involve, in addition to skin and mucous membrane, the fascia and muscles of the perineal body but not the rectal sphincter. These tears usually extend upward on one or both sides of the vagina, forming an irregular triangular injury.

Third-degree lacerations extend through the skin, mucous membrane, and perineal body and involve the anal sphincter.

Fourth-degree lacerations are third-degree lacerations with rectal wall extensions.

First- and second-degree laceration repair is straightforward. Third-degree laceration repair has many varieties. Many techniques have been recommended, but in all instances it is essential to approximate the torn edges of the rectal sphincter with sutures 0.5 cm apart. This muscular layer then is covered with a layer of fascia. Finally, the cut ends of the anal sphincter are isolated, approximated, and sutured together with two or three interrupted stitches. The remainder of the repair is the same as that for an episiotomy. If the rectal mucosa is involved, stool softeners should be prescribed for a week. Enemas should be avoided. The value of prophylactic antibiotics has not been established.[9,10]

Third- and fourth-degree extensions of median episiotomies are common. Prompt recognition and careful repair usually yield excellent results.

While maintaining exposure, a continuous suture of 4–0 chromic catgut is begun at the apex of the rectal mucosal laceration and carried to the anus, approximating submucosa to submucosa, thus inverting the mucosal edges.

Interrupted sutures are used to reapproximate more lateral submucosal tissue, further imbricating the rectal mucosa.

The fascial sheath of the rectal sphincter is then reapproximated end-to-end with interrupted 3–0 chromic catgut (or polyglycolic acid) figure-eight sutures placed circumferentially.

Once the rectal mucosa and sphincter are reapproximated, the repair proceeds as if the laceration were second degree (ie, midline episiotomy).

Management of delivery is an essential skill for ED physicians, particularly in settings where obstetricians are not immediately available. Protocol or guidelines should therefore be in place and should include provisions for availability of appropriate equipment, trained support personnel, necessary forms for documentation, and universal precaution material (mask, gowns, gloves, goggles, wall suction) needed for the prevention of human immunodeficiency virus (HIV) and hepatitis B virus transmission.

REFERENCES

1. Cunningham FG, MacDonald PC, Gant NF. Conduct of normal labor and delivery. In Williams Obstetrics, 18th ed, p 307. East Norwalk, CT: Appleton & Lange, 1989
2. Gibbs CE. Obstetrics—an overview. In Pauerstein CJ (ed): Clinical Obstetrics, p 3. New York: John Wiley, 1987
3. Patterson, RM. Episiotomy. In Pauerstein CJ (ed): Clinical Obstetrics, p 843. New York: John Wiley, 1987
4. Varner MW. Episiotomy: techniques and indications. Clin Obstet Gynecol 29:309, 1986
5. Benedetti TJ. Shoulder dystocia. In Pauerstein CJ (ed): Clinical Obstetrics, p 871. New York: John Wiley, 1987
6. Seeds JW. Malpresentation. In Gabbe SG, Niebyl JR, Simpson JL (eds): Obstetrics: Normal and problem pregnancies, 2nd ed, p 562. New York: Churchill Livingstone, 1991
7. Acker DB. A shoulder dystocia intervention form. Obstet Gynecol 78:150, 1991
8. Yasin S, O'Sullivan MJ. Breech presentation. In Plauché WC, Morrison JC, O'Sullivan MJ (eds): Surgical Obstetrics. Philadelphia: WB Saunders, 1992:325
9. Cunningham FG, MacDonald PC, Gant NF. Injuries to the birth canal. In Williams Obstetrics, 18th ed, p 415. East Norwalk, CT: Appleton & Lange, 1989
10. Blanco JD. Postpartum lacerations and hematomas. In Pauerstein CJ (ed): Clinical Obstetrics, p 943. New York: John Wiley, 1987

CHAPTER 11

Postpartum Emergencies

Daniel P. Eller and Roger B. Newman

Although women in the reproductive years are generally young and healthy, the postpartum period is a time of special risks. Postpartum emergencies occur suddenly and in many cases may be life-threatening. Having been recently discharged from the hospital, the postpartum patient will be intolerant, frightened, frustrated, distraught, and angry at further complications.

This physical and emotional vulnerability requires the physician in the emergency setting to act carefully but expediently to assess the patient's symptoms and physical signs, perform the appropriate evaluation, obtain necessary consultation, and initiate therapy. Table 11-1 lists the common complications encountered.

Infection

In the 1930s the Joint Commission on Maternal Welfare defined puerperal infectious morbidity as "a temperature of 100.4 degrees Fahrenheit (38 degrees Centigrade) or higher, to occur on any two of the first ten days postpartum, exclusive of the first 24 hours, and to be taken by mouth by standard technique at least four times daily."[1] The usual source of puerperal fever is the genital tract, including the uterus, vagina, and episiotomy site. Overall, the rate of puerperal genital tract infection ranges from 1% to 8%.[2] Risk factors for puerperal infection include those re-

TABLE 11-1
Primary Medical Problems of the Postpartum Patient When Presenting to the Emergency Department

I. Infection
   A. Genital tract
      1. Endometritis
      2. Parametritis
      3. Pelvic cellulitis (including episiotomy infection)
      4. Septic pelvic thrombophlebitis
   B. Mastitis
   C. Urinary tract
      1. Cystitis
      2. Pyelonephritis

II. Postpartum hemorrhage
   A. Early
   B. Late

III. Thrombosis and thrombophlebitis
   A. Superficial thrombophlebitis
   B. Deep venous thrombosis
   C. Pulmonary embolus

IV. Postpartum seizures
   A. Eclampsia
   B. Other

V. Postpartum psychological reactions
   A. Postpartum "blues"
   B. Postpartum depression
   C. Postpartum psychosis

lated to general infection risks (anemia, poor nutrition, lack of prenatal care, obesity, low socioeconomic status, sexual intercourse during pregnancy), factors related to labor events (prolonged ruptured membranes, intra-amnionic infection, intrauterine fetal monitoring, number of digital examinations during labor), and those related to mode of delivery (cesarean section—especially emergent, general anesthesia, manual removal of placenta, postpartum hemorrhage, forceps delivery, cervical and vaginal lacerations, and/or episiotomy).[3] The surgical injury and devitalization of tissue caused by cesarean delivery is clearly the major predisposing clinical factor that is of particular importance because of the increasing cesarean section rates nationwide.

Endometritis and Wound Infections

The most common causes of puerperal fever originate from the uterus and most commonly occur in the first 2 to 7 days after delivery. These infections have been called endometritis, endomyometritis, endoparametritis, or metritis,[4] and they tend to be polymicrobial, involving both aerobic and anaerobic organisms that have ascended from the lower genital tract. Among organisms isolated in patients with endometritis are group A and group B streptococci, enterococci, *Staphylococcus aureus*, *Gardnerella vaginalis*, *Escherichia coli*, *Enterobacter*, *Proteus mirabilis*, *Bacteroides bivius*, and other *Bacteroides* species, peptococci and peptostreptococci, *Ureaplasma urealyticum*, *Mycoplasma hominis*, and *Chlamydia trachomatis*.[4] *Chlamydia trachomatis*, an degree of anemia and the white blood cell count. Two units of blood should be cross-matched in the face of significant bleeding in the event that a transfusion becomes necessary. Coagulation studies should be performed to rule out coagulopathies. A vaginal or abdominal ultrasound may be helpful when attempting to rule out retained products of conception.[19] Many problems will require obstetric consultation, preferably with the delivering physician. If one suspects retained products of conception, obstetric consultation should be obtained and plans for dilatation and curettage should be made. If a laceration has been identified that is actively bleeding in the cervix or vagina, consultation should be obtained for surgical repair. If a hematoma is identified, consultation should be obtained to evaluate for evacuation.

If suction curettage is indicated, it must be thoroughly yet carefully performed. The suction curettage performed during the late postpartum period on a soft subinvoluted and/or infected uterus is the classic situation in which myometrial injury occurs, resulting in Asherman's syndrome.[20] If bleeding persists after adequate curettage, consultation for exploratory laparotomy for arterial ligation or hysterectomy must be considered.

Thrombosis

Fifty percent of all thromboembolic events in the United States in women under the age of 40 are related to pregnancy and the puerperium.[21] More than 100 years ago, Virchow described three factors required to initiate intravascular coagulation—injury to the vessel wall, stasis, and changes in clotting factors. Pregnancy causes changes in the blood coagulation system, in the fibrinolytic system, in venous flow, and in the vessel wall that all predispose to thrombosis. As a result, thromboembolic events occur more frequently during pregnancy, especially in the postpartum period, than in the nonpregnant state. Puerperal patients with thromboembolic disease outnumber antepartum patients approximately three to one.[22] Deep venous thrombosis most commonly occurs approximately 48 hours after delivery; however, it may occur up to 4 weeks after delivery.[23] The risk of deep venous thrombosis is magnified after cesarean section or instrumental delivery, in those with advanced maternal age or increased parity, and in those receiving estrogens for lactation suppression. Other risk factors that are not directly related to pregnancy include a history of prior thromboembolism, varicose veins, a history of trauma or infection, obesity, blood type other than type O, congestive heart failure, dehydration, shock, disseminated cancer, dysproteinemia, polycythemia vera, and anemia (especially sickle cell).[22]

Superficial Thrombophlebitis

Superficial thrombophlebitis is the most common form of thrombosis encountered during pregnancy. These patients present with pain, redness, warmth, and swelling in the affected region, usually along the course of the saphenous vein (Fig. 11-4). One can commonly palpate "cords" of thrombus within the affected superficial vein. Superficial thrombophlebitis alone poses no risk for pulmonary embolus; how-

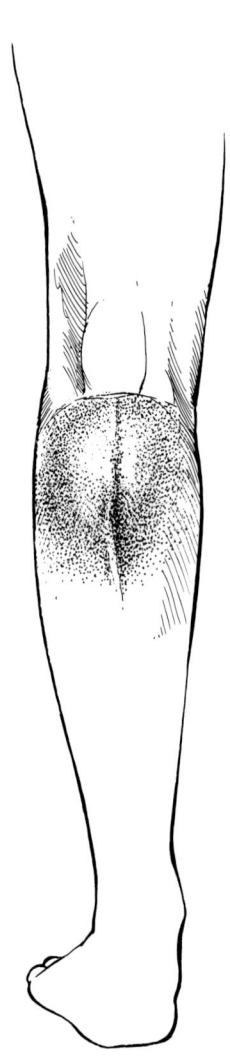

FIGURE 11-4
Superficial thrombophlebitis.

ever, one must rule out an associated deep venous thrombosis (DVT). If a low index of suspicion is present, noninvasive Doppler ultrasonography of the leg may be performed. Otherwise, venography should be performed to rule out deep venous thrombosis. In the absence of DVT, heat, elevation, and rest are the prescribed measures for treatment. Anticoagulation in these patients is unnecessary. If concomitant cellulitis is present, an antibiotic such as dicloxacillin should be prescribed to treat *Staphylococcus aureus*, the most likely pathogen. Untreated superficial thrombophlebitis can lead to deep venous thrombosis.

Deep Venous Thrombosis

A high index of suspicion must be present when evaluating a patient for possible DVT. Conversely, it would not be prudent to commit a patient to long-term anticoagulation therapy without being certain of the diagnosis.

Evaluation and Management

Patients commonly present with pain and swelling in the affected leg. Physical examination reveals tenderness, and the affected leg circumference should be greater than 2 cm larger than the contralateral leg at the same level. Homans' sign for calf deep vein thromboses may be present (pain in the calf when the foot or great toe is dorsiflexed). However, this sign is neither sensitive nor specific. Unfortunately, no clinical signs and symptoms are either sensitive or specific. Cranley and coworkers found that 45% of patients with clinically certain DVT had an entirely normal venous system by venography. Venograms performed on patients with pulmonary emboli demonstrated clots in a totally asymptomatic limb.[24] However, whenever a patient presents with suggestive symptoms, a deep venous thrombosis must be ruled out.

Common diagnostic procedures include venography, isotope scanning, impedance plethysmography, and Doppler ultrasound. Doppler flow studies are noninvasive and usually the first-line test used in pregnant patients. This procedure, which evaluates blood flow through the vein using a 5-megahertz transducer, has a 30% false-positive rate. Venography continues to be the gold standard for diagnosis. Limitations include its invasiveness, radiation exposure, expense, and difficulty to interpret if the deep veins are not adequately filled. Venography is not useful for identifying pelvic vein thromboses. The most common side-effect is phlebitis. Isotope scanning with ^{125}I fibrinogen is useful in the lower extremities below the midthigh. This method is absolutely contraindicated during pregnancy because radioactive iodine will cross the placenta and concentrate in the fetal thyroid. In the postpartum period, isotope scanning is not very useful, since most pulmonary emboli are thought to originate from deep veins in the iliofemoral region. Impedance plethysmography is only of historical interest, as most vascular laboratories have discontinued its use in favor of Doppler flow studies.

The mainstay of treatment for deep venous thrombosis is full anticoagulation with heparin. Heparin is a mucopolysaccharide that combines with antithrombin III to become a potent inhibitor of thrombin, therefore preventing the conversion of fibrinogen to fibrin. Heparin also increases the circulating level of activated factor X inhibitor.[25] Before therapy is begun, a CBC, platelet count, prothrombin time, and activated partial thromboplastin time (APTT) should be obtained. The loading dose should be approximately 5000 to 7000 units intravenously by rapid administration followed by a continuous infusion of 15 to 20 units/kg per hour. The goal is to achieve an APTT of two to two and a half times control. Continuous therapy is recommended because intermittent administration produces peaks and valleys in the heparin activity, increasing the risk of both subtherapeutic treatment and major bleeding complications. If DVT is strongly suspected on a clinical basis, heparin therapy can begin prior to diagnosis, after which a venogram should be performed. This will decrease the risk of a pulmonary embolus.

Pulmonary Embolus

The incidence of pulmonary embolism is dependent upon the adequacy of treatment of DVT. Approximately one fourth of patients with untreated DVT will have a pulmonary embolus with a 15% mortality rate.[26] The incidence drops to 4.5% if patients are adequately anticoagulated. The mortality rate in this case is reduced to less than 1%.[27] Therefore anticoagulation of DVT is essential.

Evaluation and Management

The most common presentation of a patient with pulmonary emboli is shortness of breath. The major sign is tachypnea. Other signs and symptoms of pulmonary embolism include pleuritic pain, apprehension, cough, tachycardia, hemoptysis, and fever. The differential diagnosis in these patients includes pneumonia, trauma, and myocardial infarction. Indicated laboratory studies include an electrocardiogram that most commonly reveals sinus tachycardia. Patients with extensive embolization may show a right axis shift and strain pattern. Patients with pulmonary emboli usually have an arterial partial pressure of oxygen (PaO_2) of less than 80 mmHg on room air. If signs and symptoms are strongly suggestive of a pulmonary embolus, one should strongly consider definitive diagnostic testing, even in the face of a normal PaO_2.

A ventilation-perfusion scan should be the primary diagnostic test when pulmonary embolus is clinically suspected. Pulmonary angiography is the gold standard but is usually not necessary unless surgical intervention is contemplated or if the ventilation-perfusion scan is equivocal. Therapy should be initiated once the diagnosis is made. Treatment requires intravenous heparin therapy as described for deep venous thrombosis. Patients should be admitted to the hospital and receive continuous cardiac monitoring. Oxygen should be started if the patient is hypoxic.

Seizures

The most common cause of seizures in the postpartum period is eclampsia.[28] Therefore a postpartum patient presenting with seizures must be evaluated for other signs or symptoms of preeclampsia, including hypertension, proteinuria, edema, severe headache, and visual disturbances (blurred vision and scotomata). The common belief that seizures more than 24 hours postpartum are unlikely to be eclampsia is untrue. Between 17 and 34% of the cases of eclampsia occur postpartum, and up to one half of these cases may occur more than 48 hours after delivery.[29] Interestingly, not all of these patients will be diagnosed antepartum or intrapartum, and prior treatment with magnesium sulfate does not prevent late-onset postpartum eclampsia. When a postpartum patient is admitted with convulsions more than 48 hours after delivery and is hypertensive with proteinuria or edema, late-postpartum eclampsia should be the leading diagnosis while other possible etiologies are considered.

The physician should evaluate the patient's obstetric records, specifically evaluating whether the patient carried the diagnosis of preeclampsia or had any signs or symptoms of preeclampsia during the antepartum, intrapartum, or postpartum period. If eclampsia is the most likely diagnosis, initial treatment should include all the precautions taken with any patient presenting with seizures, including establishment of an airway and prevention of injury. Magnesium is still considered the drug of choice for eclampsia in the United States.[30] Once the seizure has stopped, 4 to 6 g of magnesium sulfate (MgSO$_4$) in a 10% (not 50%) solution can be administered IV over a 15- to 20-minute period. This should be followed by a continuous MgSO$_4$ drip at approximately 2 g per hour. In addition to magnesium sulfate treatment, the patient should be watched closely for other systemic signs of preeclampsia, such as thrombocytopenia, hepatic injury, renal failure, or hypertensive encephalopathy. Treatment with magnesium sulfate should be continued for 24 to 48 hours. The differential diagnosis of late-onset eclampsia includes cerebral venous thrombosis, intracerebral hemorrhage, hypertensive encephalopathy, pheochromocytoma, space-occupying lesion of the central nervous system, such metabolic disorders as hypoglycemia, syndrome of inappropriate ADH secretion, and epilepsy.

Postpartum Psychological Reactions

Childbirth is commonly followed by a transient depression or "postpartum blues" a few days after delivery. Fifty to 70% of postpartum patients experience a transient state of tearfulness, anxiety, irritation, and restlessness. These "postpartum blues" are generally self-limited and resolve in 2 to 3 days but occasionally persist for 1 or 2 weeks.[31] Ten to 15% experience a true postpartum depression and 0.14 to 0.26% experience frank postpartum psychosis.[32] Risk factors for a true postpartum depression include an unwanted pregnancy, serious marital difficulties, or a prior history of psychiatric disturbances.[33] The mother with a high-risk pregnancy may be particularly vulnerable to postpartum psychiatric complications.[34] Women who have previously experienced a postpartum psychosis may have a recurrence risk of almost 50%.[35] The vast majority of puerperal psychoses are affective, manic, or depressive psychoses.[36] They usually present very abruptly between days 3 and 14 of the puerperium. These patients may present with delusions, hallucinations, and disturbance of behavior. A high index of suspicion for major mental illness must be present when a postpartum patient presents to the emergency department complaining of depression. These illnesses can be considered some of the most severe in psychiatry. Suicidal thoughts, paranoid delusions or thoughts of violence involving the newborn or other children should all be taken seriously. Psychiatric consultation should be employed liberally. Frequently, hospitalization is required. Some psychiatrists have recommended that the patients be admitted with their babies.[36] Fortunately, the short- and long-term prognosis is very good with these illnesses. Patients usually recover within 8 weeks.

Summary

The emergency department physician must always be alert when the postpartum patient presents with a problem. Table 11-2 describes specific problem areas. When infection is suspected, the patient should be treated with antibiotic therapy that is appropriate for the perceived problem. The initiation of broad-spectrum antibiotics immediately in the emergency department may well prevent puerperal sepsis. Post-

TABLE 11-2
Areas of Careful Consideration

1. Initiate antibiotic therapy for postpartum infection in the emergency room.
2. Carefully determine the etiology of postpartum bleeding.
3. Treat postpartum seizures as eclampsia but rule out other disorders.
4. Obtain psychiatric consultation for patients at risk for postpartum psychosis.

partum bleeding must be immediately evaluated and treated with attempts to determine the specific etiology of the bleeding. Therapy for postpartum thromboembolic phenomena should be initiated as soon as possible to prevent pulmonary embolus or death due to massive pulmonary embolus. When a patient presents with a postpartum seizure, careful evaluation must be performed to rule out organic causes. Eclampsia continues to be the most likely diagnosis, even when signs or symptoms of preeclampsia were not present in the antepartum period. Puerperal psychiatric disorders must be carefully evaluated by the appropriate consultants, as these patients may be profoundly affected and could be dangerous to themselves and their infants.

REFERENCES

1. Easterling HW. The puerperium. In Danforth DN (ed): Obstetrics and Gynecology. Philadelphia: JB Lippincott, 1982
2. Gibbs RS. Severe infections in pregnancy. Med Clin North Am 73:713, 1989
3. Eschenbach BA, Wager GP. Puerperal infections. Clin Obstet Gynecol 23:1003, 1980
4. Rosene K, Eschenbach BA, Tompkins LS et al. Polymicrobial early postpartum endometritis with facultative and anaerobic bacterial, genital mycoplasmas, and C. trachomatis: treatment with piperacillin or cefoxitin. J Infect Dis 153:1028, 1986
5. Hoyme UB, Kiviat N, Esenbach DA. Microbiology and treatment of late postpartum endometritis. Obstet Gynecol 68:226, 1986
6. Hibbard LT, Snyder EN, McVann RM. Subgluteal and retropsoal infection in obstetric practice. Obstet Gynecol 39:137, 1972
7. Svancarek W, Chirino O, Schaeffer G. Retropsoas and subgluteal abscesses following paracervical and pudendal anesthesia. JAMA 237:892, 1977
8. Gibbs RS, Blanco JD, St Clair PJ. A case-control study of wound abscesses after cesarean delivery. Obstet Gynecol 62:498, 1983
9. Emmons SL, Krohn M, Jackson M, Eschenbach DA. Development of wound infections among women undergoing Cesarean section. Obstet Gynecol 72:559, 1988
10. Hankins GD, Hauth JC, Gilstrap LC, Hammond TL, Yeoman ER, Snyder RR. Early repair episiotomy dehiscence. Obstet Gynecol 75:48, 1990
11. Marshall BR, Hepper JK, Zirbel CC. Sporadic puerperal mastitis. An infection that need not interrupt lactation. JAMA 233:1377, 1975
12. Olsen CG, Gordon RE. Breast disorders in nursing mothers. Am Fam Physician 41:1509, 1990
13. Benson EA, Goodman MA. An evaluation of the use of stilboestrol and antibiotics in the early management of acute puerperal breast abscess. Br J Surg 57:255, 1970
14. Warren JW, Platt R, Thomas RJ et al. Antibiotic irrigation and catheter associated urinary tract infection. New Engl J Med 299:570, 1978
15. Pritchard JA, Baldwin RM, Dickey JC, Wiggins KM. Blood volume changes in pregnancy

and the puerperium: II. Red blood cell loss and changes in apparent blood volume during and following vaginal delivery, cesarean section and cesarean section plus total hysterectomy. Am J Obstet Gynecol 84:1271, 1962
16. Gilstrap III, LC. Diagnosis and management of postpartum hemorrhage. ACOG Technical Bulletin 143, 1990
17. King PA, Duthie SJ, Dong ZG, Ma HK. Secondary postpartum hemorrhage. Aust NZ J Obstet Gynaecol 29:394, 1989
18. Hayashi RH, Castillo MS, Noah ML. Management of severe postpartum hemorrhage with a prostaglandin F_2 alpha analogue. Obstet Gynecol 63:806, 1984
19. Hertzberg BS, Bowie JD. Ultrasound of the postpartum uterus: predication of retained placental tissue. J Ultrasound Med 10:451, 1991
20. Schenker JG, Margalioth EJ. Intrauterine adhesions: an updated appraisal. Fertil Steril 37:593, 1982
21. Howie PW. Thromboembolism. Clin Obstet Gynaecol 4:397, 1977
22. Laros RK. Thromboembolic disease. In Creasy RK, Resnick R (eds): Maternal fetal medicine: principles and practice, p 763. Philadelphia: WB Saunders, 1989
23. Aaro LA, Juergens JL. Thrombophlebitis associated with pregnancy. Am J Obstet Gynecol 109:1128, 1971
24. Cranley JJ, Canos AJ, Sull WJ. The diagnosis of deep venous thrombosis—fallibility of clinical symptoms and signs. Arch Surg 111:34, 1976
25. Rosenberg RD. Actions and interactions of anti-thrombin and heparin. New Engl J Med 292:146, 1975
26. Wessler S. Medical management of venous thrombosis. Ann Rev Med 27:313, 1976
27. Villasanta U. Thromboembolic disease in pregnancy. Am J Obstet Gynecol 93:142, 1965
28. Sibai BM, Schneider JM, Morrison JC et al. The late post-partum eclampsia controversy. Obstet Gynecol 55:74, 1980
29. Watson DL, Sibai BM, Shaver DC, Dacus JV, Anderson GD. Late postpartum eclampsia: an update. S Med J 76:1487, 1983
30. Sibai BM. Magnesium sulfate is the ideal anti-convulsant in preeclampsia/eclampsia. Am J Obstet Gynecol 162:1141, 1990
31. Robinson GE, Stewart DE. Postpartum psychiatric disorders. Can Med Assoc J 134:31, 1986
32. Bowes WA. Postpartum care. In Gabbe SG, Niebyl JR, Simpson JL (eds): Obstetrics: normal and problem pregnancies, 2nd ed, p 753. New York: Churchill Livingstone, 1991
33. Watson JP, Elliot SA, Rugg AJ, Brough DI. Psychiatric disorders in pregnancy and the first postnatal year. Br J Psychol 144:453, 1984
34. Wohlreich MM. Psychiatric aspects of high risk pregnancy. Psychiatr Clin North Am 10:53, 1987
35. Vanderbergh RL. Postpartum depression. Clin Obstet Gynecol 23:1105, 1980
36. Oates MR. Treatment of psychiatric disorders in pregnancy and the puerperium. Clin Obstet Gynaecol 13:385, 1986

CHAPTER 12

Role of Imaging Modalities in Obstetric Emergencies

Francisco L. Gaudier
and Gerardo O. Del Valle

Pregnancy is always a possible concurrent condition in any woman of reproductive age who presents for evaluation in an emergency setting. However, with the use of current technology, such as sensitive urine or blood pregnancy tests and real-time ultrasound, the diagnosis of pregnancy can be either established or ruled out and the patient managed accordingly. The uniqueness of the evaluation of a pregnant woman in an emergency situation rests in the fact that, although she is the primary patient, the different modalities needed for her evaluation or therapy may have potentially serious effects on the fetus and therefore cannot be overlooked.

Imaging Modalities

Ultrasound is the primary imaging technology used in the evaluation of most obstetric emergencies. It is readily available and can be used to evaluate the fetus, placenta, and amniotic fluid dynamics. Ultrasound is also extremely helpful for visualization of abdominal and pelvic organs. During the first trimester of pregnancy transvaginal ultrasound is used extensively in the evaluation of the ovaries and adnexa. Ectopic pregnancies, as well as cystic and solid lesions in the ovaries, can be identified. With the transabdominal approach the liver, gallbladder, kidneys, and pancreas can be evaluated for underlying pathology.

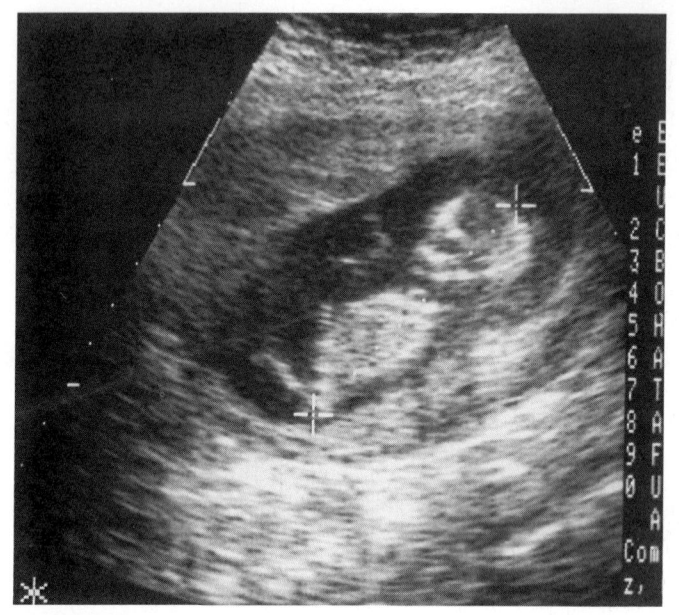

FIGURE 12–1
Ultrasound view of a first-trimester fetus. Measurement of the fetal crown–to–rump length.

Examination of the intrauterine contents should include a detailed assessment of the fetus, placenta, and amniotic fluid volume. With real-time technology, fetal cardiac activity may be identified from the sixth week of gestation. Fetal gestational age is calculated using a series of biometric parameters. The most commonly used measurements include crown-to-rump length; biparietal diameter of the head, abdominal, and head circumference; and femur length (Figs. 12-1 to 12-4). With a composite of these anthropometric measurements, an estimation of the fetal weight can be calculated using a variety of formulas.[1,2] Fetal well-being can also be assessed with the evaluation of several biophysical variables as a composite known as the Biophysical Profile (Table 12-1).[3] Evaluation of the placenta includes its location within the uterine cavity, relationship with the internal cervical os, and visualization of any abnormality (ie, retroplacental hematomas in some cases of abruptio placenta). Real-time ultrasound has added a new dimension to obstetrics, making it possible to evaluate the fetus and intrauterine contents with safe, reliable, and readily available technology.

Radiographic technology used in the evaluation of emergency conditions include x-ray films, computed tomography, radionuclide studies, and magnetic resonance imaging. Animal and human studies suggest that fetal irradiation can be associated with developmental defects, growth restriction, postnatal neoplasias, and death.[4] Although the threshold radiation dose in the human pregnancy is not completely known, most authors agree that exposure to less than 5 rad has no teratogenic or mutagenic effect.[5,6] Table 12-2 summarizes estimated fetal exposure from several radiologic procedures.[7–10] If radiographic tests are indicated in a pregnant woman, some helpful general guidelines include the following:

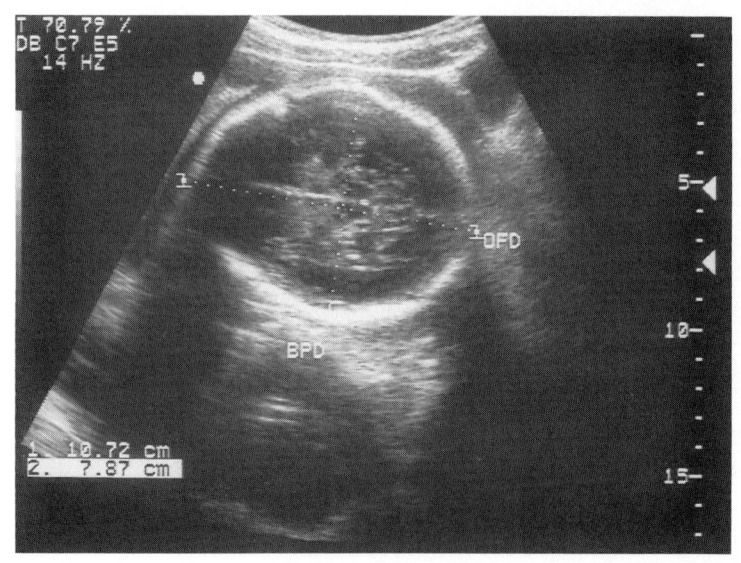

ROLE OF IMAGING MODALITIES IN OBSTETRIC EMERGENCIES ♦ 173

FIGURE 12-2
Axial scan of the fetal head at the level of the thalami. Measurement of the fetal biparietal diameter (BPD) and occipitofrontal diameters

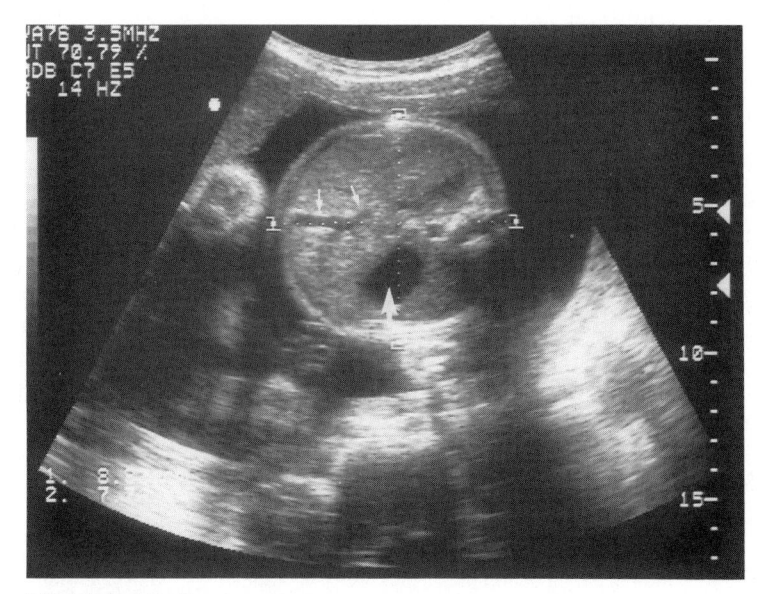

FIGURE 12-3
Transverse view of the fetal abdomen at the level of the umbilical vein (*small arrows*) and stomach (*large arrow*). Measurement of the abdominal circumference.

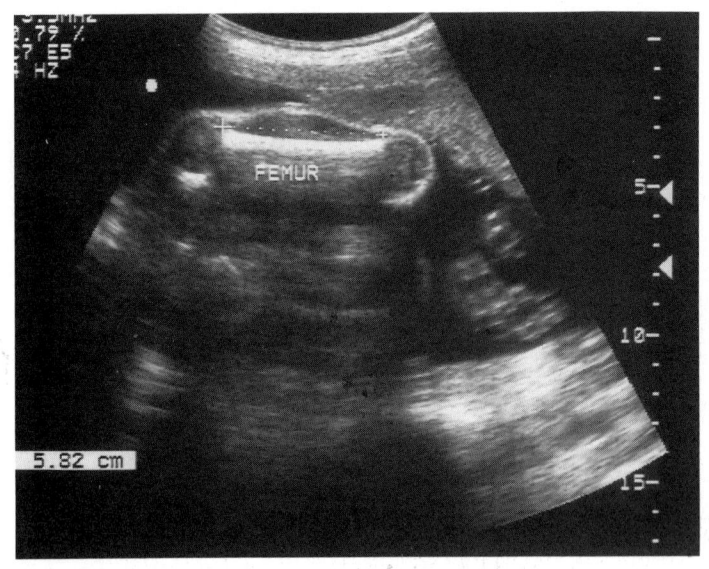

FIGURE 12-4
Ultrasound view and measurement of the femur length.

1. Limit exposure to the essential films required and use these efficiently, avoiding duplication and using abbreviated studies whenever possible (ie, single-shot intravenous pyelogram).
2. Limit fluoroscopic procedures as they are associated with a higher radiation exposure than simple x-ray films.
3. Whenever possible, use abdominal lead shield to cover the pregnant uterus from radiation exposure, especially during x-ray procedures of the head, chest, and lower extremities.

TABLE 12-1
Biophysical Profile Scoring System

Variable	Normal	Abnormal
Fetal breathing movements	At least one episode of at least 30 sec duration in 30 min	Absent FBM or none >30 sec in 30 min
Gross body movements	At least three discrete body/limb movements in 30 min	Two or fewer episodes of body/limb movements in 30 min
Fetal tone	At least one episode of active extension with return to flexion of fetal limb(s) or trunk	Absent fetal movement or slow extension with return to partial flexion or movement of limb in full extension
Qualitative amniotic fluid volume (AFV)	At least one pocket of AF that measures at least 2 cm in vertical plane	A pocket <2 cm in vertical plane
Reactive fetal heart rate (FHR)	At least two episodes of FHR acceleration of >15 bpm and of at least 15 sec duration associated with fetal movement in 20 min	Less than two episodes of acceleration of FHR or acceleration of >15 bpm min in 20 min

Modified from Manning FA, Morrison I, Lange IR, Hartman CR, Chamberlain PF. Fetal Assessment Based on Fetal Biophysical Profile Scoring: Experience in 12,620 referred high-risk pregnancies. Am J Obstet Gynecol 151:343, 1985.

TABLE 12-2
Estimated Fetal Radiation Exposure from Radiologic Studies[7-10]

Study	Estimated Fetal Exposure (Millirads)
X-rays	
Skull film	4
Chest film	8
Abdominal film	140–290
Upper GI series*	360–560
Cholecystogram	300
Barium enema*	439–800
IVP	400
Unilateral venography	305–350
Lumbar spine	275–608
Pelvic	158
Pulmonary angiography (femoral)	405–450
Pulmonary angiography (brachial)	<50
Computerized tomography	
Abdomino-pelvic	5–10,000
Radionuclide	
^{99}Tc lung scan	2–18
^{133}Xe ventilation scan	3–20
^{125}I-fibrinogen leg scan	2,000

*The use of fluoroscopy will significantly increase radiation exposure.

Although unnecessary x-ray exposure during pregnancy should be avoided, concern for safety should not prevent its use for necessary diagnosis in the pregnant patient.

Bleeding During Late Pregnancy

Vaginal bleeding during pregnancy is a frequent and potentially fatal complication that presents a diagnostic challenge to the clinician. Approximately 3 to 4% of all pregnancies are complicated with vaginal bleeding after 20 weeks.[11] Obstetric hemorrhage is also directly responsible for 13% of non-abortion-related maternal deaths in the United States.[12]

Any vaginal bleeding during the last trimester of pregnancy should be considered an obstetric emergency that demands immediate evaluation and management. Assessment of the maternal and fetal status and prompt diagnosis of the underlying cause of bleeding are imperative. Although slight vaginal bleeding can be seen during labor, active bleeding can be due to placenta previa, abruptio placenta, rupture of a fetal vessel, or lesions in the reproductive tract. Placenta previa and abruptio placenta are associated with a significant increase in both maternal and perinatal morbidity and morality. In all women with vaginal bleeding during the last trimester of pregnancy, the possibility of a placenta previa and abruptio placenta should be considered. Active bleeding during the last trimester of pregnancy requires immediate consultation with an obstetrician.

Placenta previa refers to a placenta implanted over, or in close proximity to, the internal cervical os. It affects from 0.4% to 0.6% of all deliveries. Its incidence is increased with multiple gestations, prior uterine surgeries, and advanced maternal age and with multiparity. The abnormal placental implantation is usually due to deficient endometrial vascularization with suboptimal decidualization. Painless bright red vaginal bleeding is the most characteristic clinical finding of placenta previa. The first episode of bleeding usually occurs in the early third trimester. In pregnant women with vaginal bleeding, the presence of a placenta previa should be ruled out before a digital cervical examination is performed because it may cause massive, life-threatening hemorrhage.

Ultrasound is the imaging modality of choice for placental localization, having 95% diagnostic accuracy for placenta previa. The transabdominal approach is currently the standard for the diagnosis of placenta previa.[13] For an accurate diagnosis the endocervical canal, internal os, and its anatomic relationship with the placental edge must be identified. This is achieved on a sagittal scan, with the assistance of a partially full bladder, followed by reevaluation with an empty bladder. In an emergency situation the bladder can be distended by retrograde filling through a Foley catheter. A partially distended urinary bladder provides an acoustic window for adequate visualization of the cervix, and an overdistended one can lead to false diagnosis of placenta previa. In experienced hands a transvaginal or transperineal ultrasound approach can be of help when the diagnosis is difficult for technical reasons and in the absence of acute bleeding (Fig. 12-5). Technical difficulties that may be

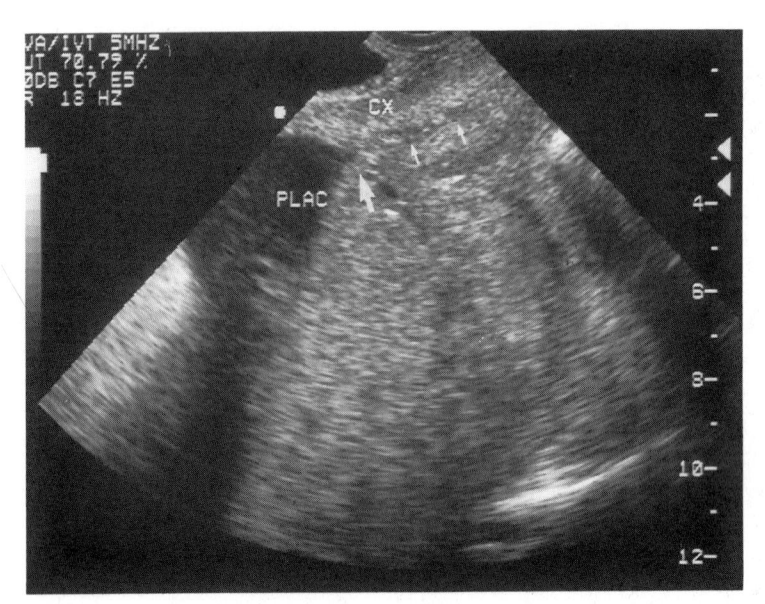

FIGURE 12–5
Transvaginal sagittal view of the cervix and a posterior partial placenta previa. The tip of the placenta is partially over the internal cervical os (*large arrow*). The endocervical canal is clearly visualized (*small arrows*).

encountered in the identification of placental location include a posteriorly implanted placenta, maternal obesity, overdistended bladder, and presence of blood clots over the internal os. The diagnosis of placenta previa has also been described with computerized tomography and magnetic resonance imaging.[14] The latter modalities are more expensive and not readily available in most emergency situations.

Abruptio placenta refers to the premature separation of the placenta from its implantation site. This acute and potentially catastrophic condition occurs with an incidence of one in 75 to one in 200 deliveries.[15] Abruptio placenta is associated with maternal hypertension, trauma, cocaine use, short umbilical cord, and sudden uterine decompression. The recurrence risk in a subsequent pregnancy is estimated to be 5 to 10%.[15] The clinical presentation of abruptio placenta varies considerably. Signs and symptoms include vaginal bleeding, hypertonic uterine contractions, uterine tenderness, labor, fetal distress, intrauterine demise, shock, and consumptive coagulopathy.

The diagnosis of abruptio placenta is clinical. Ultrasound is usually used to exclude other causes of bleeding (ie, placenta previa). Sonographic findings of abruptio placenta are inconsistently present and vary according to the time interval since the acute bleeding and to the size and location of the blood collection. With retroplacental hematomas a defined hyperechoic collection together with a thickened heterogeneous placenta can be identified.[16] With subchorionic bleeding there is an elevation of the amniotic and chorionic membranes (Fig. 12-6). It is important to emphasize that normal ultrasound findings do not exclude an abruptio placenta and that proper management of the patient suspected to have clinically significant placental separation should not be delayed awaiting sonographic confirmation.

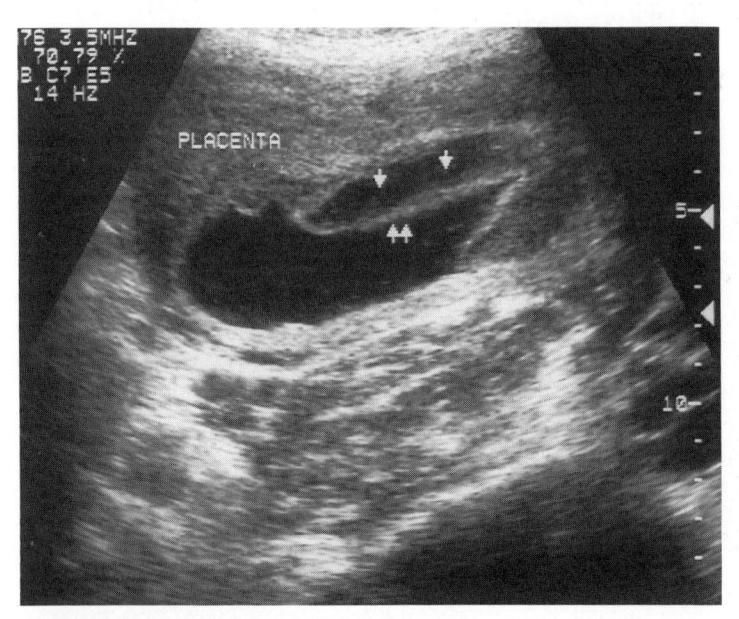

FIGURE 12–6
Transabdominal longitudinal ultrasound view of a subchorionic hematoma. The blood collection elevates the chorionic membrane (*arrows*).

Maternal Trauma

The incidence of physical injury during pregnancy ranges from 6 to 7%,[17] with an increased risk as pregnancy progresses. Trauma is a leading cause of death in women of reproductive age.[18] Although most accidental injuries during gestation have no significant sequelae, major trauma can have catastrophic consequences for both the mother and fetus. Management of pregnant women who have sustained a major injury should consist of a combined approach by the emergency department personnel, intensivist, obstetrician, trauma surgeon, radiologist, and pediatrician.

Direct assaults on the abdomen and motor vehicle accidents are the leading cause of blunt abdominal trauma during pregnancy. Rupture of the spleen is the most common cause of intraperitoneal bleeding after abdominal trauma, and retroperitoneal bleeding occurs most frequently in pregnant women. Abruptio placenta is also associated with both minor and severe traumatic injuries during gestation.

The initial evaluation and management of the pregnant woman with severe trauma should not differ significantly from that of the nonpregnant female. Immediate maternal resuscitation with establishment of an adequate airway, correction of hypoxemia, and stabilization of the maternal cardiovascular status will subsequently lead to fetal stabilization. Uterine displacement away from the inferior vena cava and aorta will improve uterine perfusion. Immediately following maternal stabilization, fetal evaluation is indicated with electronic heart rate monitoring and real-time ultrasound.

In cases of maternal abdominal trauma, diagnostic peritoneal lavage is accurate and safe during pregnancy.[19] Physical examination of the abdomen is less reliable, as the peritoneal response to trauma is minimized and delayed during pregnancy. If pelvic fractures are suspected, prompt evaluation of the extent of bone damage and urologic or vascular compromise is indicated.

Gunshot wounds are the most common type of penetrating injury during pregnancy, with the uterus being the most frequently injured organ in these cases.[20] Exploratory laparotomy should be performed after a gunshot wound to the abdomen in order to evaluate the extent of visceral damage. The evaluation of a stab wound to the abdomen should proceed as in the nonpregnant patient, with the use of peritoneal lavage, fistulograms, and observation as indicated.

The diagnostic approach in a severely traumatized pregnant woman should balance the need for invasive procedures and x-ray testing in the mother with the risk of fetal radiation exposure. Real-time ultrasound should be used to calculate fetal gestational age and to assess fetal viability and well-being. Sonography is an important tool to evaluate placental localization, the possibility of a retroplacental hematoma, and adequacy of amniotic fluid volume. Ultrasound also can be used in the diagnosis of hemoperitoneum and to guide the needle placement during paracentesis.

In case of a seriously traumatized pregnant patient, radiographic studies should be performed as needed, regardless of potential fetal exposure.[5,18] When injury to the urinary tract is suspected, an infusion pyelography, computerized tomography (CT), or magnetic resonance imaging (MRI) is indicated. Women with neurologic trauma require a detailed clinical evaluation, followed by skull films or CT or MRI of the head. Some trauma centers recommend the use of computed tomography of the abdomen and pelvis in cases of blunt trauma in order to evaluate the retroperitoneal space and renal system, although fetal exposure with this technique ranges from 5 to 10 rad.[8] Delayed traumatic rupture of the diaphragm is a rare complication of both blunt and penetrating injury. Pregnant women with major trauma should have a baseline chest radiographic evaluation.[21]

Acute Abdomen

Because of the significant physiologic and anatomic alterations normally encountered in gestation, both the evaluation and management of an acute abdomen can be markedly altered by pregnancy. A prominent pregnant uterus will make the abdominal examination more difficult and reduce the peritoneal response to visceral inflammation. Some of the conditions associated with acute abdominal pain during pregnancy are presented in Table 12-3.

Acute appendicitis is one of the most common nonobstetric causes of abdominal pain during pregnancy. Its increased mortality during gestation is mostly due to delays in both diagnosis and surgical management. The diagnosis of acute appendicitis is complicated by some of the normal changes of pregnancy. Nausea, vomiting, and leukocytosis are common during gestation. There is also a significant upward and lateral displacement of the appendix as pregnancy advances.

The role of ultrasound in the setting of acute abdominal pain includes evaluation of gynecologic, obstetric, urinary, and gastrointestinal factors. A detailed sonographic search for gallstones, dilatation of the bile duct, and pancreatic and liver involvement is important. Ultrasound evaluation of the kidneys will include search for renal calculi and ureteral and caliceal dilatation. The uterus should be examined for the possibility of myomas. An abdominal radiographic evaluation will be of help in selected cases when a renal stone and intestinal distention or perforation are suspected. If ureteral obstruction is strongly considered, a single-shot intravenous pyelogram (IVP) is preferred over a complete IVP in order to decrease fetal exposure to radiation.

TABLE 12-3
Etiologies of Acute Abdominal Pain During Pregnancy

Gastrointestinal System	Reproductive System
Appendicitis	Rupture or torsion of adnexal mass
Cholecystitis	Ectopic pregnancy
Pancreatitis	Degeneration of a myoma
Peptic ulcer disease	Abruptio placenta
Diverticulitis	Chorioamnionitis
Intestinal perforation	Uterine rupture

Urinary System
Pyelonephritis
Renal colic
Renal calculi

Thromboembolic Complications

Thromboembolic events are one of the main causes of maternal mortality. Clinical findings are nonspecific for the diagnosis of both deep venous thrombosis and pulmonary embolism. During pregnancy noninvasive and selective invasive diagnostic tests should be chosen carefully. Special consideration should be given to the use of techniques to minimize fetal radiation exposure.

Deep venous thrombosis (DVT) of the lower extremities affects between 0.2 and 3.0% of all deliveries.[22] It is more frequent during the postpartum period, especially after cesarean delivery. Clinical findings of DVT include localized pain, swelling, and tenderness of the affected extremity. Unfortunately, signs and symptoms associated with DVT lack both sensitivity and specificity for its diagnosis. Noninvasive and invasive vascular studies have been developed in order to achieve a more accurate diagnosis of DVT. The use of ^{125}I-fibrinogen is *absolutely contraindicated during pregnancy,* as it freely crosses the placenta and accumulates in the fetal thyroid gland.

Noninvasive tests for the diagnosis of DVT include impedance plethysmography and Doppler ultrasound. Impedance plethysmography evaluates electrical resistance to determine changes in blood flow. It has an excellent sensitivity and specificity for proximal vein thrombosis. False-positive results can be due to compression of the inferior vena cava by the pregnant uterus, especially in the third trimester. Doppler ultrasound evaluates resistance to venous blood flow. Unfortunately, both of these noninvasive tests are unreliable in the diagnosis of calf vein thrombosis.

Invasive tests for the diagnosis of DVT are used to confirm equivocal plethysmography and Doppler studies or when a surgical vascular procedure is contemplated (ie, embolectomy).[23] Venography is the most definitive test for the diagnosis of DVT. During venography a radiopaque contrast medium is injected into the dorsal vein of the foot. Visualization of a well-defined filling defect is diagnostic of DVT. Injection of the radiographic dye can be performed during pregnancy. The estimated fetal radiation exposure during a routine unilateral venography with abdominal shielding is below 50 mrad.[24]

Pulmonary embolism occurs in approximately one in 2000 deliveries.[23] Classical signs and symptoms include tachypnea, dyspnea, and a pleuritic chest pain. Findings on chest x-ray film and electrocardiogram are nonspecific. The diagnosis of pulmonary embolism requires either a lung perfusion and ventilation scan or pulmonary angiography. A perfusion scan uses radiolabeled compounds bound to albumin that are deposited in the pulmonary capillaries. These macroaggregates do not cross the placenta.[25] A normal perfusion scan study excludes pulmonary embolism. If the perfusion scan is abnormal, a ventilation test is performed. Ventilation scans use a gamma-emitting gas such as ^{133}Xe or ^{99m}Tc (Fig. 12-7). This radiolabeled compound crosses the placenta. The fetal radiation exposure dose of a ventilation-perfusion lung scan is approximately 50 mrad.[24] Lung fields that are ventilated but not perfused are suggestive of a pulmonary embolism.

The most definite test for the diagnosis of pulmonary embolism is angiography. This invasive test is indicated when

1. A definitive diagnosis cannot be made with a ventilation-perfusion scan (intermediate or subsegmental perfusion defects).

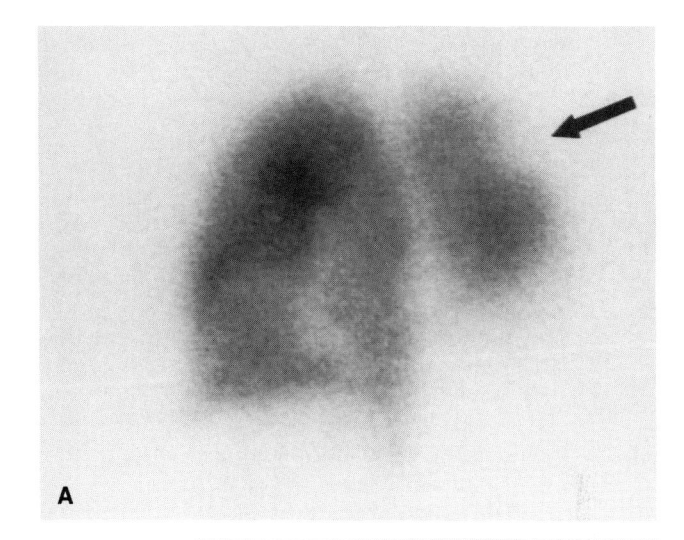

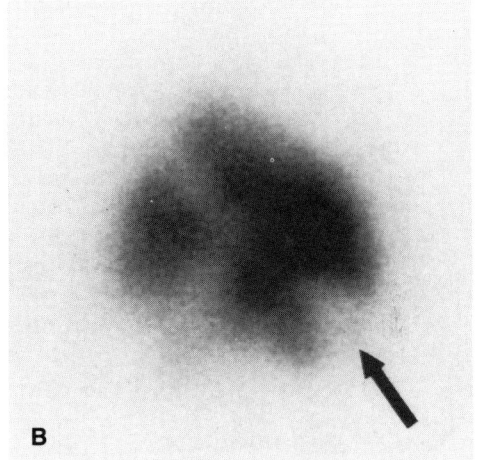

FIGURE 12-7
Views of perfusion lung scan after injection of Tc 99m MAA. There are nonmatching perfusion defects (*arrows*).

2. Pulmonary embolism is suspected in patients with other pulmonary disorders.
3. There is massive pulmonary embolism requiring suction embolectomy.
4. There is a high-probability lung scan in a patient with contraindications to anticoagulation.

If pulmonary angiography is required during pregnancy, it should be performed through the brachial route with the use of an abdominal shield and while attempting to minimize the use of fluoroscopy, in order to keep the fetal radiation exposure rate between 450 and 850 mrad.

The selection of imaging modalities for the evaluation of emergency conditions is influenced by the presence of a viable intrauterine pregnancy. The interpretation of the results obtained with these modalities may be affected by the normal anatomic and physiologic changes of pregnancy. Ultrasound is the primary imaging technology used during gestation with radiographic diagnostic studies used judiciously as necessary. In life-threatening situations the physician taking care of a pregnant woman should use all the diagnostic modalities required for an adequate evaluation.

REFERENCES

1. Shepard MJ, Richards VA, Berkowitz RL, Warsof SL, Hobbins JC. An evaluation of two equations for predicting fetal weight by ultrasound. Am J Obstet Gynecol 142:47, 1982
2. Deter RL, Hadlock FP, Havist RB, Carpenter RJ. Evaluation of three methods for obtaining fetal weight estimates using dynamic image ultrasound. J Clin Ultrasound 9:421, 1981
3. Manning FA, Morrison I, Lange IR, Hartman CR, Chamberlain PF. Fetal assessment based on fetal biophysical profile scoring: experience in 12,620 referred high-risk pregnancies. Am J Obstet Gynecol 151:343, 1985
4. Hoffman D, Felten R, Cyr W. Effects of ionizing radiation on the developing embryo and fetus: a review. Rockville, MD: US Department of Health and Human Services, Public Health Service, Food and Drug Administration, Bureau of Radiological Health, HHS Publication FDA 81, 1981
5. National Council on Radiation Protection and Measurements. Medical radiation exposure of pregnant women. NCRP Report 54. Washington, DC: NCRPM, 1977
6. American College of Obstetricians and Gynecologists. Teratology. ACOG Technical Bulletin 84, Washington, DC: ACOG, 1985
7. Ginsberg JS, Hirsh J, Rainbow A, Coates G. Risk to the fetus of radiological procedures used in the diagnosis of maternal thromboembolic disease. Thromb Haemost 61:189, 1989
8. Wagner LK, Archer BR, Zeck OF. Conceptus dose from two state-of-the-art CT scanners. Radiology 159:787, 1986
9. Brent RL. The effects of embryonic and fetal exposure to x-ray, microwave and ultrasound. Clin Obstet Gynecol 26:484, 1983
10. Mossman KL, Hill LT. Radiation risk in pregnancy. Obstet Gynecol 60:237, 1982
11. Scott JR. Vaginal bleeding in the midtrimester of pregnancy. Am J Obstet Gynecol 113:329, 1972
12. Kaunitz AM, Hughes JM, Grimes DA, Smith JC, Rochat RW, Kafrissen ME. Causes of maternal mortality in the United States. Obstet Gynecol 65:605, 1985
13. Lavery JP. Placenta previa. Clin Obstet Gynecol 33:414, 1990
14. Powell MC, Buckley J, Price H, Worthington BS, Symonds EM. Magnetic resonance imaging and placenta previa. Am J Obstet Gynecol 154:565, 1986
15. Obstetrical hemorrhage. In Cunningham FG, MacDonald PC, Gant NF (eds): Williams Obstetrics, p 695. Norwalk, CT: Appleton & Lange, 1989
16. Nyberg DA, Callen PW. Ultrasound evaluation of the placenta. In Callen PW (ed): Ultrasonography in Obstetrics and Gynecology, p 304. Philadelphia: WB Saunders, 1988
17. Patterson RM. Trauma in pregnancy. Clin Obstet Gynecol 27:32, 1984
18. American College of Obstetricians and Gynecologists. Trauma during pregnancy. ACOG Technical Bulletin 161. Washington, DC: ACOG, 1991
19. Esposito TJ, Gens DR, Smith LG, Scorpio R. Evaluation of blunt abdominal trauma occurring during pregnancy. J Trauma 29:1628, 1989
20. Dildy GA, Cotton DB. Trauma, shock, and critical care obstetrics. In Reece EA (ed): Medicine of the Fetus and the Mother, p 883. Philadelphia: JB Lippincott, 1992
21. Dudley AG, Teaford H, Gatewood TS. Delayed traumatic rupture of the diaphragm in pregnancy. Obstet Gynecol 53:25S, 1979

22. Rutherford SE, Phelan JP. Deep venous thrombosis and pulmonary embolus. In Clark SL (ed): Critical Care Obstetrics, p 150. Boston: Blackwell Scientific, 1991
23. Cowchock FS, Merli GJ. Pulmonary embolism and thrombophlebitic disorders. In Gleisher (ed): Principles and Practice of Medical Therapy in Pregnancy, p 738. Norwalk, CT: Appleton & Lange, 1992
24. Ginsberg JS, Hirsh J. Thromboembolic disorders of pregnancy. In Reece EA (ed): Medicine of the Fetus and the Mother, p 1103. Philadelphia: JB Lippincott, 1992
25. Mitchell MS, Capizzi RL. Neoplastic diseases. In Burrow GN, Ferris TF eds. Medical Complications During Pregnancy, p 540. Philadelphia: WB Saunders, 1988

CHAPTER 13

Drug Therapy in Pregnancy

Mark W. Todd

Drug exposure during pregnancy is a common occurrence.[1-3] A 1963 study determined that only 7.9% of gravid women complete pregnancy without any medication, 20.8% use more than five drugs, and 3.9% use 10 or more.[1] The average number taken was 3.6. A decade later, despite the widely publicized thalidomide tragedy of the 1960s, drug use and prescribing during pregnancy was largely unchanged. In 168 gravid women studied, all received at least two drugs, and 93% received five or more. The average number of drugs used was 11.[2] Much of this drug use was therapeutically avoidable and exposed mother and fetus to unnecessary potential risks. However, avoiding medication use during pregnancy at all cost is also unnecessary and may jeopardize the mother's health. This dichotomy clouds clinical practice.

The goal of this chapter is to review the relative safety of common medications prescribed in the emergency setting.

Principles of Teratogenesis

Approximately 25 to 30 medications are thought to be truly teratogenic.[4-6] Whether a given agent can induce congenital malformations in animals or humans is based on three fundamental principles of teratogenesis first described in 1959.[7] These include the particular dose of the substance, the susceptibility of the species, and the embryo's stage of development at the time of the exposure.

All species are not equally susceptible to teratogenic consequences. Animal studies are not indicative of expected human outcomes and should be used only as a guide. The thalidomide tragedy is a striking example. Initially, no congenital malformations were seen in mice, rats, and rabbits following thalidomide exposure. But in pregnant women, exposure to even a single dose from the 20th to the 35th day after conception produced unique birth defects consisting of deformities of the limbs and face.[8] Only after many years and thousands of malformed infants was the relationship between thalidomide and birth defects well understood. This helps to illustrate the difficulty in linking a particular drug to teratogenicity.

The timing of fetal exposure is arguably the most important determinant of teratogenesis. There are four critical periods in human development in which drugs may adversely affect the fetus.[9] Days 0–7 represent the preimplantation phase, in which fertilization and zygote formation occur. Exposure to teratogens during this period usually results either in death of the embryo or in replacement of damaged cells by undifferentiated cells that go on to develop normally. During organogenesis (days 14–60) the embryo is at its peak sensitivity to teratogens. Most morphologic congenital abnormalities are thought to be produced during this interval. As organogenesis ends, susceptibility to anatomic abnormalities declines. Minor structural malformation may still occur throughout histogenesis. Exposures during the fetal development period are associated with a much lower risk of major birth defects because most major organ systems are well developed by this time.[10,11] Problems that do occur usually involve growth or functional deviations.

Major congenital malformations occur at a rate of about 2 to 3%, whereas the rate of minor defects in newborns is close to 9%.[8-10] Of these, environmental factors (including drugs) are thought to be responsible for up to 10% and genetics or chromosomal abnormalities account for 25%.[1,8] Sixty-five percent of all reported congenital defects have no known cause.

Very few drugs are known to cause fetal harm. Nonetheless, it is virtually impossible to prove drugs safe for use in pregnancy because no well-designed studies can be ethically conducted. Therefore a huge void exists between known teratogenesis and known safety. This void is difficult to fill with available literature, but some clinically relevant conclusions can be reached (Table 13-1).

FDA Pregnancy Categories

In 1980 the FDA required that the labeling of prescription drugs include information about use in pregnancy.[12] Unfortunately, these data are usually limited to animal studies. This information can be found in the precautions section of the package insert. Five categories were established that indicate a drug's potential for causing birth defects.

> Category A. Well-controlled studies in women fail to demonstrate a risk to the fetus. Because of the nature of this research, few drugs, if any, qualify for this category.
> Category B. Drugs in this category have either not been shown to pose a fetal risk, in animal studies, or have demonstrated a slight fetal risk in animals but not in controlled studies in women.

TABLE 13-1
Pregnancy Categories for Selected Drugs*

Drug	FDA Pregnancy Category	Comments
Antibiotics		
Penicillins	B	Most safety experience with penicillin G. Little data available on mezlocillin and piperacillin.
Tetracyclines	D*	Avoid if possible, especially during last half of pregnancy.
Trimethoprim/sulfamethozole	C	Both drugs may inhibit folic acid synthesis. Sulfonamides can induce kernicterus in the newborn if used late in pregnancy. Avoid if possible.
Metronidazole	B	Conflicting data exist on safety in pregnancy. Centers for Disease Control consider the drug contraindicated during first trimester for treatment of trichomonas.
Erythromycin	B	The base is considered a relatively safe drug for use during pregnancy. No significant evidence of congenital defects reported. The estolate salt has been reported to cause hepatotoxicity in pregnant women.
Nitrofurantoin	B*	Considered safe. Theoretically, could cause hemolytic anemia in the newborn, but no cases have been reported.
Aminoglycosides	D	Streptomycin has been reported to cause congenital deafness. Serious side-effects in the fetus have not been reported with other aminoglycosides.
Vancomycin	C	No adverse fetal effects have been reported.
Anticoagulants		
Heparin	C	Does not cross the placental barrier. The anticoagulant of choice in pregnancy, but is not without risk.
Warfarin	X	A definite teratogen. Contraindicated during pregnancy. Can cause fatal hemorrhage in the fetus.
Antiasthmatics		
Theophylline	C	No conclusive reports of congenital defects.
Beta-agonists	C	Risk to fetus low, especially the aerosol forms. Opinions differ on safety of epinephrine.
Corticosteroids	C*	Appropriate for use when disease state of mother dictates (e.g., risk of severe asthma episodes greater than teratogenic risk).
Anticonvulsants		
Phenytoin/Phenobarbital	D*	Higher incidence of birth defects in children of drug-treated epileptic women. Risk of seizures outweighs risk of teratogenicity from these agents.
Trimethadione	D*	Considered a human teratogen.
Valproic acid (Depakene)	D	Considered a human teratogen.
Carbamazepine (Tegretol)	C	No convincing reports of fetal harm.
Analgesics		
Acetaminophen	B*	Analgesic and antipyretic of choice in pregnancy.
Aspirin	C*	May produce adverse effects in mother and fetus. Can inhibit labor if used late in pregnancy. Avoid if possible.
Nonsteroidal anti-inflammatories	B	Very limited data are available. No association to date with congenital malformations. Can theoretically inhibit labor if used late in pregnancy.
Pediculocides and Scabicides		
Lindane	B	Low risk for teratogenicity. The drug can be absorbed and possibly induce toxicity in the fetus. Not recommended for use during pregnancy.

(continued)

TABLE 13-1 (Continued)

Drug	FDA Pregnancy Category	Comments
Pyrethrins with piperonyl butoxide	B*	Currently recommended in place of lindane for lice treatment during pregnancy. No congenital malformations associated with its use.
Permethrin 1%, 5%	B*	Limited data are available. No fetal harm has been reported.
Antinauseants		
Prochlorperazine (Compazine)/Promethazine (Phenergan)	C	Safety data are conflicting, but there is more data to suggest their safety. If absolutely indicated, use occasionally and in low doses. Not indicated for "morning sickness."
Diphenhydramine (Benadryl)	B	A large study found no association with congenital defects.

*Not categorized by FDA; pregnancy category provided by author.

Category C. This category includes drugs for which (1) animal studies have revealed adverse effects on the fetus but no adequate controlled studies in women exist or (2) studies in women and animals are unavailable. Most drugs are placed in this category.

Category D. Drugs in this group have been shown to cause birth defects when used in humans, but the risk may be acceptable because of the potential benefits of the drug (eg, phenytoin for seizures). These drugs generally will be used for life-threatening conditions or serious illness (that may affect the mother, fetus, or both) when equally effective yet safer drugs are not available. The decision to use these drugs should be carefully reviewed with the mother and all known risks to the fetus and mother discussed. An appropriate statement must appear in the warnings section of the package insert.

Category X. Drugs in this category are known to induce fetal abnormalities in animals or humans and their potential risks clearly outweigh their therapeutic benefit (eg, isotretinoin [Accutane] for acne). These drugs are contraindicated in women who are or may become pregnant and must be stated as such in the package insert.

This classification system was an important step for assisting the clinician in identifying potential teratogenic prescription drugs. However, since so few drugs are demonstrated teratogens, the practical benefit of the system is limited. The vast majority of drugs fall into category C, leaving the clinician with many quandaries.

Antibiotics

Although *penicillins* cross the placenta, they have proven to be the safest antibiotics for use during pregnancy in the nonallergic patient.[13] A large study involving over 3546 fetal exposures to penicillin derivatives (primarily penicillin G) during the first trimester of pregnancy found no link to major or minor malformations.[8] Other reports and the wide use of this class of drugs during pregnancy support this finding.[14,15] When pregnant women with syphilis are penicillin allergic, the U.S. Public Health Service recommends hospitalization and desensitization.[16]

Data on the newer penicillins, such as mezlocillin and piperacillin, are lacking. The FDA places each of these agents in risk category B.

Less information is available on the safety of *cephalosporins*. The majority of these agents readily cross the placenta and have pharmacokinetic parameters very similar to the penicillins. No known teratogenicity has been reported. The safety of cephalosporins is thought to equal that of the penicillins.[13,15] Cephalosporins are the preferred alternative in patients with nonanaphylactic penicillin sensitivity. Erythromycin base should be used in penicillin-allergic patients demonstrating immediate type sensitivity.

Tetracyclines are known to cause numerous potential problems to mother and fetus and should be avoided during pregnancy.[8,15] Nearly all tetracyclines can readily cross the placenta and appear in significant quantities in cord blood.[13] Prior to 1961, tetracycline was thought safe for use during pregnancy and was commonly used. A case report in 1962 first described a child with the classic yellow discoloration of the teeth after exposure to the drug in utero.[17] Since then this well-known adverse effect has been well publicized and is now known to be caused by tetracycline's ability to chelate calcium orthophosphate, which becomes incorporated into bones and teeth during calcification.[15] Severe dysplasia of the teeth and inhibition of bone growth also have been demonstrated. These effects are more common when the drug is taken in the second and third trimesters, when bone mineralization occurs.[18] Tetracycline has also been reported to induce limb anomalies, inguinal hernia, and congenital cataracts.[5,15] Potentially fatal maternal liver and renal toxicities, although rare, have been attributed to tetracycline.[15]

Erythromycin base has been used during pregnancy with no known increased risk to the mother or fetus. One large study found no evidence to suggest an increased risk for malformations in 309 pregnancy exposures, 79 of which were first trimester.[8] Although the drug crosses the placenta, plasma levels are low in the fetus. One salt of erythromycin, the estolate form, is considered contraindicated during pregnancy because of a reported 10 to 15% reversible incidence of hepatotoxicity occurring in the mother.[15,19] No human data are available on the newly available erythromycin derivatives (eg, clarithromycin).

Sulfonamides cross the placenta and accumulate in significant quantities in the fetus.[13] They have been shown to be teratogenic in some animal species, but a link to human malformations has not been made.[5,13,15] In a large human study, first-trimester exposures have not led to higher than expected fetal abnormalities.[8] These drugs are potentially dangerous when administered close to delivery. Theoretically, the drug is capable of causing kernicterus in the newborn through displacement of bilirubin from albumin-binding sites, resulting in central nervous system penetration of free bilirubin.[5,15] Earlier in pregnancy, the placenta is capable of clearing this free unconjugated bilirubin. However, at birth the clearing mechanism is no longer available, placing the newborn exposed to sulfonamides at increased risk.[13] Severe jaundice and hemolytic anemia may also be seen.[20]

Trimethoprim, used alone or in combination with sulfonamides, should be avoided during pregnancy. The drug is a folic acid antagonist, a group of agents known to be potentially teratogenic.[7] However, no human case reports of congenital abnormalities have been published.

Metronidazole crosses the placenta and appears in maternal and cord blood in equal amounts. Because the drug is mutagenic in bacteria and carcinogenic in rats, most recommend avoiding it in pregnancy.[13,15] However, there are no good human data implicating metronidazole as a teratogen or carcinogen. One human study reported 31 first-trimester exposures leading to four cases of birth defects.[8] Older studies and case reports suggest that metronidazole does not adversely affect the fetus.[21-23] For the treatment of *Trichomonas vaginalis*, metronidazole has been recommended to treat severe symptoms, but only after the first trimester.[24] To date, the relative risk of metronidazole's use in pregnancy is unknown, and its use in pregnancy is controversial.

The *aminoglycosides* are frequently used to treat serious infections during pregnancy and have not caused fetal malformation.[8,13] Gentamicin, amikacin, and tobramycin all cross the placenta and appear in the fetal circulation. Highest fetal concentrations are found in the kidneys and urine. The pharmacokinetics of these agents are usually significantly altered in pregnant women. Careful maternal serum level monitoring is required to limit fetal exposure yet assure therapeutic levels in the mother. Even with widespread use, few problems have been reported.[13] Ototoxicity and deafness have been reported in infants exposed to streptomycin in utero.[5]

Data are unavailable to determine *vancomycin's* safety during pregnancy. The drug is not thought to be teratogenic.[15] Animal studies suggest the drug will cross the placenta and accumulate in the fetal circulation. Although ototoxicity and nephrotoxicity are potential problems, no cases have been documented.

Clindamycin's fetal circulation levels are about 50% of that found in the mother. Reports have not implicated clindamycin as a fetal toxin.[15]

Nitrofurantoin is frequently used for urinary tract infections. The drug appears safe for mother and fetus. Over 1700 case histories have been gathered by the Norwich-Eaton pharmaceutical company describing use of nitrofurantoin during various stages of pregnancy, with no fetal toxicity noted.[15] Theoretically, the drug could induce hemolytic anemia in newborns exposed during late pregnancy.

Nalidixic acid crosses the placenta and has been reported to cause increased intracranial pressure, papilledema, bulging fontanelles, and possibly hydrocephalus in infants exposed late in pregnancy.[15,25]

The *quinolones* (ciprofloxacin, norfloxacin, and many more to follow) are considered contraindicated during pregnancy until more data are available. These agents induce erosions of cartilage of weight-bearing joints in various species of immature animals.[26] Ciprofloxacin has led to lameness in dogs. Until these effects are better understood in humans, this class of drug should be avoided in pregnancy.

Anticoagulants

If anticoagulation is required during pregnancy, heparin is considered safer than warfarin. Heparin has a large molecular weight and does not cross the placenta to any significant degree.[4] However, risks still obviously exist for the mother and fetus.

Warfarin is widely recognized as a teratogen.[5,7] A fetal warfarin syndrome has been described, principally characterized by nasal hypoplasia, as a result of warfarin exposure during the first trimester. Other features include mental retardation, blindness, hydrocephalus, and congenital heart disease. Second- and third-trimester exposures have been associated with mental retardation, central nervous system defects, optic atrophy, and microcephaly. Use of this drug any time during pregnancy can lead to malformations or retardation.

Antiasthmatics

The incidence of asthma during pregnancy is about 1%.[27] Active asthma throughout pregnancy leads to greater infant morbidity and mortality. Therapy in the pregnant patient should not differ significantly from that of other patients. If asthma is well controlled, pregnancy outcome should not differ from that of the general population.[28] Avoidance of status asthmaticus results in a more favorable fetal outcome. A prospective study of 198 pregnancies evaluated whether carefully managed asthma resulted in increased risk of maternal or fetal complications.[29] Patients routinely received inhaled beta-agonists, ipratropium, beclomethasone, and cromolyn sodium. Theophylline and injectable corticosteroids were given as indicated. Systemic ephedrine and epinephrine were avoided based on the author's perceived danger to the fetus. Results indicated that careful supervision of asthma during pregnancy leads to maternal and fetal complication rates no greater than those found in nonpregnant patients.

Drugs considered appropriate for treatment of the pregnant asthmatic include theophylline, inhaled beclomethasone, methylprednisolone, prednisone, cromolyn sodium, and hydrocortisone.[27-31] More controversial agents include epinephrine and the beta-agonists.

Theophylline crosses the placenta. The drug's pharmacokinetics may be significantly altered in pregnant women, necessitating dosage adjustments. Plasma levels must be monitored closely to prevent unnecessary fetal exposure yet achieve therapeutic levels (8 to 20 µg/mL) in the mother. The Collaborative Perinatal Project monitored 193 first-trimester exposures to theophylline.[8] An increased incidence of malformations was not found. Use of the beta-agonists during pregnancy is more controversial. The Collaborative Perinatal Project found a statistically significant increase in major and minor malformations in 189 infants exposed to epinephrine during the first trimester.[8] An association was also found with inguinal hernia. The results could be largely due to the conditions treated instead of the drug. Because of lack of data, ephedrine and isoproterenol are best avoided. Metaproterenol, terbutaline, and albuterol have not been associated with congenital abnormalities.[15] However, they frequently induce maternal and fetal tachycardia. When used close to delivery, these agents could theoretically prolong labor by inhibiting uterine contractions. For treatment of asthma the inhaled route is preferred to limit absorption and minimize fetal exposure.

When they are clearly indicated, inhaled and systemic corticosteroids appear safe and appropriate.[27] One study indicated that systemic corticosteroids may slightly increase the incidence of mild preeclampsia in the mother and hypoglycemia in the infant.[29] Although data are limited, cromolyn sodium has not been associated with fetal toxicity.[15]

Anticonvulsants

The effect of pregnancy on seizure frequency varies. The net result is generally no change in incidence.[32] Infants born to mothers taking anticonvulsants are at two to three times the normal risk of having congenital malformations.[4,5] It is not known if this increased risk is due to the disease, the drugs, genetics, or a combination of each. However, risk to the mother and fetus is even greater if seizures are not treated and well controlled. Complications from seizures far outweigh concerns for teratogenicity. When patients are closely monitored and compliance with medication is encouraged, only a 4% to 16% increase in seizure frequency should be expected—mainly during the third trimester, because of altered drug metabolism.[32]

Serum anticonvulsant levels tend to decrease throughout pregnancy because of impaired absorption, increased volume of distribution, decreased serum albumin, induction of liver enzymes by hormones, and increased renal clearance. Because of low serum albumin, the unbound (active) fraction of phenytoin may actually increase, leading to an effective response even at a lower total drug level. Close monitoring of medication serum levels, albumin, and seizure frequency is essential.

Trimethadione, used for petit mal seizures, is strongly associated with congenital malformations and mental retardation and is therefore contraindicated during pregnancy.[5,33,34] Safer agents are available. Valproic acid should also be considered a human teratogen and avoided during pregnancy. The drug is associated with a 1% to 2% incidence of neural tube defects.[35] Other consistent defects involve facial changes, heart defects, and psychomotor dysfunction.[36]

Phenytoin use during pregnancy has been associated with a fetal hydantoin syndrome consisting of craniofacial abnormalities, limb defects, mental retardation, and impaired growth.[15] Some argue that phenytoin itself may not be the cause, suggesting genetic factors.

Phenobarbital was not found to be associated with congenital malformations in the Collaborative Perinatal Project.[8] Other reports indicate that the drug carries risks of malformations similar to phenytoin.[15] Other risks to the fetus include hemorrhagic disease of the newborn (possibly due to depletion of vitamin K stores) and addiction.

The safety of carbamazepine remains largely unknown. First-trimester exposures in more than 600 cases suggest a potential for malformations similar to those seen with phenytoin use. However, the incidence appears lower.[15] Some consider carbamazepine a teratogen[37]; others believe it to be the prophylactic agent of choice.[32]

Management of status epilepticus during pregnancy is the same as that for nonpregnant women.[32]

The American Academy of Pediatrics Committee on Drugs makes the following recommendations:[33]

1. Withdraw seizure medication prior to pregnancy if the patient has been seizure-free for many years.
2. Advise a pregnant woman on anticonvulsants that she has a 90% chance of having a normal child, but the chance the child will be mentally retarded is two to three times greater than normal, because of either the drugs or the disease.

3. Women asking for advice after the first trimester should be reassured rather than urged to seek an abortion. Medication should be continued, since the major malformation would have already occurred.
4. There is no reason to change from phenytoin to phenobarbital.
5. Discontinuing the drugs and resultant prolonged seizures may have a worse fetal outcome than continuing the medications.

Analgesics

Acetaminophen has been widely used during pregnancy, and only a few cases of possible adverse effects to the fetus have been reported.[15] The drug does cross the placenta. For short-term use in therapeutic doses, acetaminophen is considered to have a very low risk and should be considered the antipyretic and analgesic of choice during pregnancy.[37–39] Aspirin, on the other hand, is more controversial. The Collaborative Perinatal Project failed to associate 14,864 first-trimester fetal exposures to aspirin with malformations.[8] Other studies and reports contradict these findings.[15,39] Another potential problem includes an increased incidence of stillbirths because of early intrauterine blockade of the ductus arteriosus.[37] Aspirin also has been reported to affect the intelligence quotient of children adversely if exposure occurs during the first half of pregnancy.[39] A similar study refutes these findings.[15] Used late in pregnancy, aspirin can induce neonatal bleeding due to platelet inhibition, increased chance for maternal blood loss, and prolongation of labor due to prostaglandin inhibition. Aspirin should be avoided, especially late in pregnancy. Although teratogenicity caused by aspirin may not be of great concern, other fetal and maternal adverse effects are.

The nonsteroidal anti-inflammatory drugs (e.g., ibuprofen, naproxen, ketorolac) have not been linked with congenital malformations. However, since they are prostaglandin inhibitors, like aspirin, they can inhibit labor when used late in pregnancy and should be avoided.

For severe pain meperidine and morphine appear equally safe. Both have been weakly associated with inguinal hernia.[15] There is more experience with using meperidine during pregnancy. Like all narcotics, both rapidly cross the placenta and can induce maternal and fetal addiction if used in high doses or chronically.

Pediculocides and Scabicides

The treatment of pregnant patients with lice or scabies is a common dilemma. Most authors agree that lindane (Kwell) should be avoided.[15] The drug has not been reported to cause malformations but can induce central nervous system toxicity in the fetus. Lindane can be absorbed, especially when used inappropriately in excessive doses or for long periods of time. Either pyrethrins with piperonyl butoxide (eg, Rid, R&C) or permethrin shampoo (Nix) should be used. These agents are minimally absorbed. For scabies, permethrin 5% cream (Elimite) or crotamiton (Eurax) is preferred.

Gastrointestinal Agents

Interestingly, nausea and vomiting during early pregnancy has been associated with a lower incidence of spontaneous abortion.[5] About 60% of women experience these symptoms during the first trimester.[40] To avoid unnecessary drug exposure, these symptoms should be managed without drug therapy. Antiemetics should only be considered when the vomiting persists, leading to dehydration, weight loss or electrolyte disturbances. The efficacy of these agents has not been well studied, nor has one agent proved more effective than another.[40] The safety of these agents during pregnancy is not clear. The Perinatal Collaborative Project found the phenothiazines overall not to be associated with increased risk for congenital malformation.[8] Specifically, promethazine and prochlorperazine were most commonly used. Another large, prospective study found no teratogenic potential for phenothiazines and meclizine.[41] Trimethobenzamide, however, was found to be slightly suggestive of an excess of abnormalities at the 5-year follow-up. The true risk appears small.

The antihistamine meclizine does not appear to be teratogenic in humans, based on results of large observational studies. Diphenhydramine and dimenhydrinate also appear relatively safe when used in low doses for short periods.[15,41]

For treatment of indigestion, standard aluminum/magnesium antacid preparations are appropriate. Sodium bicarbonate should not be used because it can be easily absorbed. For constipation, bulk-forming laxatives are indicated when diet therapy fails. Stimulants should be avoided.

REFERENCES

1. Peckman CH, King RW. A study of intercurrent conditions observed during pregnancy. Am J Obstet Gynecol 87:609, 1963
2. Doering PL, Stewart RB. The extent and character of drug consumption during pregnancy. JAMA 239:843, 1978
3. Hill M. Drugs ingested by pregnant women. Clin Pharmacol Ther 14:654, 1973
4. Hill R, Stern L. Drugs in pregnancy: effects on the fetus and newborn. Drugs 17:182, 1979
5. Hays DP. Teratogenesis: a review of the basic principles with a discussion of selected agents: Part II. Drug Intel Clin Pharm 15:542, 1981
6. Hays DP. Teratogenesis: a review of the basic principles with a discussion of selected agents: Part III. Drug Intel Clin Pharm 15:639, 1981
7. Schardein JL. Chemically induced birth defects. New York: Marcel Dekker, 1985
8. Heinonen OP, Slone S, Shapiro S. Birth defects and drugs in pregnancy. Littleton, MA: Publishing Sciences Group, 1977
9. Moore KL. Causes of congenital malformations. In The Developing Human: clinically oriented embryology, 3rd ed. Philadelphia: WB Saunders, 1982
10. Beely L. Adverse effects of drugs in the first trimester of pregnancy. Clin Obstet Gynecol 8:261, 1981
11. Hayes DP. Teratogenesis: a review of the basic principles with a discussion of selected agents: Part I. Drug Intel Clin Pharm 15:544, 1981
12. Pregnancy labeling. FDA Drug Bulletin. Sept 1977:23.
13. Chow AW, Jewesson PJ. Pharmacokinetics and safety of antimicrobial agents during pregnancy. Rev Inf Dis 7:287, 1985

Obstetric and Gynecologic Emergencies, edited by
Guy I. Benrubi. J.B. Lippincott Company,
Philadelphia © 1994.

CHAPTER 15

Equipment Needs in The Emergency Department

D. Scott Wells

Obstetric and gynecologic problems constitute a significant percentage of emergency department visits. Their diagnosis and treatment depend on a few critical pieces of equipment. The most valuable diagnostic tool is the bimanual pelvic examination. It requires no equipment but is enhanced by the use of equipment specific for the presenting condition. This brief chapter will address the equipment needs crucial in the evaluation and subsequent treatment of obstetric and gynecologic problems seen in the emergency department.

Complications of First-Trimester Pregnancy

Among the conditions most common and potentially life-threatening are complications of ectopic and abortive first-trimester pregnancies. Evaluation for ectopic pregnancy begins with the *rapid pregnancy test* (urine or serum). *Real-time transvaginal* or *transabdominal ultrasonography* is invaluable in assessing the contents of the uterus and the anatomy of the adnexas in early pregnancy. Culdocentesis allows for rapid diagnosis and confirmation of a hemoperitoneum. Culdocentesis requires a large *Graves speculum, Betadine swab, single-tooth tenaculum, 18- to 20-gauge spinal needle*, and a *10-mL syringe*.

The diagnosis of incomplete or inevitable abortion is largely determined by ex-

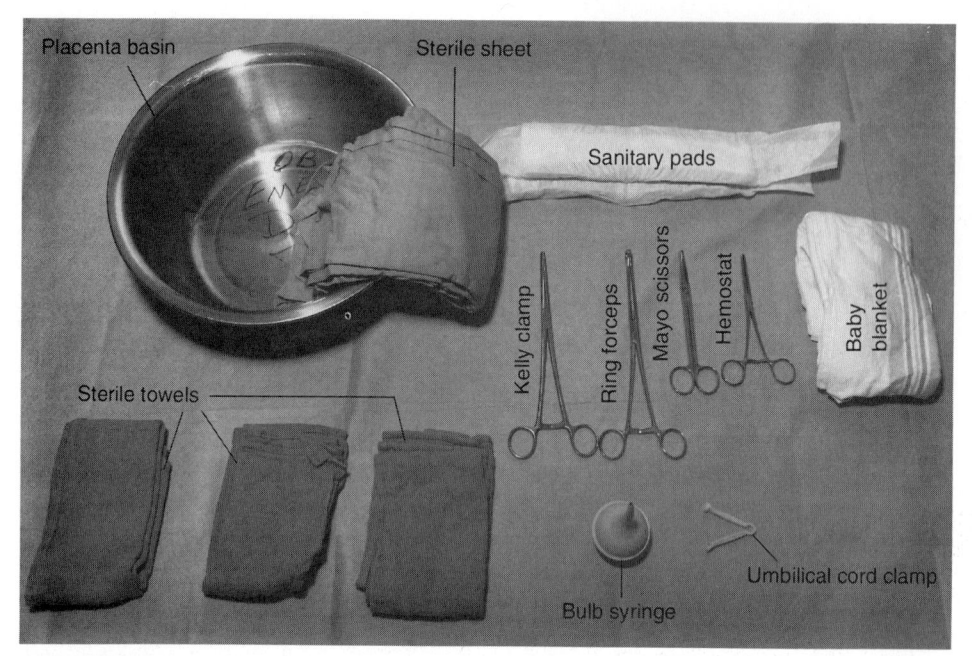

204 ♦ OBSTETRIC AND GYNECOLOGIC EMERGENCIES

FIGURE 15-1
Prepackaged trays can improve efficiency in emergency situations. Pictured here is a precipitous delivery tray. *Clockwise from top left:* placenta basin, sterile sheet, sanitary pads, Kelly clamp, ring forceps, Mayo scissors, hemostat, baby blanket, umbilical cord clamp, bulb syringe, and three sterile towels.

amination, with no specific equipment. However, because of the amount of hemorrhage that accompanies incomplete or inevitable abortions, it is imperative that suction curettage be rapidly available. The equipment needed to perform a suction curettage includes a *portable suction machine* capable of generating 60 to 80 cm of water pressure, *suction cannulas* ranging in size from 6 to 14 cm, *sterile suction tubing*, a large *Graves speculum, single-tooth tenaculum, ring forceps, cervical dilators* (Hagar or Pratt), and *sharp curettes*. Suction curettage is performed in the emergency department, frequently under paracervical block with or without intravenous sedation.

Precipitous Delivery: Neonatal Resuscitation

Precipitous deliveries frequently provoke anxiety in emergency departments, especially where equipment to aid in the delivery and possible neonatal resuscitation is not readily available. This uneasiness can be partially alleviated by preparing a vaginal delivery pack consisting of a *sterilely wrapped wash basin* containing *towels, suction bulb,* two *Kelly clamps,* plastic *umbilical cord clamp, scissors, ring forceps,* and a *needle holder*. Absorbable suture and 1% lidocaine should also be available for the repair of lacerations and/or episiotomy. *Pitocin* should be administered after placental deliv-

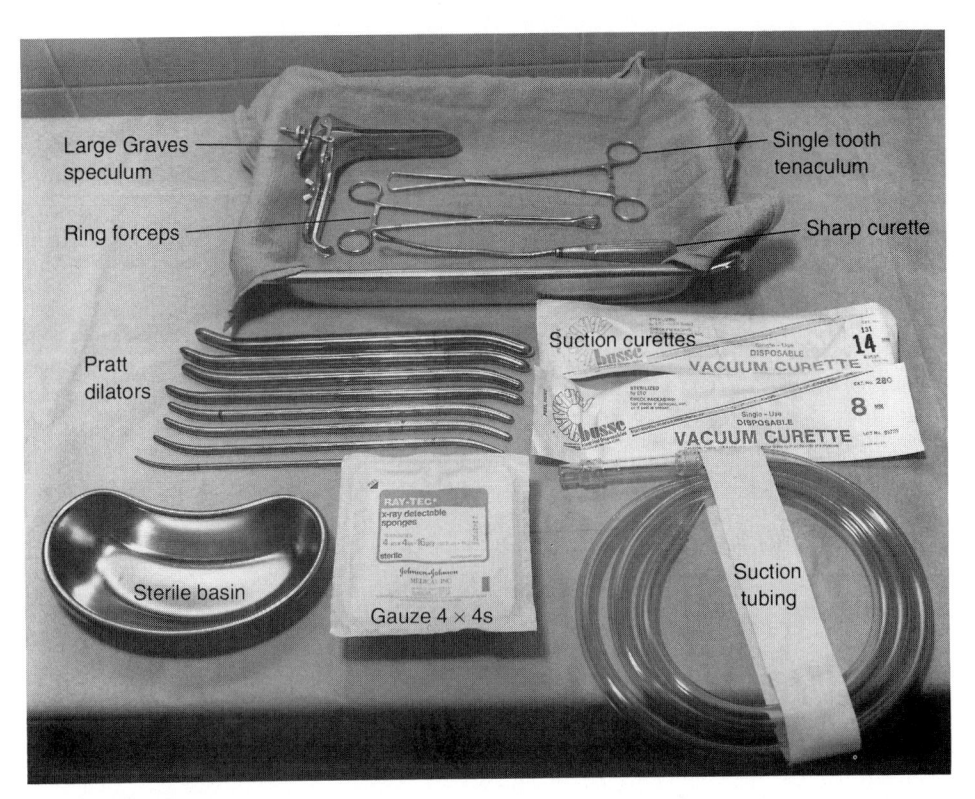

FIGURE 15–2
D&E tray includes (*clockwise from top left*) large Graves speculum, single-tooth tenaculum, ring forceps, sharp curette, suction currettes, suction tubing, gauze 4 × 4s, sterile basin, and Pratt dilators.

ery to decrease uterine bleeding. *Methergine* and synthetic *prostaglandins* should also be available for marked postpartum hemorrhage. Delivery of a depressed neonate may require only vigorous stimulation and assisted ventilation; however, an emergency department physician must be prepared for an extensive neonatal resuscitation. Neonatal resuscitation supplies include a *radiant warmer*, *neonatal concentrations* of resuscitation drugs (naloxone, epinephrine, bicarbonate, and atropine), *neonatal AMBU bag*, *masks* (infant and neonate sizes), uncuffed *endotracheal tubes* (sizes 2.0, 2.5, 3.0, and 3.5), *Deli-suction* tubing, neonatal *laryngoscope* with straight and curved number 0 blades, and a neonatal *transport system*.

Sexual Assault

Although most larger cities have facilities and personnel to care for victims of sexual assault, the emergency department is frequently the place of initial evaluation and examination. This examination is extremely important both psychologically, for the patient, and legally, because evidence for potential criminal prosecution is best gathered during the initial examination. Supplies needed for performing a sexual assault

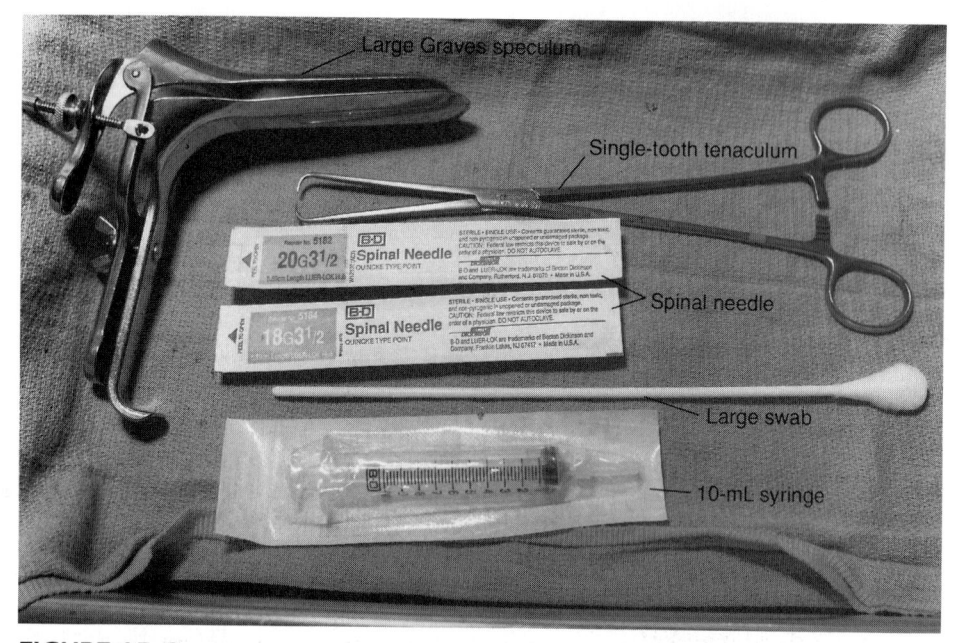

FIGURE 15–3
Culdocentesis tray includes (*from top to bottom*) large Graves speculum, single-tooth tenaculum, spinal needles, large swab, and 10-mL syringe.

evidence collection examination include *questionnaire* and *examination forms*, a physician *checklist*, small and large *evidence collection containers* (envelopes, bags, bottles), *glass slides*, *comb*, and gonorrhea and chlamydia *culture media*. Medical *photographic equipment* and a *Wood's lamp* should also be available.

Minor Emergencies

Emergency departments, instead of the appropriate primary-care facilities, are frequently used (misused) by patients for nonemergent conditions. Because of this, emergency department personnel must be equipped to evaluate and diagnose common obstetric and gynecologic problems. They should have supplies such as *Ward catheters* for Bartholin's cysts and abscesses; *biopsy instruments* for vulvar, vaginal, or cervical lesions; *pap smear spatulas and fixatives; culture transport media* for gonorrhea and chlamydia; *nitrazene paper* to aid in the diagnosis of rupture of the fetal membranes; and battery-powered *ultrasound transducers* for detection of fetal heart rate.

Conclusion

In light of the frequency with which obstetric and gynecologic problems present to the emergency department, advanced preparation of examination rooms with appropriate equipment maximizes patient care and minimizes physician frustration.

The basic equipment can be maintained in a variety of ways. Efficient *prepackaged trays* for specific problems greatly improve patient care. Examples include trays for *precipitous delivery, D&E, culdocentesis,* and *sexual assault.* Each tray contains the sterilely prepackaged equipment outlined earlier. Time wasted looking for individual items is eliminated. Once the equipment is assembled and available, it must be maintained. The examination rooms must be periodically restocked. Successful management of the problem begins with accessibility of appropriate equipment.

PART II

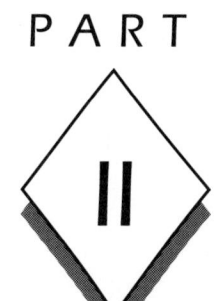

GYNECOLOGY

Obstetric and Gynecologic Emergencies, edited by
Guy I. Benrubi. J.B. Lippincott Company,
Philadelphia © 1994.

CHAPTER 16

Sexually Transmitted Diseases

I. Keith Stone

Pelvic Inflammatory Disease

Any discussion of gynecologic infectious emergencies should begin with a review of pelvic inflammatory disease (PID). PID accounts for approximately 2.5 million outpatient visits, 200,000 hospitalizations, and over 100,000 surgical procedures annually.[1,2] Aside from the personal, physical, and emotional distress associated with PID, the financial cost to the individual and to society is staggering. The total cost for PID in 1990 has been estimated to be $4.2 billion in the United States. By the year 2000 costs associated with PID are projected to approach $10 billion.[3]

Because the clinical presentation of PID may be subtle, it is important for the clinician to recognize certain risk factors that may be associated with increased risk. A major risk factor is that of age. Young women are at greater risk of acquiring this disease because of the greater prevalence of sexually transmitted diseases in the younger population. In addition, younger females have a lower prevalence of protective chlamydial antibodies, larger zones of cervical ectopy, and greater penetrability of cervical mucus.[4] Sexually active adolescents are three times more likely to be diagnosed with PID than women who are 25 to 29 years old.[5] Multiple sexual partners, high frequency of sexual intercourse, and the rate of new partner acquisition within the previous 30 days all appear to increase the risk of acquiring PID.[6] One contraceptive device that appears to increase the risk of PID is the intrauterine device (IUD). Though studies suggest an increased risk of PID with the IUD, the greatest risk may occur around the time of insertion of the IUD and within the first 4 to 5 months after insertion.[7] It is presumed that this increased temporal association is secondary to the introduction of vaginal and cervical pathogens into the endometrium during IUD insertion. Other factors that appear to be associated with an increased risk of PID include douching, smoking, and proximity to menses. It has been observed that women with chlamydial or gonococcal salpingitis develop symptoms significantly more frequently within 7 days of menses than at other times during the cycle.[8]

Though *Neisseria gonorrhea* and *Chlamydia trachomatis* are considered to be the primary pathogens in PID, other organisms are also isolated from tubal and peritoneal fluid. These organisms include aerobes (*Streptococcus* species, *Escherichia coli*, and *Haemophilus influenzae*) and anaerobes (*Bacteroides bivius*, *Bacteroides fragilis*, *Peptostreptococcus*, and *Peptococcus*).[9] Other organisms that have been isolated but whose significance is still indeterminate include *Mycoplasma* and *Actinomycosis*. Finally, tuberculosis is a remote consideration in patients at risk (Third World countries and immunosuppressed patients). Though PID may be caused by a single agent, infection is frequently polymicrobial. Polymicrobial PID results when more than one primary pathogen infects the oviductal epithelium, or after damage caused by a single primary pathogen creates altered host immune defense mechanisms in the oviduct. Secondary invading organisms may be normal inhabitants of the upper vagina that become pathogenic upon exposure to damaged tubal epithelium.

Pelvic inflammatory disease has always posed a diagnostic dilemma for the examining physician. Mild disease may be diagnosed as functional bowel syndrome or gastroenteritis. Occasionally, cystitis is the presumptive diagnosis. On the other end of the spectrum, severe disease may be diagnosed as ovarian torsion, diverticulitis, or perhaps most commonly appendicitis. Frequently this diagnostic dilemma results from the lack of sensitivity and specificity of the patient's complaints, physical findings, and laboratory evaluation. A patient complaint of fever and chills has been noted to have a sensitivity of 41% and a specificity of 80%.[10] A temperature of more than 38°C has been observed to have a sensitivity ranging from 24% to 40% and a specificity ranging from 79 to 91%. The presence of a palpable mass has been noted to have a sensitivity of 24 to 49% and a specificity of 74 to 79%. A sedimentation rate of more than 25 mm per hour has been associated with a 55% sensitivity and an 84% specificity. Given the lack of sensitivity and specificity of these signs, symptoms and laboratory findings, rigid criteria for the diagnosis of PID have been established. Currently accepted criteria include three major physical findings (all of which must be present): (1) abdominal tenderness, (2) cervical or uterine tenderness, and (3) adnexal tenderness. One of the following five minor criteria must be present in addition to the three major criteria: (1) a temperature of more than 38°C, (2) a white blood cell count of more than 10,000, (3) an adnexal mass consistent with a tuboovarian abscess, (4) a Gram stain of cervical material demonstrating gram-negative intracellular diplococci, and (5) purulent material obtained by culdocentesis.[11]

It must be understood when using this fairly rigid diagnostic scheme that patients with mild PID may present without significant abdominal tenderness. It has recently been suggested that a new diagnostic approach be established to correct the inadequacy in the established scheme.[10] Since abdominal tenderness is nonspecific and often lacking, the copresence of adnexal tenderness and cervical motion tenderness may prompt a presumptive diagnosis of PID. Minor criteria, or diagnostic indicators, from which the presence of one indicator would support the presumptive diagnosis, include (1) abnormal vaginal discharge, (2) elevated C-reactive protein, (3) elevated erythrocyte sedimentation rate, (4) endometritis by biopsy, (5) gram-negative intracellular diplococci on cervical Gram stain, (6) positive chlamydial assay, (7) elevated temperature, (8) palpable adnexal mass, and (9) laparoscopic evidence of PID. If the patient is presumed to be at risk for a sexually transmitted disease and has physical findings suggestive of mild disease, then it may be more appropriate to overtreat than undertreat her and cause significant damage to the oviducts resulting in infertility or a future ectopic pregnancy.

Ultrasonography and computerized tomography scanning may be useful in examining the patient with severe rebound tenderness upon whom an adequate pelvic examination is impossible to perform. Ultrasonography may demonstrate echogenic fluid in the pelvis consistent with pus (Fig. 16-1). CT scanning may demonstrate abscess formation with fluid and air collection (Fig. 16-2).

Where significant uncertainty exists concerning the diagnosis, the gold standard has been the performance of a diagnostic laparoscopy. One major study of patients presenting with signs and symptoms of PID who underwent laparoscopic examination demonstrated that the preoperative diagnosis was confirmed in 65% of the patients, 23% had normal pelvic anatomy, and 12% had other pathology diagnosed (appendicitis or endometriosis).[12]

The decision to admit the patient to the hospital for further evaluation or treatment should be based upon certain well-established criteria. These include (1) significant peritoneal signs or upper quadrant rebound tenderness, (2) the presence of an IUD, (3) pregnancy, (4) an adnexal mass consistent with a tubo-ovarian abscess (on pelvic examination or diagnostic imaging), (5) gastrointestinal symptoms

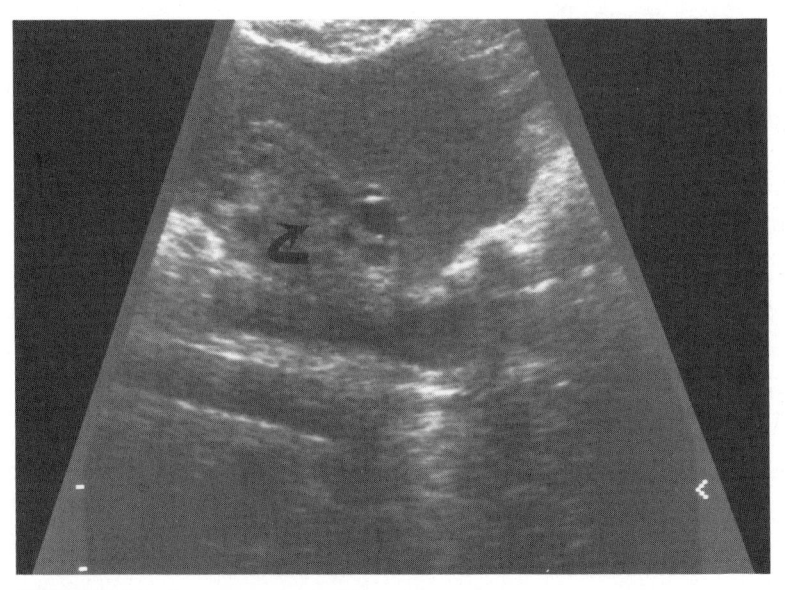

FIGURE 16–1
Transvaginal probe demonstrating ovary with follicles (**arrow**) surrounded by echogenic fluid (pus).

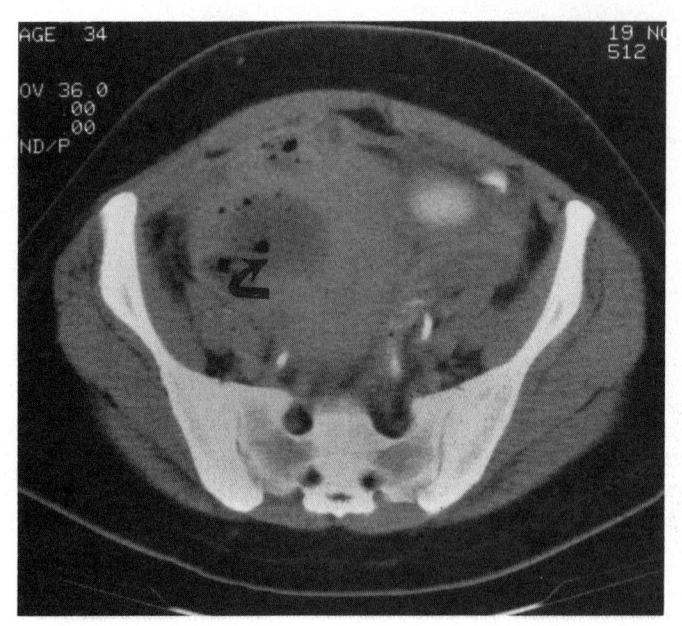

FIGURE 16-2
CT scan demonstrating tubo-ovarian abscess with fluid collection and gas (**arrow**).

precluding appropriate outpatient therapy or suggestive of bowel pathology, (6) failed outpatient therapy, (7) a nulliparous patient, and (8) an uncertain diagnosis. Patients with an uncertain diagnosis will require further evaluation and institution of therapy. The decision to perform laparoscopy to delineate the disease process may be based upon the patient's severity of symptoms upon admission or upon her response to antibiotic therapy. If the decision is made to treat with antibiotics and no resolution of symptoms occurs in 24 to 48 hours or if symptoms increase in severity during this time frame, a laparoscopy should be considered.

Treatment regimens recommended by the Centers for Disease Control for PID are outlined in Tables 16-1 and 16-2.[13] Appropriate follow-up should be obtained when patients are treated with the outpatient regimen to assure compliance and resolution of symptoms.

Of dire consequence is the possibility of a ruptured tubo-ovarian abscess or a leaking tubo-ovarian abscess presenting as an emergent threat to life. Mortality from a ruptured tubo-ovarian abscess ranges from 10 to 15%. Appropriate diagnosis and therapy are mandatory. When a tubo-ovarian abscess ruptures, endotoxin is released into the systemic circulation. The lipid-A portion of the lipopolysaccharide results in release of numerous factors or mediators: beta-endorphins, bradykinin, activators of the complement and coagulation cascades, plasminogen, and histamine. Decreased systemic resistance, a low pulmonary artery occlusive pressure and increased cardiac output are noted in the initial stage of shock, known as "warm shock." As shock progresses, systemic vascular resistance increases and cardiac output decreases, resulting in "cold shock." Microvascular hypoperfusion secondary to microembolization from fibrin degradation products and precapillary sphincteric dilatation secondary to hypoxia result in arterial venous shunting and loss of effective intravascular volume. Myocardial depression results in a diminution of effective car-

TABLE 16-1
In-patient Treatment for PID

Regimen A	Regimen B
Cefoxitin IV 2 g every 6 h or Cefotetan IV 2 g every 12 h	Clindamycin IV 900 mg every 8 h plus Gentamicin loading dose IV or IM (2 mg/kg) followed by a maintenance dose (1.5 mg/kg) every 8 h
plus Doxycycline 100 mg every 12 h orally or IV	

Continue regimen for at least 48 h after clinical improvement. Following hospital discharge, continue doxycycline 100 mg orally two times a day for 10 to 14 days.

diac output. Inadequate perfusion of vital organs results in renal dysfunction and accentuated acidosis. It is imperative that the managing physician recognize the presence of septic shock and respond appropriately. The hypotensive, tachycardiac patient with abdominal findings suggestive of a diffuse peritonitis, secondary to a ruptured tubo-ovarian abscess, should be managed aggressively with fluid resuscitation. Large volumes of crystalloid should be administered intravenously through two large-bore catheters. If there is a failure to correct hypotension with fluid administration, intravenous sympathomimetic amines should be initiated. Dopamine is the primary agent of choice. When administered in a dose of 1 to 3 µg/kg per minute, dopamine causes minor inotropic and chronotropic effects on the heart with concomitant dilatation of mesenteric, cerebral, coronary, and renal arteries.[14] At dosages between 4 and 10 µg/kg per minute there is a further increase in cardiac output and increased heart rate. Dosages beyond 15 µg/kg per minute result in increased vasoconstriction and a deleterious effect due to a markedly increased heart rate. As the heart rate increases there is less effective time for filling, and though cardiac energy consumption is increased, output is not increased. The decision to initiate invasive monitoring for fluid resuscitation should be based upon the patient's response to crystalloid administration and urine output. If blood pressure fails to respond to intravascular volume repletion and sympathomimetic amines and

TABLE 16-2
Out-patient Treatment for PID

Cefoxitin 2 g IM*
or
Ceftriaxone 250 mg IM
plus
Doxycycline 100 mg orally two times a day for 10 to 14 days
or
Tetracycline 500 mg orally four times a day for 10 to 14 days
For patients who cannot tolerate doxycycline: substitute erythromycin, 500 mg orally four times a day for 10 to 14 days.

*Plus Probenecid, 1 gram orally, concurrently

urine output is not appropriate (>30 mL per hour), then pulmonary capillary wedge pressure monitoring should be considered to prevent the development of adult respiratory distress syndrome (shock lung). An effort should be made to keep the pulmonary capillary wedge pressure in the range of 10 to 12 mmHg. As pulmonary capillary wedge pressure approaches 18 to 20 mmHg, the risk of developing pulmonary extravasation of intravenously administered fluids increases. Broad-spectrum antibiotic therapy should be initiated promptly to cover the polymicrobial gamut of pelvic pathogens (see Regimen B in Table 16-1). Preparation should be made for emergency admission to the hospital and laparotomy to remove the ruptured abscess and irrigate the peritoneal cavity. Blood should be sent for type and crossmatch, coagulation panel, electrolytes, and blood gases. The decision to use monoclonal antibodies for septic shock should be considered when signs of organ failure are present. This expensive form of therapy will require further evaluation before its role in the management of septic shock due to ruptured tubo-ovarian abscess is defined. It is imperative that the physician managing the patient in septic shock, secondary to a ruptured tubo-ovarian abscess, understand that this is a surgical disease and pharmacologic intervention is supportive and preparatory to laparotomy.

Gonorrhea

Neisseria gonorrhea, the cause of the most frequently reported sexually transmitted disease in the United States, is accorded emergency care in two situations: (1) when it is associated with acute PID and (2) when it is the cause of a disseminated gonococcal infection. Pelvic inflammatory disease has been discussed earlier in this chapter. Only 1 to 2% of patients with gonorrhea develop disseminated gonococcal infections. Women appear to be more commonly affected by this presentation then men. This may be explained by the relative lack of symptoms in women harboring *Neisseria gonorrhea* in the lower reproductive tract, specifically the cervix. Men more commonly seek medical therapy for a mucopurulent urethral discharge, whereas women may have no symptoms in association with gonococcal cervicitis. With a breakdown in host immune defense, gonococcemia may occur. With invasion of the bloodstream, symptoms will be noted, including fever, chills, and arthralgias. Eventually the gonococcal dermatitis–arthritis syndrome will develop within 2 to 3 weeks of the primary genital infection. Cutaneous manifestations usually consist of fewer than 25 lesions, usually on the distal extremities and in various stages of development. Lesions begin as pinpoint erythematous macules that progress to papules, vesicular pustules, or hemorrhagic bullae. Advanced lesions contain a necrotic-appearing center surrounded by an erythematous halo. Cultures of cutaneous lesions rarely are positive for *Neisseria gonorrhea*; however, immunofluorescent tissue stains may be of assistance in demonstrating organisms. Blood cultures and urethral, cervical, pharyngeal, and rectal cultures may be of assistance in defining the etiology of the rash. A high index of suspicion is imperative (Fig. 16-3).[15] With dissemination the patient may present with an acutely inflamed septic joint. The typical age of the patient is the early 20s. Disseminated gonococcal disease is the most common cause of septic arthritis in patients under the age of 30. The arthritis may be mono- or oligoarticu-

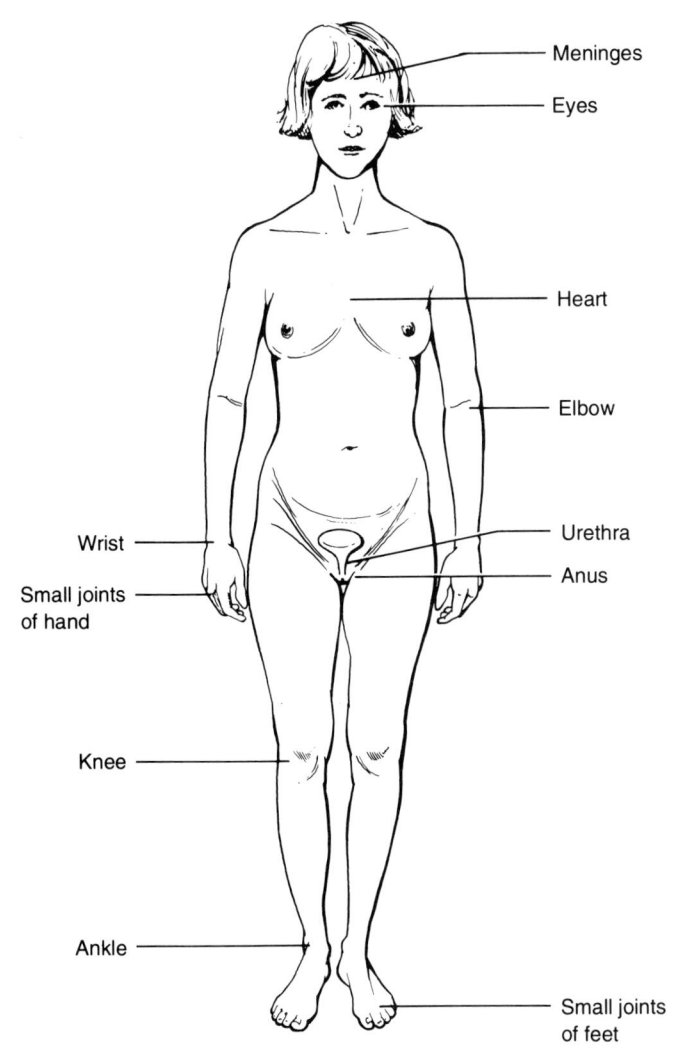

FIGURE 16–3
Sites of desseminated GC infection.

lar. Joints most commonly affected are the knees, elbows, ankles, wrists, or small joints of the hands and feet.[16] The knee is the most commonly involved joint from which the gonococcus is recovered, but this may reflect the relative ease with which this joint is aspirated. The fluid withdrawn from the involved joint will usually contain polymorphonuclear neutrophils, but a Gram stain for gram-negative intracellular diplococci will be positive only 10 to 30% of the time. Cultures likewise are positive in approximately 20 to 30% of cases. Once again, it is imperative that appropriate cultures be obtained from blood, urethral, pharyngeal, rectal, and cervical sites.

With dissemination of the gonococcus to the heart, endocarditis may be observed. Patients may complain of symptoms for several weeks and may present with fever, chills, arthralgias, malaise, fatigue, dyspnea, and chest pain. Most patients will have a murmur, and evidence of embolization may be present (conjunctival petechiae, Osler's nodes, splinter hemorrhages). Occasionally, splenomegaly and arthritis may be noted. Depending on the degree of cardiac compromise, congestive heart failure may be manifested by rales, ascites, edema, or a gallop rhythm on auscultation of the heart. The chest x-ray may demonstrate cardiomegaly as a manifestation of congestive heart failure. The electrocardiogram may demonstrate left ventricular hypertrophy, bundle branch block, or intraventricular conduction delay. Usually blood cultures are positive for *Neisseria gonorrhea*. Echocardiography is useful in determining whether vegetations exist on the heart valves. The most common involvement is of the aortic and mitral valves. Without treatment the endocarditis is almost always fatal.[3]

Rarely, *Neisseria gonorrhea* may disseminate to the meninges and cause manifestations of meningitis. Fever and nuchal rigidity in a patient complaining of headache, general malaise, and arthralgias should prompt a lumbar puncture to evaluate for organisms. As with synovial fluid, Gram stain and cultures may be negative, and therefore it is imperative to perform appropriate blood, cervical, urethral, rectal, and pharyngeal cultures for *Neisseria*.

Hospitalization is recommended for patients with disseminated gonococcal infection. Endocarditis and meningitis should be ruled out. When bacteremia and arthritis are present, the recommended therapy is ceftriaxone 1 g IV daily for 7 to 10 days. Meningitis should be treated with ceftriaxone 2 g IV daily for at least 10 days. Endocarditis should be treated with ceftriaxone 2 g IV daily for at least 3 to 4 weeks. Depending upon the severity of the valvular involvement with vegetations, cardiac surgery with valvular replacement may be necessary. Consultation should be obtained early with the appropriate specialist.[17]

Acquired Immune Deficiency Syndrome (AIDS)

Though the decade of the 1980s began with human immunodeficiency virus as a male-specific entity, it ended as a non-gender-specific entity. Women now account for more than 11% of patients with AIDS in the United States. It has been estimated that worldwide over 3 million women will die of AIDS in the 1990s.[18] Physicians cannot avoid the potential for exposure to patients infected with human immunodeficiency virus, whether the patients' infectivity status is known or unknown. The infected patient may present to the emergency room as a consequence of a number of infectious complications of the disease, or as a consequence of the therapy used to ameliorate the disease.

The human immunodeficiency virus (HIV) is an RNA virus, specifically a retrovirus, which utilizes reverse transcriptase to transcribe DNA from RNA. It has a propensity to target the CD4 molecule on the surface of the T_4 lymphocyte. After being incorporated in the T_4 lymphocyte and using the reverse transcriptase to transcribe DNA, it is integrated into the host genome and production of viral RNA. The T_4 cells are comprised of inducer and helper cells. The inducer cells stimulate maturation of the T lymphocytes from precursor cells, and the T_4 helper cells help cytotoxic T cells destroy foreign cells. The T_4 cells comprise approximately 60% to 80% of the circulating T-cell population. As a result of the infection and depletion of the T_4 lymphocytes by the invading HIV, the B cells cannot produce antibody to HIV or other microorganisms. There is a depression of the cytotoxic response. There is decreased secretion of interleukin-2, and T_4 cells are incapable of antigen recognition. Not only does HIV attack the T helper cells, but the virus may also attack macrophages and other target cells, resulting in direct infection of bowel, nervous tissue, heart and lung.[19] It is well recognized that the infected host may transmit HIV to susceptible individuals through blood or body fluids, including vaginal secretions, semen, peritoneal fluid, and amniotic fluid.[20] Once infected with HIV, seroconversion may not occur for a mean of 18 months with a range of 3 to 42 months.[21] The latency period from seroconversion to the immune deficiency syndrome is usually a mean of 10 to 11 years. Once the immune deficiency syndrome has developed, death is inevitable. As the disease progresses in the female patient, a number of opportunistic infections may result in infections that prompt the need for emergent therapy.

Since AIDS is a sexually transmitted disease, the AIDS patient is prone to acquire other sexually transmitted disease. In one study of women admitted to the hospital for treatment of PID, approximately 14% were found to be seropositive for human immunodeficiency virus. These women were significantly more likely to have admission white blood cell counts of less than 10,000. There was also a greater trend toward surgical intervention in the seropositive women than in the seronegative women.[22] (The presentation and management of PID are discussed earlier in this chapter.) It is important for the clinician to understand that the patient presenting with signs and symptoms of PID may not demonstrate a leukocytosis because of immunocompromise by the infecting virus. For this very reason strong consideration should be given to admitting the AIDS patient with signs and symptoms of PID, so that maximum therapeutic benefit may be realized with inpatient intravenous antibiotic therapy. Those antibiotic regimens used to treat seronegative women should provide the same beneficial polymicrobial coverage in the seropositive HIV patient. Currently, there appears to be no basis to provide treatment regimens other than those currently recommended by the Centers for Disease Control for acute PID.[18]

In addition to suspecting HIV in the patient who presents with signs and symptoms of acute PID, the observant physician should be alert to clinical manifestations of AIDS in any patients seen in an emergency setting. Such manifestations include enlarged lymph nodes, night sweats, fevers, oral candidiasis, chronic cough, paresthesias, Kaposi's sarcoma, nausea, vomiting, diarrhea, weight loss, and skin ulcerations.

The primary pulmonary emergency in the patient with AIDS is *Pneumocystis carinii* pneumonia. This most common of the opportunistic infections in patients with AIDS poses the greatest risk to those who have CD4 T-lymphocyte counts of less than 200. Patients may present with shortness of breath and may appear septic. Physical examination demonstrates diminished breath sounds and dullness to percussion. Chest x-ray will show a diffuse bilateral interstitial pneumonia (Fig. 16-4). Blood gases may show a diminished PO_2 and acidosis. If the presumptive diagnosis is *Pneumocystis carinii* pneumonia with evidence of pulmonary compromise, then the pa-

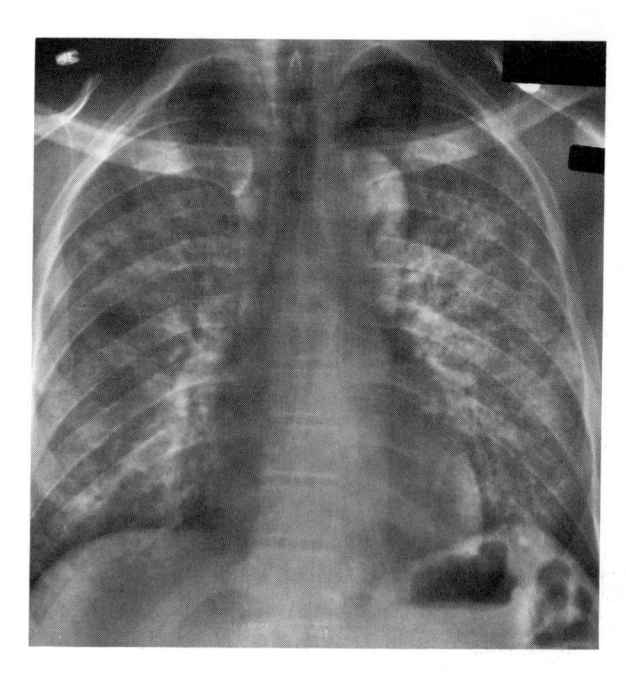

FIGURE 16-4
Extensive, bilateral pulmonary infiltrates in a patient with *Pneumocystis carinii* pneumonia complicating AIDS.

tient should be admitted for trimethoprim-sulfamethoxazole therapy. The medication may be given orally or intravenously as 15 to 20 mg/kg per day in three to four doses for 21 days.[23]

Tuberculosis is becoming an increasing concern in AIDS patients and should be considered in any pulmonary emergency in a seropositive or at-risk individual. Typical symptoms include cough, fever, night sweats, and weight loss. PPD testing should be considered in at-risk patients unless there is a known history of tuberculosis or a prior positive PPD. A reaction of 5 mm in an immunocompromised person suggests exposure to tuberculosis; chest x-rays and sputum stains should be obtained for confirmation.[24] Standard therapy consists of isoniazid, rifampin, and ethambutol. Other considerations in patients with pulmonary symptoms would include community-acquired bacterial and viral pneumonias, and fungal pneumonias (cryptococcosis, coccidiomycosis, and histoplasmosis). A final consideration in the patient with emergency pulmonary compromise is that of pneumothorax associated with aerosolized pentamidine. Pathogenesis for the pneumothorax is presumed to be related to bronchopleural fistulae resulting from pneumocystis infection. Significant pneumothorax demonstrated on chest x-ray requires insertion of a chest tube and admission to the hospital. All HIV-infected patients who suffer pneumothoraces during aerosolized pentamidine therapy should be admitted and examined for evidence of *Pneumocystis carinii* pneumonia.[24]

In addition to pulmonary complications that may result in significant compromise in the AIDS patient, the examining physician must recognize the frequent abdominal manifestations of AIDS that may obscure the etiology of the patient's underlying condition. The female AIDS patient with an acute abdomen presents a diagnostic dilemma. Does she have PID or does she have primary bowel involvement by HIV or an opportunistic infection? Right upper quadrant pain associated with either jaundice or abnormal liver function tests suggests the possibility of cytomega-

Obstetric and Gynecologic Emergencies, edited by
Guy I. Benrubi. J.B. Lippincott Company,
Philadelphia © 1994.

CHAPTER 17

Vulvar and Vaginal Disease

Benson J. Horowitz

Diseases of The Vulva

Many factors complicate the diagnosis of vulvar disease. First, located at the apex of the vagina is the cervix, with its transitional glandular epithelium, which is attractive to bacterial invasion. Second, vaginal inflammations and infections promote vulvar symptomatology because of the drainage path. Discharge from the microaerophilic milieu of the vagina carries organisms to the aerobic environment of the vulva. Third, the vulva is composed of integument and is subject to all dermatologic afflictions. Finally, the skin of the vulva is the site of the gradual transition of fully appendaged and keratinized skin to the nonkeratinized and nonappendaged mucous membrane of the vagina. The vagina is richly supplied with minor and major glands; because of this transitional and glandular composition, it is a frequent site of microbiologic disease. Therefore the ambulatory care physician must be cognizant of both vaginal and dermatologic disease.

Bartholin Gland Cysts and Abscesses

The Bartholin gland, also known as the major vestibular gland, is located beneath the labia minora and is exterior to the vaginal constrictor musculature. The gland is located between the superficial and deep layers of the urogenital diaphragm, deep to the bulbocavernosus muscle, with the bulb of the gland resting on the deep transverse perineal muscle. It is a compound racemose gland with a tortuous 2- to 2.5-cm duct that opens on each side of the vestibule just exterior to the hymenal ring. During the late excitement and plateau stage of sexual arousal, a mucoid secretion is produced that aids in lubrication prior to penile entry.[1]

Obstruction of the duct leads to cyst and abscess formation. Though disease of this structure should not be misinterpreted as prima facie evidence of a venereal infection,[2] gonococcus may be isolated from an abscessed gland. Rarely, pain is noted upon sexual arousal due to an obstructed Bartholin gland duct orifice.[3] Excision or marsupialization of the gland is curative in this usual circumstance.

Treatment of a Bartholin gland cyst or abscess consists of correcting the glandular enlargement. This can be accomplished by incision and drainage, marsupialization, insertion of a catheter, laser ablation, or glandular excision. Although cystic enlargement of the gland without infection is not an emergency, experience suggests a drainage procedure prior to the formation of an abscess. If they are left unattended, most cysts form abscesses.

Incision and drainage of a Bartholin gland cyst or abscess are not recommended for permanent cure but only as a temporary method of relief of symptoms, not as a permanent cure. In almost all cases the patient will return at a later date in need of more definitive therapy. Marsupialization of the gland is accomplished by incising the swelling at the approximate location of the orifice of the duct and then suturing the cut edge of the cyst wall to the skin of the vestibule or packing the gland with iodoform gauze for 3 to 4 weeks.[2] In 1964, Word described a catheter that is inserted through a small stab wound on the vaginal side of the swelling.[4] The catheter, which lies in the vagina, is left in place for 4 to 6 weeks and then removed (Fig. 17-1). Davis created a new ostium in a vestibular gland cyst with the use of a CO_2 laser,[5] and Lashgari described a method of ablation of a Bartholin duct cyst after incision and drainage, by vaporizing the cyst wall from the inside.[6] Finally, the entire gland can be removed surgically. This technique is difficult because of the deep extension of the gland and possible hemorrhage and postoperative infection. Nonetheless, when the other techniques have failed, surgical excision becomes the only available option; regardless of the technique employed, recurrences are common.

Vulvar Dermatoses

Seborrheic Dermatitis

Seborrheic dermatitis is a papulosquamous disorder of the skin. Its incidence is greatest in young adulthood but is also found in newborns and in late adult life. Approximately 2 to 5% of the population is afflicted; the disease is more common in males than in females.[7] The lesions of this dermatosis appear symmetrically as raised red or brown papules with fairly distinct borders and scaling surfaces. The borders are less defined in the vulvar areas. Lesions are commonly found in areas of hair follicles with active sebum production. The scalp, eyelids, eyebrows, retroauricular, and paranasal areas are commonly affected. The exanthem is seen less commonly on the trunk, axillae, groin, and vulva. The etiology of this condition is largely un-

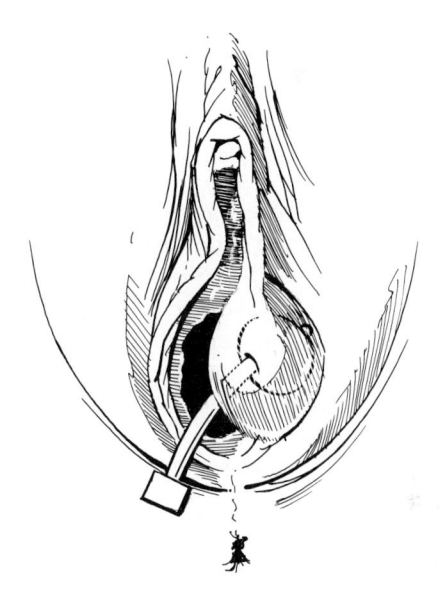

FIGURE 17–1
Use of Word catheter for Bartholin gland swelling.

known; however, it is frequently associated with the organism *Pityrosporum ovale*.[8] Decreased levels of T lymphocytes and diminished levels of IgG antibodies to this organism are found in affected patients. Increased incidence, prevalence, and severity in AIDS patients corroborate evidence of exacerbations associated with defects in cell-mediated immunity.[9]

The observation of a reddish, symmetric papulosquamous eruption with surface scaling unassociated with pruritus establishes the diagnosis. The most effective treatment of seborrheic dermatitis is 2% ketoconazole cream applied once daily for 4 weeks.[10] Frequent exacerbations and remissions are common.

Psoriasis

Psoriasis is a papulosquamous, inflammatory, chronic, and relapsing skin eruption characterized by sharply demarcated red raised patches covered by silvery scales. It is most frequently found on the scalp, elbows and knees and not uncommonly on the vulvar skin.[11] Characteristically, the patches are symmetric, although isolated vulvar lesions are also observed. The reddened raised patch has a thick, silvery scale that leaves punctate bleeding points when removed (Auspitz sign).

Approximately one third of patients report a family history of psoriasis. The disease is transmitted by an autosomal dominant gene with 60% dominance. Recent evidence suggests that psoriasis is associated with specific antigens of class I histocompatibility group types B13, B17, BW16 and CW6. Psoriasis is one of the papulosquamous skin eruptions seen in the early stages of the acquired immunodeficiency syndrome (AIDS). Pityriasis rosea, varicella zoster, tinea pedis, onychomycosis, candidiasis, and extensive molluscum contagiosum are some of the other illnesses observed in AIDS.[9] Psoriasis is associated with an arthropathy (psoriatic arthritis) and dystrophic changes of the nail and nailbed. The clinical appearance in most cases is diagnostic. Nevertheless, confusion with other papulosquamous disorders leads to diagnostic errors. Current therapy consists of coal tar preparations, salicylates, corticoids, and retinoids. Severe cases respond well to methotrexate.[12]

Pityriasis Rosea

Pityriasis rosea is an acute, benign, self-limiting, papulosquamous dermatosis that is believed to be viral in origin. It occurs with equal frequency in both sexes and is seen in the 10- to 30-year-old patient. The onset of the disease begins with fever, malaise, and occurrence of the "herald patch." This lesion is raised reddish, or salmon-colored, 3 to 5 cm in diameter, with light peripheral scaling. Within 15 days, coinlike salmon-colored lesions occur along Langers' lines of the trunk. This appearance is described as a Christmas tree pattern. The distribution of the rash is in the "T shirt" area of the front and back of the trunk. The eruption lasts 4 to 8 weeks and is benign in course and symptomatology. Lesions extending to the vulva are common and the diagnosis can be missed by not examining the remainder of the torso.[13,14]

Lichen Simplex Chronicus

Three "lichens" appear on the vulva: lichen simplex chronicus (LSC), lichen planus, and lichen sclerosus. *Lichen simplex chronicus, neurodermatitis, nodular neurodermatitis, vulvar hyperplastic dystrophy,* and *squamous hyperplasia of the vulva* are probably synonymous terms. Clinically, the condition is characterized by thickened, white keratinized plaques exhibiting lichenification of the skin surface. Pathologically, there is enlargement of rete pegs and a dermal inflammatory infiltrate. Women are affected more than men, and the average age of incidence is 30 to 60 years. Pruritus is the most common complaint, and it is believed that the lichenlike appearance is created by persistent scratching. The border of the affected area is indistinct and is frequently surrounded by papules. In addition to the vulva, LSC can be found on the scrotum, nape of the neck, eyelids, scalp, wrists, foot, thighs, and ears.

It has been suggested that the etiology of this condition is related to neuroses best described as manifestations of anxiety. Phobias of parasitosis or systemic illnesses have also been described.[12] Dermatologists frequently associate LSC with atopy.[15]

Treatment is directed to the itch/scratch cycle. Intralesional, systemic and topical steroid preparations have been used effectively. Antihistamines, antianxiety, and sedative preparations have also been of value. Other papulosquamous disorders and fungal diseases can confound diagnosis. Fungal KOH preparations and cultures are useful in this regard.

Lichen Planus

Lichen planus is a papulosquamous mucocutaneous disorder of unknown etiology. Skin, the oral cavity, and the vulva are primarily affected. Cutaneous manifestations include flat, polygonal, violaceous, or brownish papules that frequently coalesce to form plaques on the extensor surfaces of the legs and flexor surfaces of the forearm. Approximately 33% of patients have oral lesions of a reticular appearance (Wickham's striae), or plaques, ulcers, or erosions on the buccal mucosa. Any part of the oral cavity can be involved, including the gingiva or tongue.[16] Vulvar lesions consist of pruritic plaques, ulcers, or papules in the vestibule or the perineum. Lesions are symmetric and in the vestibule have the appearance of brawny reddened and scaly skin. Immunologic abnormalities of class II major histocompatibility group antigens HLA-B7, HLA-A3, HLA-5, HLA-28 and HLA-DR have been described.[17,18] The differential diagnosis includes the other papulosquamous disorders, secondary syphilis, pemphigus, and pemphigoid. A tissue biopsy revealing the characteristic pathologic changes of a subepithelial lymphocytic infiltration—vacuolar degeneration; an intense, bandlike infiltrate with eosinophilic bodies (Civatte bodies) in the area of the stratum spinosum; necrotic keratinocytes; para- and hyperkeratosis—is considered by trained dermatopathologists as diagnostic.[19]

In the oral cavity and vagina an erosive form of the disease is also infrequently present. In the vulva, the appearance of erosive lichen planus is that of almost total denuding of the vulvar epithelium from Hart's line internally to the hymenal ring.[20]

The treatment of vulvar lichen planus is topical corticosteroids. Clobetasol 0.05% is effective when applied sparingly twice a day until symptoms disappear. Erosive vulvovaginitis also responds to suppositories of hydrocortisone acetate 25 mg twice a day inserted vaginally for several months. In some cases oral prednisone, up to 70 mg per day has been prescribed with beneficial results.[21] Drugs implicated in lichenoid eruptions include arsenic, antimalarial agents, beta blockers, thiazides, and gold salts. Less frequently implicated are aminosalicylic acid, phenothiazines, methyldopa, streptomycin, tetracycline, mercury, and iodides.[22,23]

Lichen Sclerosus

Lichen sclerosus (LS) is a benign vulvar condition of unknown etiology that was formerly classified as hypoplastic vulvar dystrophy. Wallace quotes the incidence of the disease as between one in 300 and one in 1000 in the general population.[24] The disease is more frequent in women than in men, and genital sites are more commonly involved than nongenital sites. Pruritus and other symptoms of vulvar irritation cause much of the discomfort. The clinical signs of LS are atrophic, white vulvar epithelium, with the absence of the labia minora and the clitoral folds. Vulvar adhesions are the most diagnostic feature of the disease; even in the presence of epithelium of normal color, absence of labial and clitoral folds, and vulvar adhesions suggest the presence of the disease. LS affects prepubertal, menstruating, and postmenopausal women. Approximately two thirds of prepubertal girls will remit spontaneously at menarche.[25]

The etiology of LS is unknown. HLA types A31, B40, A29, and B44 have been reported with increased frequency in this disease.[26] The findings of a homogenization of collagen in the upper dermis, with an inflammatory exudate, thinning of the epithelium, and loss of rete ridges are characteristic pathologic findings found on a directed tissue biopsy. Friedrich reported a defect in conversion of testosterone to dihydrotestosterone in vulvar skin and reported good therapeutic results with the application of 2% testosterone ethanate in white petrolatum base applied two or three times daily until relief was obtained.[27] Paslin observed reversal of architectural changes on this regimen but little symptomatic relief.[28] Clobetasol ointment 0.05% applied sparingly twice a day for symptomatic relief appears more efficacious. In prepubertal girls, progesterone 100 mg/oz formulated in a cream base is safe and effective.

Secondary Syphilis

Secondary syphilis presents as a papulosquamous skin eruption approximately 6 to 8 weeks after the initial infection or 3 to 4 weeks after the development of the primary chancre. The rash of secondary syphilis is symmetric and can be muscular, papular, pustular, or follicular. "Moth-eaten" alopecia with the loss of eyelashes and the lateral third of the eyebrows is common. In moist areas, such as vulva and rectum, the epithelium forms raised flat plaques (condylomata lata). In the mouth, similar findings are described as "mucous patches." These signs are associated with generalized lymphadenopathy and splenomegaly. In secondary syphilis, serologic tests are always positive and diagnostic. Early syphilis (less than 1 year's duration) is treated with benzathine penicillin G 2.4 million units, intramuscularly, weekly for 2 consecutive weeks. Recognition of one sexually transmitted disease always requires investigation for others.

Ulcerative Disease of the Vulva

Herpes Simplex Virus

Herpes simplex virus (HSV) is the most common cause of genital ulceration. The ulcers of HSV infection occur individually or in groups of painful, punched-out lesions, frequently surrounded by a red halo. The initial infection is often secondarily invaded by bacteria, producing an extremely painful, purulent, and inflamed vulva covered with serosanguineous exudate. The painful, ulcerated vulva leads to urinary retention, which may require hospitalization. Subsequent attacks are usually mild and marked by infrequent and less painful ulcerations. The diagnosis is made by culture of the suspected lesion. Titers to HSV virus are only useful in determining the initial infection. A negative titer followed by a rising titer after a positive vaginal culture documents an initial attack. Oral acyclovir five times daily until symptoms have disappeared is the most effective therapy. Maintenance regimens of three to four tablets per day have been described.[29] Herpes simplex infection is a sexually transmitted disease, and when it is accurately diagnosed it requires a search for other diseases of similar transmission.

Regional Enteritis

In 1932 Crohn, Ginsberg, and Oppenheimer reported a disease of the terminal ileum characterized by a subacute or chronic necrotizing or cicatrizing inflammation.[30] Vaginal ulceration caused by fistulization from the small bowel is often the first sign of the disease. The fistulous lesions can be single or multiple and often are described as chronic draining sinus tracts. These findings also lead to other diagnostic considerations, such as granuloma inguinale, lymphogranuloma venereum, hidradenitis suppurativa, follicular abscess, Behçet's disease, and tuberculosis. Radiographic confirmation of disease of the ileum establishes the diagnosis.

Behçet's Disease

In 1937 Behcet described a triad of symptoms consisting of oral ulcerations, genital ulcerations and uveitis.[31] In 1946 Curth described a form in which only oral and genital ulcerations were present.[32] Other manifestations of this disease include peripheral neuropathy, encephalitis, arthritis, ulcerative colitis, nodules of the extremities, and thrombophlebitis.[33] However, oral ulcerations are present in all cases. Oral and penile ulcerations are very painful; vaginal ulcerations are not.

The etiology of Behçet's disease is unknown. Viral and autoimmune antibody theories have been proposed. Vasculitis is the predominant pathologic finding; necrotizing angiitis has been described. Strachan and Wigzell comment that Behçet's syndrome or disease is rarely diagnosed in the United States.[34] The diagnosis is established by the symptoms triad. Treatment with corticoids, immunosuppressants, and blood transfusions has had variable therapeutic success. No fatalities occurred in O'Duffy's series of patients, attesting to the fact that Behçet's disease is a benign vasculitis.[33]

Lymphogranuloma Venereum

Lymphogranuloma venereum (LGV) is a sexually transmitted disease caused by *Chlamydia trachomatis* serotypes L1, L2, and L3. The lymphatic system is the primary site of involvement. Three stages are recognized: the primary phase of vulvar ulceration; the lymphatic stage, characterized by buboes; and the anorectal stage, with eventual rectal stricture and fistula formation. The primary papule or ulcer of LGV is usually single but may be multiple. Although originally painful, healing is quite rapid, and the illness is often dismissed without consultation. In 1 to 4 weeks, inguinal adenopathy, which is unilateral in two thirds of cases, appears. Rapid lymphatic spread causes inflammation of both inguinal and femoral nodes. The inguinal ligament crossing the area of matted nodes creates the classical "groove" sign, which is considered to be pathognomonic of LGV (Fig. 17-2).[35] Continued lymphatic involvement results in grossly hypertrophied and edematous vulvar tissue and coloproctitis leading to scarring and stenosis. Diagnosis is established by culture of infected tissue or positive serologic test for LGV. However, culture techniques either from vaginal ulcers or material aspirated from inguinal buboes, yield positive results in only 24 to 30% of cases. Sowmini and colleagues recommended the use of minocycline 300 mg as a loading dose followed by 200 mg bid for 10 days to treat inguinal and femoral adenopathy as well as anorectal disease.[36] Chloramphenicol, erythromycin, and rifampin have also been advocated.[37]

Chancroid

Chancroid is an ulcerative disease of the vulva produced by the organism *Hemophilus ducreyi*. The characteristic vulvar lesions are ulcers that are soft and painful and that have a necrotic, purulent base. They are more frequently multiple than single and no induration is present adjacent to the ragged edges of the ulcer. The incubation period is 2 to 10 days. Chancroid is not a disease indigenous to Western culture, but endemic pockets now exist in both New York and Miami. This disease is spread by prostitutes, and outbreaks can be traced to these reservoirs of infection. As vaginal ulcerations persist, inguinal adenopathy becomes evident. The bubo is usually uni-

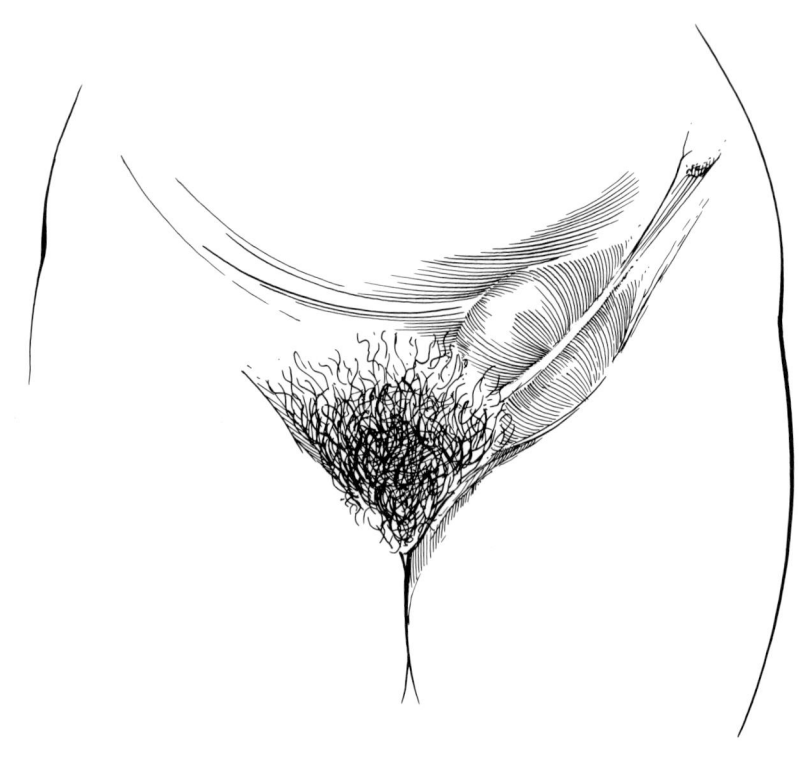

FIGURE 17–2
"Groove sign" in lymphogranuloma venereum.

lateral and if left untreated will rupture and discharge purulent necrotic material. A Gram stain of necrotic material from the base of an ulcer may show the characteristic "school of fish" or "railroad track" pattern of the coccobacillus (Fig. 17-3).[38] The organism is fastidious and requires hemin for growth. Exposure of the organism without favorable culture media will result in its death in 2 to 4 hours. Consequently, a culture must be obtained by directly plating material from the base of the ulcer to a specially enriched chocolate agar plate impregnated with vancomycin. In contrast, aspiration of material from a bubo will not result in laboratory confirmation of the disease. Recent advances in culture media and techniques have added significantly to our diagnostic abilities. The current recommendations from the Center for Disease Control for the treatment of chancroid include ceftriaxone 250 mg IM single-dose therapy; erythromycin 500 mg four times daily for 7 days; trimethoprim and sulfamethoxazole (160 and 800 mg), double strength, given twice a day for 7 days; and amoxicillin/clavulanic acid, 500 mg three times a day for 7 days. Recent studies have shown that ciprofloxin 500 mg bid for 3 days is effective.[39,40] There is evidence that chancroid and other ulcerative vaginal disease facilitate the transmission of the HIV virus.[39]

Granuloma Inguinale (Donovanosis)

Granuloma inguinale is an ulcerative disease of the vulva infrequently found in developing countries and found regularly in Asia and Australia. The causative organism is *Calymmatobacterium granulomatis,* an organism difficult to grow on artificial

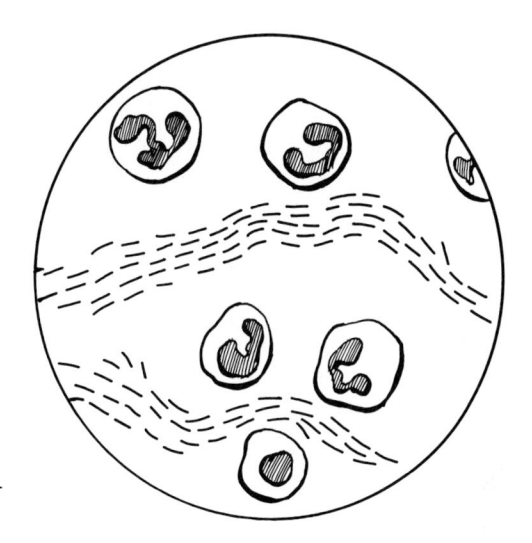

FIGURE 17-3
"Railroad track" pattern of cocco bacillus in chancroid.

media and therefore of uncertain classification. The organism gains entry into the host either from rectal contamination, autoinoculation, or sexual contact. The initial lesion is a papule that erodes to form an ulcer, increasing in size and penetration, extending laterally, and healing centrally with scarring. The process extends into lymphatics, causing swelling, elephantiasis and necrosis. Pseudobuboes are formed that resemble pustular inguinal adenopathy. Ironically, the process is generally painless and indolent. The diagnosis is made by creating a "crush" preparation of vulvar tissue. This is accomplished by obtaining a small amount of tissue by pressing a slide to the infected area or by taking a small tissue biopsy and "crushing" it between two slides. The tissue is spread thinly and then stained with Wright's stain. The pathognomonic sign of Donovanosis is the presence of blue or black bodies in the cytoplasm of large mononucleated cells (Fig. 17-4).[41] These are the Donovan bodies, which are vacuoles containing 20 to 30 organisms that are liberated after cell rupture. Established therapy is tetracycline 500 mg every 6 hours until all signs of the

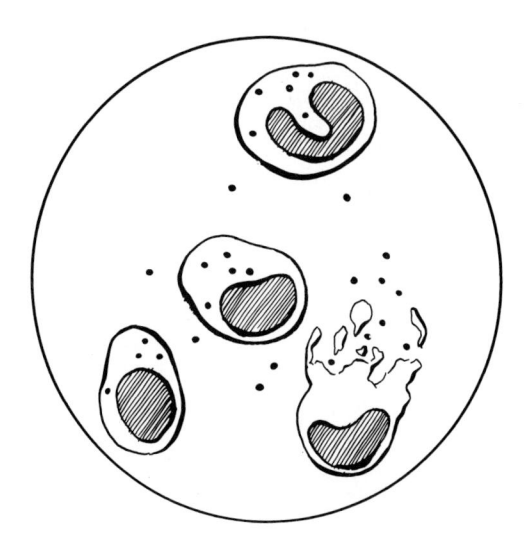

FIGURE 17-4
Donovan bodies.

disease have disappeared. Ampicillin 500 mg every 6 hours or erythromycin 500 mg every 6 hours is effective therapy during pregnancy. Chloramphenicol 500 mg every 8 hours and gentamicin 1 mg/kg every 12 hours is successful.[42] Saltzstein, Woodruff, and Novak have reported an increased incidence of carcinoma in patients with granuloma inguinale, as has Collins;[43,44] however, prophylactic vulvectomy has not been advocated.

Diagnostic Identification of Vulvar Ulcerative Disease

Herpes virus infection is characterized by multiple, painful, superficial ulcerations frequently surrounded by a red halo. The ulcers of chancroid are multiple, soft, deep, necrotic, and purulent. Syphilis produces a single, deep ulcer that is hard, painless, and indurated. The papule or ulcer of LGV is fleeting, and the disease is identified more easily by its large and matted lymph nodes. Granuloma inguinale is identified by its beefy, indurated, infected, healing, painless ulcerations and vulvar anatomic distortions. Syphilis is confirmed by a serologic test, LGV and HSV by culture; Granuloma inguinale, by a "crush" slide preparation stained with Wright's stain; and chancroid, by culture and complement fixation tests. Behcet's disease is suspected by a history of oral ulcers and ocular inflammation and Crohn's disease by a history of inflammatory bowel disease (Table 17-1).

Vaginitis and Vaginosis

Bacterial Vaginosis

Bacterial vaginosis (BV) is the most common cause of abnormal vaginal symptoms. The term *vaginosis* is more applicable than *vaginitis* because this condition is characterized by the displacement of the normal bacterial milieu of the vagina by a predominantly anaerobic bacterial flora. Symptoms of profuse vaginal discharge—milky in consistency or frothy, grayish in color, and foul in odor—are common,

TABLE 17-1
Clinical Characteristics of Vulvar Ulcers

	HSV	Syphilis	LGV	Chancroid	Granuloma
Appearance of lesion	Vesicles	Indurated hard, chancre	Ulcer	Soft, ulcer	Papule eroding to ulcer
Single or multiple	Multiple	Single	Single	Multiple	Variable
Painful or painless	Painful	Painless	Painful	Painful	Painless
Adenopathy	Firm, bilateral tender	Firm, bilateral nontender	Large buboes, "groove sign" unilateral	Unilateral	Pseudobubo
Laboratory identification	Culture	Serology	Complement fix or culture	Culture on special medium	"Crush" slide for Donovan bodies

although 50% of patients with BV have no abnormal symptoms. BV is present in nearly 20 to 30% of women attending gynecologic outpatient clinics.[45]

The condition was first described by Gardner and Dukes in 1955.[46] At that time, it was believed that the infection was caused by a single bacterium, *Haemophilus vaginalis*. Currently, the basis of the vaginal symptomatology is believed to be the conversion of the normal mixed aerobic and anaerobic bacterial symbiosis to a predominantly anaerobic vaginal flora. The etiology of this conversion has not been discovered.

The four criteria for the diagnosis of BV as described by Amsel[47] are

1. A thin homogeneous vaginal discharge
2. Vaginal pH of more than 4.7
3. Positive amine odor test
4. Presence of "clue" cells in a vaginal saline wet mount preparation.

The diagnosis of BV is suspected in the presence of a vaginal discharge with a foul odor. This symptom may be produced by a vaginal foreign body (usually a tampon) or by carcinoma; however, a careful pelvic examination excludes these diagnoses. The diagnosis is confirmed by examination of a saline wet mount from the vaginal discharge. A saline wet mount preparation is performed by mixing a sample of the vaginal discharge with one or two drops of saline on a glass slide, which is then covered by a cover slip. A second slide is prepared with 10% KOH and mixed with another sample of the discharge. After a few seconds of mixture with 10% KOH, the foul odor of the diamines, putrescine and cadaverine, is evident and the "whiff" test is considered positive. The first slide is examined microscopically under 400× magnification for the presence of "clue cells." These cells are vaginal squames with bacteria attached to their surface. Bacteria apparently "hanging off" the edge of the squamous cell constitute the pathognomonic finding of a true "clue cells." Most clinicians accept the positive "whiff" test and the observation of the "clue cells" as diagnostic of BV. The treatment of BV is metronidazole 500 mg orally twice a day for 7 days or clindamycin 300 mg orally twice a day for 7 days.[48] Partners of women with recurrent or intractable disease should be concomitantly treated. Both metronidazole and clindamycin have been formulated in vaginal creams and are now available commercially. The treatment of BV in pregnancy is complicated by the mutagenic and carcinogenic potential of metronidazole and is therefore controversial.

Candidiasis

Candidiasis is the second most frequent cause of vaginitis. In the United States, 13 million cases of mycotic vulvovaginitis occur annually.[49] No other type of vaginitis causes as much physical discomfort as does candidal vulvovaginitis. Signs and symptoms include a thick, curdy, white discharge associated with burning, itching, irritation, and vaginal pain. These symptoms are most likely caused by alcohol produced by the yeast in its anaerobic metabolic cycle. The organism is found on mucosal body surfaces predominantly in the mouth and gastrointestinal tract and in the seminal vesicle of the male. These body cavities in the sexual partners may be reservoirs of infection from which the vagina is colonized.[50] From 1963 to 1987, *Candida al-*

bicans was the most frequent pathogen present in candidal vulvovaginitis (84.2%) followed by *C. tropicalis* (5.3%) and *C. glabrata* (5.5%).[51] However, the incidence of non*albicans* species has been increasing. The importance of this selection becomes apparent in aspects of therapy because of the resistance of the non-*albicans* species to antimycotic therapy.[52]

The diagnosis of candidiasis is suspected by observation of the organism on saline wet mount or KOH preparations and is established by candidal culture. Attempted diagnosis by observation of the vaginal discharge leads to error. Anaerobic *lactobacilli, mobiluncus* spp., and *actinomycosis* all produce similar vaginal discharges. Sabouraud's dextrose media impregnated with chloramphenicol is streaked with the vaginal discharge and incubated at room temperature. In the nonrecurrent, infrequent vaginal yeast infection, therapy begins immediately while awaiting culture results. In the recurrent, or relapsing mycotic vulvovaginitis, cultures are obtained of the mouths, rectums, ejaculate, and vagina of the sexual partners. Therapy is then directed to the area of colonization. Vaginal therapy includes the imidazoles and more currently the triazoles; oral therapy, clotrimazole oral troches or nystatin pastilles. Therapy for gastrointestinal candidiasis consists of nystatin tablets or powder or ketoconazole; that for ejaculate candidiasis, ketoconazole, itraconazole or fluconazole tablets.

Trichomoniasis

Trichomoniasis is the third most frequent cause of vaginitis; its incidence and prevalence are declining. *Trichomonas vaginalis* affects approximately 3 million American women annually.[53] The symptoms of this disease are vaginal itching, burning, and discharge, which is often described as green and frothy. Pelvic examination discloses abnormal vaginal discharge with minimal vaginal or vulvar reddening or other signs of irritation. The cervix exhibits reddened punctate spots, the so-called strawberry cervix or colpitis macularis (Fig. 17-5). In active disease, the saline wet mount preparation displays the active flagellated protozoan, many white blood cells and relatively less squamous cells. However, in many studies of trichomoniasis, the wet prep is diagnostic in less than 50% of cases. Consequently, other tests, such as culture, direct immunofluorescence, direct immunoassay, and latex agglutination tests, have been utilized.[54] An inflammatory saline wet mount preparation should prompt the following diagnostic considerations: trichomoniasis, herpes, gonorrhea, chlamydia, or other sexually transmitted diseases.

The treatment of trichomoniasis has been facilitated with the introduction of the nitroimidazoles. Conventional treatment is 250 mg of metronidazole orally three times a day for 1 week. A single 2-g dose is effective in women but is less so in men. Although metronidazole is the only nitroimidazole available in the United States, other compounds (eg, tinidazole, ornidazole, nimorazole and others) are available worldwide. Metronidazole resistance is treated initially by increasing dose. Maximum doses of 3 to 3.5 g of metronidazole have been given daily, and intravenous doses of 2 g every 6 to 8 hours for 3 days are also effective. In very high doses metronidazole is toxic. Peripheral neuropathy can occur especially in patients with collagen disease. Metronidazole crosses the placenta, and although there is no evidence

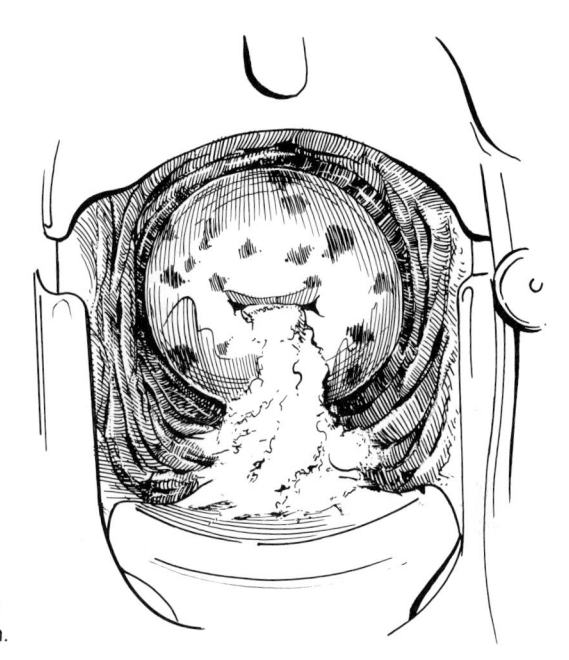

FIGURE 17–5
"Strawberry cervix" in trichomonas infection.

of teratogenicity, the oncologic potential to the developing fetus has not been adequately evaluated. Metronidazole should not be used in the first trimester of pregnancy, but a single 2-g dose in the second or third trimester appears safe.

Mobiluncus Vaginitis

Mobiluncus spp. is a tiny flagellated bacterium that is present in the vagina in association with other anaerobic organisms found in bacterial vaginosis. Three species have been described: *M. curtisii*, *M. holmesii*, and *M. mulieris*. Morphologically, these organisms are comma or sausage shaped, with a varying number of flagella arising from their concave surface.[55] Phase contrast microscopy is required to identify these organisms. Cultures are available but are generally unnecessary because the characteristic tumbling motion of these organisms seen under the phase contrast microscope is diagnostic. The short curved rod (SCR), the *M. curtisii* organism, is 1 to 2 millimicrometers in length; the long curved rod (LCR), the *M. mulieris* species, is 3 to 4 millimicrometers in length. *M. curtisii* is treated with clindamycin 300 mg three times a day for 7 days. Therapeutic failures respond to rifampin 600 mg in a single, oral, daily dose for 14 days or applications of 2% *aqueous* gentian violet applied as a vaginal paint every 2 to 3 days for three doses. *M. mulieris* is treated with 500 mg of metronidazole four times a day for 7 days or clindamycin vaginal cream. *Mobiluncus* spp. can be found in seminal fluid from infected consorts, and therefore partners should be treated with similar dosages.

Although *Mobiluncus* vaginitis is seldom seen as an isolated infection, because of its association with bacterial vaginosis, a pure culture of *M. curtisii* can result when BV is treated with metronidazole. Since this organism is resistant to metronidazole, bacterial selection creates a pure culture of the SCR. In this circumstance the discharge is white, creamy, and glistening, and to the trained observer it is diagnostic.

Vaginal Foreign Bodies

The ambulatory care physician is frequently required to treat patients with symptoms caused by vaginal foreign bodies. Unusual case histories of misplaced vaginal objects are common. The symptom complex of a very foul vaginal odor with profuse discharge makes the diagnosis likely. The odor is extremely fetid and is recognizable to experienced medical attendants. Although the forgotten tampon is the most common foreign body found in the vagina, the type of foreign body most often relates to the age of the patient. In childhood, playthings such as crayons or small pieces of toys, marbles, and so on, are more common; in the menstrual years, tampons, diaphragms, cervical caps, sponges, condoms, IUDs, applicator tips, or sexual devices predominate; in later years, pessaries or sexual aids are encountered.

Discovery of a vaginal foreign body rests on the pelvic examination. In adult women, the examination is not difficult; in a child, sedation or anesthesia may be necessary. Nevertheless, in a child of any age, vaginal discharge with foul odor requires a complete pelvic examination. General anesthesia, and vaginal examination with a small nasal speculum and dressing forceps is all that is needed (Fig. 17-6). The natural reluctance to administer general anesthesia to a small child should not deter the physician from performing a proper gynecologic examination. If no foreign body is found, smears and cultures can be obtained to establish the correct diagnosis.

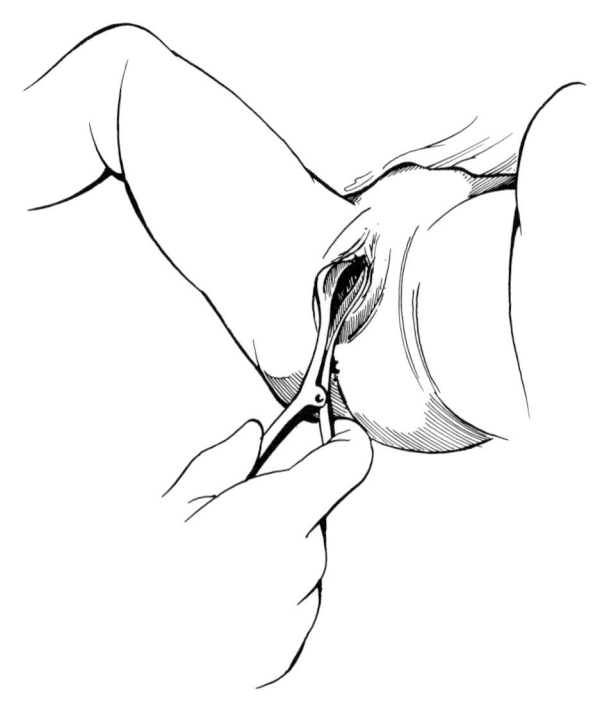

FIGURE 17-6
Nasal speculum for examination of child's vagina.

The treatment of a vaginal foreign body is its removal. In almost all cases the use of vaginal creams or douches is unnecessary. If the odor is particularly offensive, cleansing with a commercial douche product is permissible. In most cases odor and discharge disappear rapidly after the removal of the foreign object and no further therapy is required.

In some instances, however, the presence of a vaginal object exacerbates infection with a preexisting vaginal pathogen. The most common of these are gonorrhea, chlamydia, and bacterial vaginosis, including mobiluncus. If removal of the extraneous matter does not effect rapid resolution, then attention to other causes of vaginal inflammation or infection is required. Rarely, vaginal foreign bodies have created major complications. Neglected foreign bodies have produced vesicovaginal fistulas with urinary incontinence and cystitis.[56] Unusual cases of pelvic trauma due to vaginal foreign bodies include a report of periarticular irritation of the hip joint due to pervaginal wooden sticks inserted in an abortion attempt,[57] erosion of a pessary through the bladder with a large vesicovaginal fistula, and stone formation due to both intravesical and intravaginal nonabsorbable suture material with subsequent vesicovaginal fistula formation.[58]

REFERENCES

1. Masters W, Johnson V. Human sexual response, p 43. Boston: Little, Brown, 1966
2. Davies JW. Bartholin cyst. Surg Gynecol Obstet 86:329, 1948
3. Sarrel PM, Steege JF, Maltzer M et al. Pain during sex response due to the occlusion of the Bartholin gland duct. Obstet Gynecol 62:261, 1983
4. Word B. New instrument for office treatment of cyst and abscess of Bartholin's gland. JAMA 190:777, 1964
5. Davis GD. Management of Bartholin duct cysts with the carbon dioxide laser. Obstet Gynecol 65:279, 1985
6. Lashgari M, Chong A, Bruno R. Bartholin duct cyst revisited. J Gynecol Surg 5:381, 1989
7. Gardner SS, McKay M. Seborrhea, psoriasis and the papulosquamous dermatoses. Prim Care 16:739, 1989
8. Bergbrant IM, Faergemann J. The role of *Pityrosporum ovale* in seborrheic dermatitis. Semin Dermatol 9:262, 1990
9. Sadick NS, McNutt NS, Kaplan MH. Papulosquamous dermatoses of AIDS. J Am Acad Dermatol 22:1270, 1990
10. McGrath J, Murphy GM. The control of seborrheic dermatitis and dandruff by antipityrosporal drugs. Drugs 41:178, 1991
11. Menter A, Barker JN. Psoriasis in practice. Lancet 338:231, 1991
12. Robertson IM, Jordan JM, Whitlock FA. Emotions and skin. II: The conditioning of scratch responses in cases of lichen simplex. Br J Dermatol 92:407, 1975
13. Murtagh J. Patient education. Pityriasis rosea. Aust Fam Physician 19:576, 1990
14. Graham R. What is pityriasis rosea? Practitioner 233:555, 1989
15. Singh G. Atopy in lichen simplex (neurodermatitis circumscripta). Br J Dermatol 898:625, 1973
16. Jungell P. Oral lichen planus. A review. Int J Oral Maxillofac Surg 20:129, 1991
17. Walsh LJ, Savage NW, Ishii T, Seymour GJ. Immunopathogenesis of oral lichen planus. J Oral Pathol Med 19:389, 1990
18. Katzenelson V, Lotem M, Sandbank M. Famila lichen planus. Dermatologica 180:166, 1990

19. Patterson JW. The spectrum of lichenoid dermatitis. J Cutan Pathol 18:67, 1991
20. Oates JK, Rown D. Desquamative inflammatory vaginitis. A review. Genitourin Med 66:275, 1990
21. Kaufman RH, Friedrich EG. Erosive lichen planus of the vulva. In: Horowitz BJ, Mardh PA (eds): Vaginitis and Vaginosis, p 159. New York: John Wiley, 1991
22. Burgess JA, Johnson BD, Sommers E. Pharmacological management of recurrent oral mucosal ulceration. Drugs 39:54, 1990
23. Dabski C. Lichen planus. Am Fam Physician 39:120, 1989
24. Wallace HJ. Lichen sclerosis et atrophicus. Trans St Johns Hosp Dermatol Soc 57:9, 1971
25. Tremaine RD, Miller RA. Lichen sclerosis et atrophicus. Int J Dermatol 28:10, 1989
26. Purcell KG, Spencer LV, Simpson PM et al. HLA antigens in lichen sclerosis et atrophicus. Arch Dermatol 126:1043, 1990
27. Friedrich EG, Kalra PS. Serum levels of sex hormones in vulvar lichen sclerosis, and the effect of topical testosterone. N Engl J Med 310:488, 1984
28. Paslin D. Treatment of lichen sclerosis with topical dihydrotestosterone. Obstet Gynecol 78:1046, 1991
29. Mann MS, Kaufman RH. Erosive lichen planus of the vulva. Clin Obstet Gynecol 34:605,1991
30. Crohn BB, Ginsburg L, Oppenheimer GD. Regional ileitis. JAMA 99:1323, 1932
31. Behçet H. Uber rezidivierende apthose durch ein Virus verusauchte Geschwure am mund, am Auge, und an den Genitalien. Dermatol Wochenschr 105:1152, 1937
32. Curth HO. Behçet's syndrome, abortive form (?) (recurrent oral aphthous lesions and recurrent genital ulcerations). Arch Dermatol 54:481, 1946
33. O'Duffy JD, Carney A, Deodhar S. Behçet's disease. Am Intern Med 75:561, 1971
34. Strachan RW, Wigzell FW. Polyarthritis in Behçet's multiple symptom complex. Ann Rheum Dis 22:26, 1963
35. Schachter J. Lymphogranuloma venereum and other non-ocular *Chlamydia trachomatis* in non-gonorrheal urethritis. In: Hobson D, Holmes KK (eds): Washington, DC: American Society for Microbiology, 1977
36. Sowmini CN, Gopalan KN, Rao GC. Minocycline in the treatment of lymphogranuloma venereum. J Am Vener Dis Assoc 2:19, 1976
37. Perine PL, Osaba AO. Lymphogranuloma venereum. In: Holmes KK, Mardh PA (eds): Sexually Transmitted Diseases, 2nd ed, p 195. New York: McGraw-Hill, 1990
38. Willis SE. Chancroid. Primary Care 17:145, 1990
39. Schmid GP. Treatment of chancroid, 1989. Rev Infect Dis 12:S580, 1990
40. Megran DW. Quinolones in the treatment of sexually transmitted diseases. Clin Invest Med 12:50, 1989
41. Hart G. Donovanosis. In: Holmes KK, Mardh PA (eds): Sexually Transmitted Diseases, 2nd ed, p 273. New York: McGraw-Hill, 1990
42. Faro S. Lymphogranuloma venereum, chancroid and granuloma inguinale. Obstet Gynecol Clin North Am 16:517, 1989
43. Saltzstein SL, Woodruff JD, Novak ER. Postgranulomatous carcinoma of the vulva. Obstet Gynecol 7:80, 1956
44. Collins CG, Collins JH, Nelson EW, Smith RC, MacCallum EA. Malignant tumors involving the vulva. Am J Obstet Gynecol 62:1198, 1951
45. Larsson PG. Bacterial vaginosis. Linkoping, Sweden: Linkoping University Medical Dissertations, 339:5, 1991
46. Gardner HL, Dukes CD. *Haemophilus vaginalis* raginitis: a newly defined specific infection previously classified "nonspecific" vaginitis. Am J Obstet Gynecol 69:962, 1955
47. Amsel R, Totten PA, Spiegel CA, Chen KCS, Eschenbach DA, Holmes KK. Nonspecific vaginitis. Diagnostic criteria and microbial and epidemiological considerations. Am J Obstet Gynecol 74:14, 1983

48. Thomason JL, Gelbart SM, Scaglione NJ. Bacterial vaginosis. Current review with indications for asymptomatic therapy. Am J Obstet Gynecol 165:1210, 1991
49. Weisberg M. Considerations in therapy for vulvovaginal candidiasis: when and whom to treat. In: Sobel J (ed): Clinical Perspectives: Terconazole, an Advance in Vulvovaginal Candidiasis Therapy, p 2. New York: McGraw-Hill, 1988
50. Horowitz BJ, Mardh PA (eds): Vaginitis and Vaginosis, p 227. New York: Wiley-Liss, 1991
51. Horowitz BJ. Mycotic vulvovaginitis: a broad overview. Am J Obstet Gynecol 165:1188, 1991
52. Horowitz BJ. Candidiasis: speciation and therapy. Curr Probl Obstet Gynecol Fertil 12:233, 1990
53. Kent HL. Epidemiology of vaginitis. Am J Obstet Gynecol 165:1168, 1991
54. Lossick JG, Kent HL. Trichomoniasis: trends in diagnosis and management. Am J Obstet Gynecol 165:1217, 1991
55. Fox A, Phillips I. Two curved rods in non-specific vaginitis. In: Mardh PA, Taylor-Robinson (eds): Bacterial Vaginosis, p 93. Stockholm: Almqvist & Wiksell, 1984
56. Binstock MA, Semrad N, Dubow L, Watring W. Combined vesicovaginal-ureterovaginal fistulas associated with a vaginal foreign body. Obstet Gynecol 76:818, 1990
57. Bhosale PB, Dhir RS, Tejwani NC. An unusual case of hip disability. J Postgrad Med 35:232, 1989
58. Goldstein I, Wise GJ, Tancer ML. A vesicovaginal fistula and intravesical foreign body. A rare case of the neglected pessary. Am J Obstet Gynecol 163:589, 1990

Obstetric and Gynecologic Emergencies, edited by Guy I. Benrubi. J.B. Lippincott Company, Philadelphia © 1994.

CHAPTER 18

Menorrhagia and Abnormal Vaginal Bleeding

Steven J. Sondheimer

An adolescent faced with her first menstrual period may perceive menorrhagia (excessively heavy menstrual bleeding) as dangerously heavy, whereas a woman with a life-long history of heavy menstrual periods might reach fairly severe iron-deficient anemia without actually recognizing her condition. There is no simple way to measure menstrual blood loss, and so this is a subjective observation of the patient that either her periods are much heavier, are lasting more days, or have changed color or type of flow. The development of anemia is a criterion for diagnosis. Women who consistently have greater than 80 mL of blood loss during menstruation will have lower serum iron levels and will often be anemic. Menorrhagia has been clinically defined as menses lasting for longer than 7 days or menstrual blood loss exceeding 60 mL.[1] The emergency department physician faced with the acute complaint of a heavy menstrual period has to evaluate the patient as he or she would any patient with acute blood loss. If the patient shows evidence of hypovolemia or severe anemia, then acute management is necessary. The gynecologist commonly deals with abnormal vaginal bleeding or chronically heavy periods leading to the slow development of iron deficient anemia. Not all the menstrual effluvium is blood, and heavy endometrial fluid and tissue loss can occasionally occur without much actual blood loss.

Normal Menstruation

The interval from ovulation to menstruation, the luteal phase, prepares the endometrium for pregnancy or orderly sloughing. Controlled by the ovarian corpus luteum, it is also called the secretory phase because progesterone secretion by the corpus luteum changes the endometrium from mitotically active proliferative to mitotically inactive secretory endometrium receptive to embryo implantation. The first issue of the journal *Fertility and Sterility* in 1950 described the sequential and repetitive events occurring in the endometrium during this secretory phase.[2] Menstruation itself is an abnormal event, since it does not occur during pregnancy or lactation.

If pregnancy does not occur, the corpus luteum regresses. The fall in estrogen and progesterone initiates the series of vascular events within the endometrium that lead to the separation of the functional from the ever-present basal layer of endometrium. The bleeding, the sloughing of endometrium, and the release of prostaglandins are all part of normal menstruation from this sequentially prepared endometrium. Artificial destruction of the corpus luteum causing a fall in estrogen and progesterone or the use of a progesterene receptor blocker (Ru486) will lead to premature menstruation. Administration of prostaglandin F_2-alpha will also lead to endometrial necrosis and vaginal bleeding.

The fall in estrogen and progesterone causes prostaglandins to initiate vasospasm. The vasospasm leads to cell necrosis, cell death, bleeding, and separation of the functional from the basal endometrium.

The term *dysfunctional uterine bleeding* (DUB) traditionally has been used to describe acute heavy bleeding that we now call menorrhagia. Dysfunctional bleeding was considered the acute event. With a more complete understanding of the hormonal events related to menstrual bleeding and more precise characterization of the etiology of most episodes of menorrhagia, the use of the term *dysfunctional uterine bleeding* is anachronistic. More descriptive terms such as *abnormal vaginal bleeding, heavy abnormal vaginal bleeding,* or *menorrhagia* appear to be more useful as descriptions of the symptom that then evokes the differential diagnosis. When the term *dysfunctional uterine bleeding* is used today, it usually connotes an episode or episodes of heavy bleeding due to anovulation.[1] Since anovulation is only one of a number of causes of menorrhagia, it is probably best not to use DUB to describe the event.

Anovulation

Failure of ovulation, and therefore lack of progesterone effect on the endometrium, can generally be divided into two broad and overlapping categories, low estrogen and normal estrogen. As a general rule, low estrogen causes amenorrhea or light infrequent bleeding, whereas normal estrogen anovulation can cause either amenorrhea, infrequent bleeds, or menorrhagia. Anovulation with heavy vaginal bleeding is most often associated with polycystic ovarian syndrome, obesity, postpubertal cycles, or cycles in women in their later reproductive years as FSH levels begin to rise and ovarian reserve decreases. Patients with polycystic ovarian syndrome (PCO) have normal estrogen anovulation. Their symptoms begin shortly after puberty and often (but not always) include androgen excess symptoms, such as hirsutism or acne. The diagnosis is made by looking at the total clinical and laboratory picture and not at the results of a single test. The diagnosis is made by excluding less frequent disorders such as 21-hydroxylase deficiency, adult onset congenital adrenal hyperplasia, estrogen-producing ovarian tumors, adrenal tumors, or Cushing syndrome—all of which can cause irregular or heavy bleeds.

Excessive weight gain and obesity may cause anovulation independent of an underlying PCO. These patients often have heavy anovulatory bleeds, since they have normal estrogen levels. Liver disease and renal failure patients can occasionally have heavy bleeds due to both anovulation and clotting defects, but they may respond to treatment of anovulation. Thyroid disease also has been recognized as a cause of anovulatory bleeding. Weight loss, stress, exercise-induced hyperprolactinemia and incipient ovarian failure are all common causes of anovulation but most often without menorrhagia. However, with milder forms of these problems or during the recovery phase of treatment there may be a PCO-like heavy anovulatory bleed.

Hypothyroidism

Severe hypothyroidism (myxedema) often results in anovulatory intermenstrual bleeding and menorrhagia. Most patients with early or mild hypothyroidism will have normal periods. However, one report found 20% of menorrhagic women to have early or potential hypothyroidism, and these women responded to thyroid replacement with the disappearance of their menorrhagia within 6 months.[3] This study was not controlled; a larger, better designed study is needed to determine the role of mild primary, subclinical hypothyroidism in menorrhagia. Clearly, there is no place for routine use of thyroid replacement therapy for treatment of abnormal vaginal bleeding, but at least a TSH level should be obtained. Thyroid stimulatory hormone assay is now accurate and when even slightly elevated, with normal thyroxine levels and no overt symptoms of hypothyroidism, may be found with mild primary hypothyroidism. A TRH stimulatory test (increased TSH response) will diagnose others with mild primary hypothyroidism.

Pregnancy

Pregnancy and its complications most commonly cause abnormal vaginal bleeding in the reproductive-age woman and should always be considered in the differential diagnosis. Pregnancy tests, both urine and blood, detect human chorionic gonadotropin (HCG) produced by the placenta and are often positive (or at least equivocal) even before the missed period. Placental HCG is not produced until after implantation. Enzyme-linked immunoassays that assay the whole HCG molecule are sensitive to 25 mIU/mL or less. If first morning or concentrated urine is used, the urine tests (RAMP, Monoclonal Antibodies—Sunnyvale, CA; or ICON, Hybritech—San Diego; and others) are comparable to serum assays. The UCG has been reported to be positive in 95% of cases in which the serum is between 5 and 25 mIU/mL. Fortunately, almost all ectopic pregnancies will have a positive pregnancy test.[1,4]

Bleeding in pregnancy and its treatment differ by gestational age, so in addition to determining whether the patient is pregnant or not, it is important to determine approximately how large the uterus is and how far the pregnancy has progressed. If the patient is in the late second or third trimester of pregnancy the differential diagnosis includes placenta previa and abruption. Both of these are acute obstetric emergencies and need to be handled in the delivery room. Pelvic examination should be avoided in the late second or third trimester because of the possibility of disrupting a placenta previa. Abdominal ultrasound is central to the diagnosis of third-trimester bleeding.

A rare cause of bleeding in pregnancy is cervical pregnancy presenting as painless uterine bleeding in a pregnant woman, with a softened enlarged cervix usually as big as the fundus, with a snug internal os and a partially opened external os. Ultrasound shows an empty uterus with well-defined uterine stripe and the gestational sac in the cervix (Fig. 18-1).[5]

Though hysterectomy is often required to treat the hemorrhage associated with cervical pregnancy, a number of techniques have been described to attempt to prevent this. Preoperative angiographic uterine artery embolization, methotrexate chemotherapy, uterine artery ligation, hypogastric artery ligation, intercervical balloon tamponade, and placement of a circlage with an intercervical obturator have all been reported to be successful in selected cervical pregnancies.[1,2]

Endovaginal ultrasound is an exciting tool to help diagnose abnormal vaginal

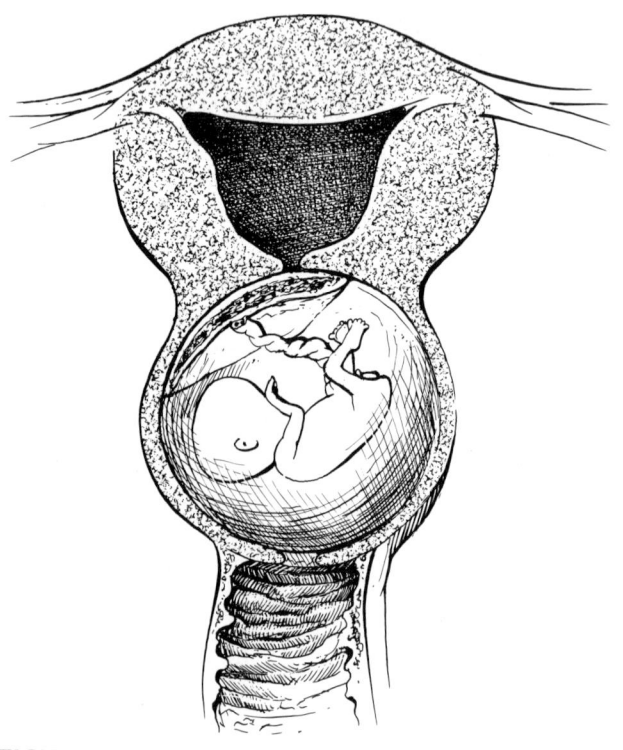

FIGURE 18–1
Cervical pregnancy.

bleeding. Its precise use has not been determined, but it may become a routine part of most gynecologic examinations. Its value increases when used by a person with skill. But a nonradiologist, particularly an experienced gynecologist, can master endovaginal ultrasound. For example, the uncommon but potentially disastrous condition of cervical pregnancy can be diagnosed preoperatively. With preoperative diagnosis there is a better chance of preparation possibly preventing the need for hysterectomy.

Bleeding Disorders

Bleeding disorders need to be considered as a cause of ovulatory menorrhagia, particularly among adolescents.[1] Even without a prior history of bleeding problems, menorrhagia can be the first clue to von Willebrand's disease or, less commonly, prothrombin deficiency, idiopathic thrombocytopenic purpura, or platelet disorder. Easy bruisability with menorrhagia is occasionally the first sign of acute leukemia. Iatrogenic menorrhagia may be due to chemotherapy, anticoagulants, or excess aspirin ingestion.

Patients with coagulopathies either from malignancy or platelet dysfunction who present with acute heavy bleeding still need a diagnostic evaluation, including pregnancy test and endometrial sampling. Use of platelet replacement will stop the acute bleeding; then the endometrium can be chronically suppressed with either danazol, a GnRH analog, or a progestational agent. The woman on an anticoagulant whose bleeding cannot be stopped presents a difficult dilemma. Often the bleeding will stop spontaneously, but occasionally operative intervention with D&C and endometrial ablation is necessary. Once bleeding is controlled, endometrial suppression is begun.

In adolescents with bleeding heavy enough to require hospitalization, 75% of the time the etiology is anovulation. The second most common cause is primary coagulopathy. Other cases are due to pregnancy complications, oral contraceptives, trauma, systemic illness (e.g., liver or renal disease), and rarely, malignancy.[6] Since DES use in pregnancy ceased after 1971, clear cell adenocarcinoma of the cervix or vagina in young women has become rare. In adolescents trauma needs to be considered in the differential diagnosis, but if it is the etiology, the laceration is usually readily identifiable. Birth control pills cause decreased menstrual flow, or irregular light to moderate flow. They are an uncommon cause of heavy bleeding.

Fibroids

Ovulatory heavy menstrual bleeding is often due to an anatomic disorder and so is not "dysfunctional" and can be due to adenomyosis, endometrial polyp, submucous fibroid, or endometritis. Intramural or submucous fibroids are the most common of these causes. Fibroids are suspected by history and examination and diagnosed by hysteroscopy, hysterosalpingogram, ultrasound, or pelvic magnetic resonance imaging.

GnRH agonist therapy has been reported to produce amenorrhea in two thirds of women with fibroids and gives relief to 30% of these women who present with menorrhagia. Increased or more frequent administration of agonist to bring estradiol below 20 pg/mL often causes amenorrhea, but severe vaginal hemorrhage due to necrosis of a submucous fibroid is reported to occur in 2% of women with submucous fibroids.[1,2,7]

Unfortunately, with the cessation of agonist therapy fibroids regrow and the bleeding symptoms usually return; however, agonist therapy may give the patient an opportunity to rebuild her hemoglobin, donate autologous blood, and possibly have a vaginal or laparoscopically directed vaginal hysterectomy rather than an abdominal hysterectomy.

The finding of an enlarged myomatous uterus does not eliminate anovulation as a coexisting condition. If the menorrhagia is regular, predictable, and associated with premenstrual awareness, then the patient is probably ovulating, and bleeding is due to fibroids. A serum progesterone approximately a week before the menses or a basal body temperature chart will help diagnose ovulation. If the cycles are anovulatory, long-term medical therapy may be successful. Failure to control bleeding with cyclic oral contraceptives suggests the need to investigate if a submucous fibroid is present.

Hysterectomy should be reserved for those with vaginal bleeding severe enough to cause anemia, to cause hypovolemia, or to affect the patient's quality of life. Hysterectomies are often done for heavy menstrual bleeding supposedly in response to failure of medical treatment, even though the patient is not anemic and no pathology is present. The patient may have a fear of cancer. An attempt should be made to explain to these patients prior to surgery that this bleeding is not due to cancer. If myomas are the cause of the bleeding, myomectomy—either abdominally or, if possible, by hysteroscopically directed resection—will reduce menstrual flow.[8]

Essential Menorrhagia

Essential menorrhagia is defined as heavy periods without an etiology that occurs in ovulatory patients without coagulopathy or uterine pathology. These women are not hormonally different from those with normal blood loss, and some women who complain of menorrhagia will not actually have excess menstrual loss. Those with proven ovulatory menorrhagia probably have an as yet unidentified problem with prostaglandin dynamics, endometrial regeneration, or steroid receptor activity.[1]

Women with an inert or copper-containing intrauterine device, such as the Paraguard, will have an average cyclic blood loss of 60 mL and will occasionally need iron to prevent anemia.

Birth control pills will decrease blood loss by 50% in most of these patients. Nonsteroidal anti-inflammatory agents (though their use may seem counterintuitive), such as mefenamic acid, ibuprofen, and naproxen, when used four times a day throughout menstruation all have been shown to have some effect on essential or IUD menorrhagia not due to fibroids.[1,2,7] Antifibrinolytic agents such as epsilon-amino caproic acid and tranexamic acid have GI side-effects and carry a risk of intra-arterial thrombosis, which keeps them from being considered as alternatives. Ergot derivatives do not work in the nonpregnant uterus and should not be used to treat menorrhagia.

A 20-year-old patient with essential menorrhagia after liver transplant and with normal coagulation studies was successfully treated with a daily subcutaneous GnRH analog, creating a hypoestrogenic amenorrheic state. Then transdermal estrogen and cyclic medroxyprogesterone acetate were added back to prevent short- and long-term hypoestrogenic side-effects.[1] This is an example of the modern use of analogs, but there is still no prospective study of how frequently this will be effective and in which situation heavy bleeding might occur and be difficult to control without surgery.

Pharmacologic induction of an amenorrheic state is possible both with a GnRH analog and with oral danazol. Danazol, an androgenic steroid, besides inhibiting pituitary gonadotrophs and directly inhibiting ovarian steroidogenesis, also directly suppresses endometrial growth. The anabolic effects of danazol have also been used to stimulate platelet and blood count. Approximately 85% of women using danazol have side-effects, most commonly weight gain. Other androgenic side-effects occur in less than 10% of patients. Just as with agonist therapy, menorrhagia can occur or worsen. The usual dose of danazol is 600 to 800 mg daily.

GnRH analogs suppress estradiol levels more markedly than danazol, and so hot flushes, vaginal dryness, and mood changes are more common. Chronic administration increases the risk of osteoporosis. Adding back a small amount of estrogen and progesterone may be an approach to overcoming this problem in those patients who require long-term GnRH analog therapy. GnRH analogs are available as daily subcutaneous, monthly intramuscular depot, or twice daily intranasal administration. In patients with coagulation problems the intranasal spray can be used.

Endometrial Cancer

Adenocarcinoma of the endometrium is the most important consideration in the postmenopausal patient with any vaginal bleeding.[1] When endometrial hyperplasia with atypia or adenocarcinoma develops in women before 40, it is usually associated with obesity or chronic anovulation due to polycystic ovarian syndrome. Risks for endometrial cancer include early menarche, late menopause, obesity, chronic anovulation, estrogen-secreting ovarian tumors, long-term exposure to unopposed estrogen (not birth control pills, which are actually protective), or a history of breast cancer. Premenopausal women who have menorrhagia, a decreased menstrual interval, or intermenstrual bleeding need to be evaluated for endometrial carcinoma or a premalignant endometrium. The Pap smear cannot be used as a tool to evaluate the endometrium reliably, though the finding of atypical endometrial cells in a nonpregnant woman's Pap smear requires endometrial sampling. In premenopausal women office endometrial sampling can usually replace the D&C. However, the postmenopausal patient requires both endometrial biopsy and endocervical curettage.

The American College of Obstetricians and Gynecologists (ACOG) lists the outpatient office evaluation of women suspected of having endometrial cancer (Table 18-1).

Endometrial sampling can be performed in the office or emergency department. Disposable endometrial suction curettes such as the Pipelle are reliable, well tolerated, and safe.[1,2]

TABLE 18-1
ACOG List of Outpatient Office Evaluation

Complete speculum and bimanual pelvic examination including rectovaginal examination
Pap smear
Biopsy of any suspicious genital lesion
Stool test for occult bleeding
Endometrial sampling (biopsy)

Cervical dysplasia and early cervical cancer may be associated with postcoital or abnormal bleeding. This is probably due to cervicitis. Cervical lesions causing menorrhagia usually are grossly visible and need to be directly biopsied.

Abnormal Vaginal Bleeding

Patients with abnormal vaginal bleeding less than menorrhagia do not need treatment for their bleeding per se but do need evaluation to help diagnose possible pregnancy and its complications, such as ectopic pregnancy; vaginal, uterine, or ovarian malignancy; gonorrhea; chlamydia; pelvic inflammatory disease; or endometriosis.

As a minimum a complete history, physical examination, pregnancy test, complete blood count, Pap smear, and culture for gonorrhea and chlamydia should be done. Vaginal ultrasound for evaluation of the uterus and ovary is helpful. Endometrial sampling if the pregnancy test is negative and the patient is over 35, or when under 35 with a life-long history of anovulation, such as polycystic ovarian syndrome, is part of the diagnostic work-up.

Patients can use a menstrual calendar and basal body temperature chart to record their episodes of bleeding. This will help differentiate ovulatory from anovulatory bleeding. Cyclic ovulatory menses with interval abnormal bleeding suggests uterine polyps, cervicitis, endometritis, or endometriosis.

Sexual abuse is presently recognized as a common cause of bleeding in children and can be disclosed by a sensitive interview.[1]

In women at high risk for sexually transmitted disease—such as the young, unmarried, or those of lower socioeconomic status or with a new sexual partner—irregular menses may motivate them to seek evaluation, and this is a good opportunity to screen for gonorrhea and chlamydia of the cervix and to look for clinical evidence of pelvic inflammatory disease (PID).[1] Though cervicitis, PID, and endometriosis may cause abnormal, irregular, or prolonged bleeding, they are seldom a cause of acute menorrhagia.

Evaluation

The initial laboratory evaluation establishes the degree of blood loss and the possibility of pregnancy with a blood count and pregnancy test. If the bleeding is recurrent or severe, additional tests to obtain include thyroid function tests, both T_4 and

TSH; coagulation studies, such as prothrombin time (PT); partial thromboplastin time (PTT); platelet count; bleeding time; and liver function tests. Particularly in the adolescent a bleeding time may eventually be necessary to determine if von Willebrand's disease is present. Evaluation for polycystic ovarian syndrome or other endocrinopathies requires thyroid function tests, testosterone, prolactin, LH, and FSH levels, but not necessarily at the time of the evaluation for the acute bleed. Vaginal and abdominal probe pelvic ultrasound will suggest and diagnose anatomic abnormalities. Magnetic resonance imaging (MRI) is a sensitive radiologic technique to localize fibroids or uterine anomalies. Uterine endometrial sampling must be done where endometrial hyperplasia or cancer is possible. This is also an opportunity to obtain a GC and chlamydia culture and possibly a Pap smear. A cervical lesion should be directly biopsied, and a pap smear should not be used to diagnose it. Hysteroscopy has added to the diagnostic accuracy of dilation and curettage.

Treatment

Anovulation most often can be treated medically (Table 18-2). Acute anovulatory menorrhagic bleeding often is self-limited. In these situations no acute treatment may be necessary, and initiation of a long-term treatment, such as oral contraceptive pills, can be used to prevent recurrence. Because they contain a progestational agent, birth control pills change the estrogenized anovulatory proliferative endometrium to a secretory endometrium. Stopping the birth control pills during the pill-free week allows for a self-limited withdrawal flow.

Estrogen is useful to stop acute heavy anovulatory bleeding. Estrogen causes mitotic activity, cell division, and growth of the endometrium. This estrogen-induced endometrial growth induces a clotting and healing mechanism of the basal endometrium that will stop acute bleeding. Sometimes progestational agents alone will stop bleeding. However, if there has already been considerable sloughing of the endometrium with little remaining proliferative endometrium, progestational agents may not be successful and may exacerbate the bleeding by causing a more decidualized atrophic endometrium that prevents estrogen-induced healing. Therefore, though progestational agents such as those found in birth control pills are optimal for long-term maintenance of a regular bleeding pattern in anovulatory patients, acute use of them is often not as successful as estrogen alone. The high dose estrogen needs to be followed by a progestational agent to prevent later uncontrolled bleeding.

Occasionally, a patient on oral contraceptives (OCP) complains that she has abnormal or irregular bleeding similar to her prepill problem. This breakthrough bleeding on the OCP is a side-effect that has no pathologic significance and is unrelated to the dysfunctional bleeding she experienced prior to the pill. It is not a continuation of the previous problem; it should not be viewed as a failure of birth control pill use and should not lead to surgical intervention. It however may be a sign of cervicitis due to gonorrhea or chlamydia.[9]

Initial treatment for menorrhagia includes acute high-dose estrogen, such as oral conjugated estrogens (Premarin) 2.5 mg every 8 hours or intravenous conjugated estrogens (Premarin) 25 mg IV every 4 hours until the bleeding stops or slows, or the use of a 50-µg ethinyl estradiol OCP three or four times a day. If there is no response in 12 to 24 hours, then a curettage (D&C) is indicated. If the bleeding slows, then

TABLE 18-2
Etiology of Menorrhagia

Pregnancy

Anovulation
  Perimenarcheal
  Perimenopausal
  Stress
  Obesity
  Androgen excess syndrome, polycystic ovarian syndrome
  Hypothyroidism

Low estrogen anovulation less likely to cause heavy bleeding
  Prolactinoma, hyperprolactinemia
  anorexia, weight loss, exercise, stress

Bleeding disorder
  von Willebrand disease
  Idiothrombocytopenia
  Leukemia
  Iatrogenic thrombocytopenia (chemotherapy or bone marrow suppression)
  Anticoagulation

Anovulation and bleeding disorder
  Severe hepatic disease
  Chronic renal failure

Lesions
  Fibroid uterus
  Trauma
  Endometrial hyperplasia or cancer
  Cervical cancer, sexual abuse
  Vaginal, vulvar, tubal, or ovarian cancer
  Infection, endometritis (cervicitis alone usually causes postcoital or spotting-type bleeding)
  Intrauterine contraceptive device
  Estrogen-producing tumor of the ovary
  Estrogen medications (possibly digitalis)
  Uterine or cervical polyps

OCP are used for a total of 7 days. At the end of 7 days a withdrawal bleed will occur and then cyclic OCPs are restarted. Standard 35-mcg ethinyl estradiol pills are sufficient, and higher estrogen-containing pills are not necessary for long-term therapy. Hospitalization or at least prolonged observation in the emergency department is indicated when there is evidence of hypovolemia or a hemoglobin below 7 g/100 mL.[1]

Besides OCPs, cyclic oral progestational agents—including the 19-nor-testosterone derivatives, such as norethindrone, norethindrone acetate, or levonorgestrel; 21-hydroxyprogesterone derivatives, such as medroxyprogesterone acetate or Megace; or physiologic but more short-acting oral micronized progesterone—can be used to regulate bleeding in the patient with chronic anovulation. Longer-acting progestins—such as depomedroxyprogesterone injections (Depoprovera), injectable norethindrone enanthate, or levonorgestrel subdermal implants (Norplant)—are associated with amenorrhea or irregular light bleeding or less frequently with heavy bleeding. When these long-acting agents are used in the anovulatory patient and are associated with irregular bleeding, this is not a recurrence of the original vical epithelium, minimal bleeding or discharge, and deviation of the cervical os suggest a primary pelvic mass rather than a primary cervical neoplasm. Sarcomas of the uterus are rare (less than 1%) and have few specific signs that differentiate them from myomas.[2] The infrequent mixed mesodermal malignancy may present with bleeding and polypoid lesions protruding through the cervical os.

3. *Developmental abnormalities of the uterus.* These may cause a pelvic mass, most often due to incomplete fusion of the müllerian ducts. This may be noted in unicornate or bicornate uteri where an exaggerated development of one horn is misinterpreted as an adnexal mass. Acute symptoms are rare, although it may be difficult to differentiate the mass from an adnexal mass requiring more immediate attention.

4. *Fallopian tube.* Fallopian tube masses are primarily inflammatory or due to pregnancy. Rarely is the diagnosis of fallopian neoplasm made preoperatively. A unilateral adnexal mass associated with a bloody intramenstrual discharge (hydrops tubae profluens) is suggestive of fallopian tube neoplasm.[3]

5. *Ovary.* The most common cause of an adnexal mass is the ovary. Most ovarian masses are either functional or benign neoplastic cysts with a definite relationship to the age of the patient. Patients should be categorized into three groups: (1) infancy to puberty; (2) puberty to menopause; and (3) postmenopause. In the first group (infancy to puberty), almost all adnexal/ovarian masses are neoplastic, may be malignant, and require urgent evaluation and treatment. Ovarian tumors are the most common genital neoplasm in this age group. In group 3 (postmenopausal), palpable adnexal masses are primarily neoplastic in origin and must also be evaluated promptly. Varying diagnostic modalities and controversial therapeutic options will be discussed in detail later. Group 2 consists of the reproductive-age group (approximately ages 14 to 54); it is in this group that most functional or benign masses occur. Functional and benign masses include cystic masses associated with anovulation, manifestations of endometriosis, and benign neoplasms such as benign cystic teratoma (dermoid). Benign cystic teratoma is the most common neoplasm between the ages of 1 and 20 years.[4] Serous and mucinous cystadenomas occur throughout the reproductive years as well as the postmenopausal years. Mucinous cystadenomas may reach gigantic size and are the most likely cause of a huge pelvic mass.[5] Physiologic cysts—such as follicle cyst, corpus luteum cyst, germinal inclusion cyst, theca-lutein cyst, and sclerocystic ovaries (polycystic ovaries)—occur throughout the reproductive years and may masquerade as pregnancy, inflammatory masses, or neoplasms. Special mention should be made of theca-lutein cyst associated with marked elevation of human chorionic gonadotropin. Usually these cysts, which reach 20 cm in diameter, are found in association with gestational trophoblastic disease and will spontaneously regress with serum clearance of the chorionic gonadotropin. Care must be taken during an examination to avoid converting a benign, spontaneously resolving problem to an operative emergency secondary to rupture of the cyst.

Approximately 22,000 women will develop ovarian malignancies, and 13,300 will die of this disease during 1993.[6] A woman at birth has a one in 70 chance of developing ovarian carcinoma.[7] In the prepubertal age group, germ cell neoplasms are seen most frequently, with dysgerminoma being the most common cell type. Endodermal sinus tumors and embryonal cell carcinomas are seen less frequently.[8] In the early stages, germ cell tumors are primarily unilateral. Gonadal stromal tumors, primarily granulosa/theca cell tumors, occur infrequently (approximately 5%) before puberty and are usually limited to one ovary. Tumor markers—such as alpha-fetoprotein, β-HCG, and CA-125—are of limited value and availability (except β-HCG) during the initial evaluation. They are, however, important in management and follow-up if initially positive.[9] A negative test is of no significance. Epithelial cell malignancies account for 85% of all ovarian malignancies and increase in incidence until age 80. For a complete histologic classification of ovarian neoplasms, see Table 19-2.

6. *Nongynecologic causes of pelvic masses.* These must always be considered in the differential diagnosis of a pelvic mass. Often the patient has a long history of symptoms referable to the gastrointestinal or genitourinary tract. A distended bladder, gaseous intestinal distention, or stool in the colon have all been misinterpreted as pelvic masses. Awareness of these possibilities should prompt the physician to consider them. Inflammatory processes, such as appendiceal or diverticular abscess, usually present with a history of pain, fever, and gastrointestinal symptoms. Lymphomas may occasionally present as a pelvic mass, either a unilateral or bilateral pelvic sidewall mass, with hard, irregular, fixed, nontender features.

7. *Other diagnostic considerations.* Therapeutic radiation treatment to the pelvis in the recent or distant past may be associated with a diffuse or discrete pelvic mass. Diffuse, symmetric, smooth fibrosis is more likely to be associated with benign posttherapy changes, whereas nodular, asymmetric, discrete masses are more likely to be due to recurrence of the primary neoplasm or complications of therapy. A finding occasionally seen in patients who receive pelvic radiation is subcutaneous thickness of the abdominal wall that mimics a pelvic mass. This is secondary to intense fibrosis of the superficial fatty tissue. Finally, lymphocysts may occur secondary to surgery, including pelvic lymphadenectomy with or without postoperative radiation.

Initial Evaluation

A detailed history and comprehensive physical examination with special attention focused on the abdomen and pelvis should be correlated with the age groupings noted in the previous discussion.

History

Important historical features include the acuteness of symptoms, and significant past medical, surgical, and radiation history. Chills and fever are usually associated with inflammatory disorders and seldom occur with either benign or malignant ovarian neoplasms. Torsion of a pelvic mass may present with pain, fever, nausea, and vomiting; torsion is a surgical emergency discussed in more detail in a separate

TABLE 19-2
Modified World Health Organization Comprehensive Classification of Ovarian Tumors*

I. Common "Epithelial" Tumors
    Benign, borderline, or malignant potential
        Serous
        Mucinous
        Endometrioid
        Clear cell
        Brenner
    Mixed epithelial
    Undifferentiated
    Mixed mesodermal tumors
    Unclassified

II. Sex-Cord Stromal Tumors
    Granulosa stromal cell
        Granulosa cell
        Thecoma-fibroma
    Androblastomas; Sertoli-Leydig cell tumors
        Well-differentiated (Pick's adenoma, Sertoli cell tumor)
        Intermediate differentiation
        Poorly differentiated
        With heterologous elements
    Lipid cell tumors
    Gynandroblastoma
    Unclassified

III. Germ Cell Tumors
    Dysgerminoma
    Endodermal sinus tumor
    Embryonal carcinoma
    Polyembryoma
    Choriocarcinoma
    Teratomas
        Immature
        Mature (dermoid)
        Monodermal (struma ovarii, carcinoid)
    Mixed forms
    Gonadoblastoma

IV. Soft-Tissue Tumors Not Specific to the Ovary

V. Unclassified Tumors

VI. Secondary (Metastatic) Tumors

VII. Tumorlike Conditions (e.g., Pregnancy, Luteoma)

*International Histologic Classification of Tumors. No. 9 World Health Organization, Geneva, 1973.

chapter. Ascites with a pelvic mass is usually a manifestation of ovarian or fallopian tube malignancy but can be seen in benign situations (Meigs' syndrome).[10] Rarely is it necessary to do a paracentesis of the ascites for diagnostic purposes. Malignant ovarian neoplasms are often associated with nonspecific symptoms such as anorexia, indigestion, and dyspepsia. A pelvic mass produced by gastrointestinal disease is usually associated with more specific and localized symptoms, such as left lower quadrant pain, mucus and blood in the stool, alternating consistency of the stool, and often a history of previously diagnosed gastrointestinal disease. Menstrual dysfunction is seldom associated with nongynecologic disorders unless there are significant systemic manifestations of the disease. Abnormal uterine bleeding may be associated with uterine, tubal, or ovarian disease. However, it may be absent in all gynecologic causes of pelvic masses. Postmenopausal bleeding in association with a pelvic mass strongly suggests endometrial cancer.

Physical Examination

The examination should concentrate on the location and the features of the mass. A mass noted in a patient at the extremes of life must be considered malignant. Signs that favor benignity include unilateral location, smooth surface, mobility, cystic consistency, and symmetric shape. Features that suggest malignancy are a bilateral location, solid consistency, nodular and irregular surface, ascites, and nodularity and fixation of the cul-de-sac. Myomas of the uterus, although they show some features of malignancy (solid, bilateral, nodular, irregular), rarely have the characteristics of fixation, associated ascites, or other systemic signs of malignancy. Extremely large masses that fill the entire abdomen are usually benign or low-grade ovarian neoplasms. Exquisitely tender masses with or without peritoneal signs are usually inflammatory or pregnancy related. Torsion of a mass with or without rupture may produce similar findings. Masses located anterior to the broad ligament are most frequently benign cystic teratomas or endometriotic cysts.[11] Most functional cysts are unilateral and rarely exceed 10 cm in size. Functional cysts are not among the differential diagnosis in the postmenopausal patient, but benign cysts of all cellular types, including endometriotic cysts, may be encountered in this age group. Lymphocysts are generally firm, cystic, adherent to the sidewall, unilateral, or bilateral and have variable degrees of tenderness to palpation.

Although a careful history and physical examination are essential, further diagnostic studies are usually required. The selection of these studies depends on the acuteness and severity of the symptoms, age of the patient, physical findings, and available facilities.

Special Studies

At the time of the pelvic examination, a wet smear, Pap smear, and appropriate vaginal bacterial cultures should be considered (see the Chapters 16 and 17 on PID and vaginitis for more detail). Vulvar, vaginal, cervical, or endometrial biopsies should be performed if the findings warrant these procedures. Gross lesions should be biopsied rather than awaiting cytologic reports. The large, barrel-shaped cervical lesion should be sampled using both an Eppendorfer-type biopsy forceps and an endocervical curettage. The endometrium can easily be sampled in an outpatient setting using the aspiration biopsy, such as the pipelle cannula. Culdocentesis is an easily accomplished procedure that should be considered, especially where inflammatory, pregnancy, or ruptured masses are considered. The appearance and laboratory evaluation of aspirated fluid are often diagnostic. Serous peritoneal fluid of significant volume may occur in normal situations or in association with benign or malignant masses. Unfortunately, cytologic evaluation is inconsistently interpreted. An unequivocally positive cytologic smear may be helpful, but the absence of malignant cells has little significance. Purulent fluid is usually noted with pelvic inflammatory disease or an abscess of any cause. Blood is usually indicative of a ruptured viscus, such as an ectopic pregnancy or a bleeding ovarian cyst or neoplasm. The absence of fluid, however, has little significance, since "dry" taps occur for a variety of reasons. Fluid should be analyzed for hematocrit determination, culture, Gram stain, and cytology.

Laboratory Studies

A complete blood count, urinalysis, and β-HCG should be done in all cases. Serum electrolytes, renal function studies, and blood groupings and cross-match are performed if clinically indicated. Highly sensitive, rapidly performed β-HCG tests are now universally available and mandatory in the evaluation of pregnancy related masses. Quantitative methods, while not required for the initial evaluation, may be useful in the expectant management of ectopic pregnancy (see Chapter 3) and the management of pelvic masses secondary to gestational trophoblastic disease. Serum tumor markers, such as β-HCG, alpha-fetoprotein, and CA-125, should be drawn when ovarian neoplasms are suspected.

Imaging

Plain films of the abdomen and pelvis are readily available, are easily interpreted, and may provide definitive information. Air/fluid levels suggesting bowel obstruction or free intraperitoneal air mandate immediate attention and possible surgical intervention. Calcifications are primarily seen in benign cystic teratomas but may also be present in other ovarian neoplasms (fibroadenomas, papillary serous tumors, gynandroblastoma, Brenner tumor) and uterine myomas. Contrast studies of the lower intestinal tract are required when the differential diagnosis includes colonic lesions. Upper gastrointestinal studies are often warranted when ovarian malignancy or metastatic disease is considered. In premenopausal women gastric carcinoma may metastasize to the ovary. Intravenous pyelography (IVP) is a useful diagnostic study. The uncommon occurrence of a pelvic or horseshoe kidney can be diagnosed. If upper urinary tract obstruction is present, prompt management is required to minimize renal damage. Abnormalities in the normal course of the ureter may help localize the origin of the mass and provide useful information if retroperitoneal exploration is required. If individuals have a history of a reaction to intravenous contrast, consultation with a radiologist is indicated. Patients may be pretreated with steroids, or nonionic contrast agents may be used.[12,13] Retrograde pyelography can be performed if the expected findings warrant the increased effort and potential morbidity. In all cases, the potential nephrotoxic effects of contrast must be considered, particularly where history or laboratory findings suggest impaired renal function.

Other Imaging Studies

Ultrasonography, both transabdominal and transvaginal; magnetic resonance imaging; and computed tomography are useful diagnostic studies. Recently, pulsed and color Doppler, combined with transvaginal ultrasonography, have been recommended to improve ultrasonographic diagnostic assessment of benign and malignant masses. Because of its high sensitivity (more than 90%) in identifying pelvic masses, ultrasound has its greatest value in the confirmation or identification of masses in patients who are difficult to examine.[14] The difficulties caused by obesity in transabdominal sonography can be overcome by transvaginal sonography. However, in transvaginal ultrasonography there are problems in older patients, whose less elastic vaginas limit probe maneuverability. The specificity of ultrasound with regard to diagnosing lesions does not approach its high sensitivity. Despite the fact that ultrasound can differentiate between solid and cystic, uniloculated and multiloculated, the correct diagnosis is made in less than 70% of the cases.[15] Transvaginal ultrasonography offers greater resolution and greater detail of the internal morphology of pelvic masses. The additional information supplied by transvaginal color flow Doppler sonography should enhance the ability to distinguish between benign and malignant masses. Both Fleischer and colleagues and Kawai and colleagues report encouraging findings in differentiating benign and malignant masses with transvaginal ultrasonography, although further evaluation in larger series is needed to evaluate the specificity and sensitivity of the procedure.[16,17] Currently, it appears that the main value of ultrasonography in the evaluation of pelvic masses is to confirm size, consistency, and a tentative origin of the mass.

Magnetic resonance imaging (MRI) is advantageous in that it does not require ionizing radiation or contrast dyes. Disadvantages include expense and the inability to use it on patients with pacemakers, cerebral aneurysm clips, or intraocular metallic fragments. The sensitivity and specificity of pelvic MRI are similar to those of ultrasound. Further, MRI does not provide a specific diagnosis. MRI cannot distinguish hemorrhagic fluid from fat or a hemorrhagic solid component from a solid malignant lesion. Andreotti and colleagues suggest the following indications for MR imaging: differentiating uterine from adnexal pelvic masses where ultrasound is inconclusive; distinguishing a simple from a hemorrhagic cyst when endometriosis is suspected; and confirming a sonographically suspicious, benign cystic teratoma.[18]

Computerized tomography (CT) has the disadvantages of expense, intravenous and gastrointestinal contrast dyes, and exposure to ionizing radiation. CT is superior for depicting the presence of fat and is excellent for evaluating the retroperitoneum.[19] It is the imaging technique of choice for diagnosing benign cystic teratomas[20] and for evaluating undiagnosed abdominal-pelvic masses and peritoneal or retroperitoneal ovarian metastasis.

Diagnostic Laparoscopy

It has become the standard of care to treat ectopic pregnancies through laparoscopy. The use of laparoscopy as a diagnostic modality to evaluate pelvic masses is well accepted. The vast majority of time, however, this is accomplished in an operating room setting and is frequently associated with therapeutic procedures. The role of operative laparoscopy in the management of pelvic masses is yet to be determined. In the context of this discussion, only general principles will be addressed. Further information regarding this controversial approach to management may be found in the references.[21-26] Essential minimal requirements for a laparoscopic evaluation of pelvic masses include careful patient selection, operator experience and expertise, adequate facilities, appropriate equipment, and experienced personnel. In patient selection, several factors should be considered: age, clinical examination, ultrasonographic findings, and tumor marker values, especially CA-125.[21] Relative contraindications to the use of laparoscopy include the evaluation of pelvic masses in postmenopausal women with an elevated CA-125, ultrasonographic findings of multilocular masses, masses of more than 10 cm, masses with irregular borders, solid areas, or matted bowel. Since these are strongly suggestive of malignancy, laparotomy remains the preferred approach.[21]

Diagnostic Aspiration of Cysts

Aspiration of pelvic cysts is also controversial. Although to date ovarian tumor rupture has not been shown to affect long-term prognosis, controversy remains. Despite the perceived negative effects of fluid aspiration and spill, in reality the problem lies in the evaluation of the cyst aspirate. Ten to 65% of cyst aspirates are misinterpreted, with cells interpreted as benign when a malignancy actually exists.[27] This high false-negative rate makes laparoscopic cyst aspiration unreliable as a definitive diagnostic procedure.

Management

The management of a pelvic mass depends largely on the same features cited earlier: acuteness and severity of symptoms, age, physical findings, and results of laboratory and special studies. Pregnancy should either be diagnosed or be eliminated from the differential diagnosis through a rapid beta-HCG on all women of child-bearing age (see Chapter 3).

Immediate intervention is required almost universally in patients who present with symptoms associated with complications (rupture, infection, torsion, hemorrhage, severe pain, and peritoneal signs). Vascular access and volume expansion with crystalloid are mandatory. Blood transfusions may also be required.

The patient with fever, peritoneal signs, or purulent material aspirated on culdocentesis should have intravenous access established. Appropriate laboratory studies include blood cultures, urine culture, cervical cultures, complete blood count, and chest and possibly abdominal plain films. Parenteral antibiotics with both aerobic and anaerobic coverage should be considered. Effective initial combinations include ampicillin/sulbactam, gentamicin and clindamycin, penicillin, gentamicin, metronidazole, or ceftriaxone and clindamycin. Antibiotic therapy can be modified once cultures and sensitivities become available. The patient should be admitted for continued antibiotic therapy and monitoring. Rarely is surgery indicated before several hours of parenteral antibiotic therapy are administered.

The patient with hemodynamic instability should be considered for a culdocentesis or emergency laparoscopy/laparotomy. A patient with a clinical picture consistent with torsion should be stabilized and prepared for immediate surgery.

Incidental pelvic masses with no acute symptoms may be evaluated on an outpatient basis. The exception is the prepubertal and postmenopausal female presenting with a large pelvic mass. A mass in these two age groups must be considered malignant; inpatient evaluation with prompt surgical intervention is desirable; a gynecologic oncologist should be consulted if possible. A patient of reproductive age may receive an expeditious outpatient evaluation if malignancy is considered. The result of the imaging techniques described earlier and laboratory studies will determine whether surgical intervention is required and the most appropriate route (laparoscopy or laparotomy). Pelvic masses of a cystic nature, unilateral, between 5 and 10 cm in size in menstruating females, may be observed expectantly for 2 to 3 months. If the mass does not resolve, laparoscopic evaluation is an accepted approach. Masses considered to have a gastrointestinal or genitourinary tract origin should be referred to the appropriate specialist for management.

In all cases of pelvic masses, the etiology (see Table 19-1) determines the urgency and type of management. The main consideration is the possibility of malignancy, either primary or metastatic, regardless of organ of origin. Needless delays in therapy should be avoided. Persistent pelvic masses will require surgical intervention for appropriate histologic sampling despite a variety of noninvasive diagnostic modalities. Exploratory laparotomy is almost always the preferred approach when malignancy is considered. The surgical approach should allow for extensive evaluation of the entire abdomen (generally a vertical incision performed by an individual with the training and experience). As most causes of pelvic masses are gynecologic in nature, this evaluation is usually done by a gynecologist. If malignancy is a possibility, the surgical team should include a gynecologic oncologist. In summary, several points should be emphasized.

1. Spurious masses caused by retained urine or feces must be considered.
2. Ectopic pregnancy must always be considered in ovulating females, which includes patients in the extremes of reproductive age.
3. Ruptured tubal or ovarian abscesses may present without a systemic febrile response.
4. Ovarian carcinoma is commonly associated with gastrointestinal symptoms of a prolonged, chronic, annoying nature.
5. Ovaries decrease in size with advancing age and a palpable normal-sized ovary (3.5 × 2 × 1.5 cm) in the postmenopausal patient is abnormal.[28]
6. Ovarian functional cysts do not occur in postmenopausal patients.
7. Pelvic masses in children present as abdominal structures that are usually neoplastic and most likely malignant.
8. Ovarian cysts, especially theca-lutein cysts, are often thin-walled and may rupture with vigorous palpation; this results in potentially serious complications.
9. Ultrasound examination in nonpregnant patients is of no value in accurately diagnosing pelvic masses as to histology, malignancy, or site of origin.
10. Location, size, and consistency are helpful findings to determine immediate and subsequent treatment.
11. Laparoscopy remains controversial in its diagnostic and therapeutic roles.
12. There are no totally reliable noninvasive diagnostic procedures.
13. Malignancy is a primary concern in the evaluation of pelvic masses. The diagnosis of malignancy usually requires a surgical procedure.

REFERENCES

1. Merrill JA, Creasman WT. Lesions of the Corpus Uteri. In: Danforth DN, Scott JR (eds): Obstetrics and Gynecology, 5th ed, p 1073. Philadelphia: JB Lippincott, 1986
2. Merrill JA, Creasman WT. Lesions of the corpus uteri. In: Danforth DN, Scott JR (eds): Obstetrics and Gynecology, 5th ed, p 1075. Philadelphia: JB Lippincott, 1986
3. Merrill JA, Creasman WT. Lesions of the corpus uteri. In: Danforth DN, Scott JR (eds): Obstetrics Gynecology, 5th ed, p 1102. Philadelphia: JB Lippincott, 1986
4. Parsons L, Sommers S. Tumors in childhood. In: Parsons L, Sommers S (eds): Gynecology, 2nd ed. Philadelphia: WB Saunders, 1978
5. Symmonds RE, Spraitz AF, Koelshe GA. Large ovarian tumors. Obstet Gynecol 22:473, 1963
6. Boring CC, Squires TS, Tong T. Cancer statistics, 1993. CA 43:7, 1993
7. DiSaia PJ, Creasman WT. Advanced epithelial ovarian cancer. In: DiSaia PJ, Creasman WT (eds): Clinical Gynecologic Oncology, 3rd ed, p 325. St Louis: CV Mosby, 1989
8. Barber HRK. Diagnosing and managing the adnexal mass. In: Barber HRK (ed): Ovarian Carcinoma, 2nd ed, p 114. New York: Masson, 1982
9. Finkler NI, Bast RC, Knapp RC. Tumor markers in gynecologic cancer. Contemp OB/GYN 30:29, 1987
10. Meigs JV, Cass JW. Fibroma of the ovary with ascites and hydrothorax with report of 7 cases. Am J Obstet Gynecol 33:249, 1938
11. Morrow CP, Townsend DE. Tumors of the ovary. In: Morrow CP, Townsend ED (eds): Synopsis of Gynecologic Oncology, 3rd ed, p 242. New York: John Wiley, 1987
12. Lasser EC, Berry CC, Talner LB et al. Pretreatment with corticosteroids to alleviate reactions to intravenous contrast material. N Engl J Med 317:845, 1987
13. McClennan BL. Ionic and nonionic iodinated contrast media: evolution and strategies for use. Am J Roentgenol 155:225, 1990
14. Sanders RC, McNeil BJ, Finberg HJ et al. A prospective study of computed tomography and ultrasound in the detection and staging of pelvic masses. Radiology 146:439, 1983
15. Bennacerraf BR, Finkler NJ, Wojciechowski C et al. Sonographic accuracy in the diagnosis of ovarian masses. J Reprod Med 35:491, 1990
16. Fleischer AC, Rogers WH, Rao BK, Kepple DM, Jones HW. Transvaginal color Doppler sonography of ovarian masses with pathological correlation. Ultrasound Obstet Gynecol 1:275, 1991
17. Kawai M, Kano T, Kikkawa F, Maeda O, Oguchi H, Tomoda Y. Transvaginal Doppler ultrasound with color flow imaging in the diagnosis of ovarian cancer. Obstet Gynecol 79:163, 1992
18. Andreotti RJ, Zusmer NR, Sheldon JJ et al. Ultrasound and magnetic resonance imaging of pelvic masses. Surg Gynecol Obstet 166:327, 1988
19. Sawyer RW, Vick CW, Walsh JW et al. Computed tomography of benign ovarian masses. J Comput Assist Tomogr 9:784, 1985
20. Buy JN, Moss AA, Ghossian MA. Cystic teratoma of the ovary: CT detection. Radiology 171:697, 1989
21. Parker WH. Management of ovarian cysts by operative laparoscopy. Contemp OB/GYN 136:47, 1991
22. Maiman M, Seltzer V, Boyce J. Laparoscopic excision of ovarian neoplasms subsequently found to be malignant. Obstet Gynecol 77:563, 1991
23. Nezhat C, Winer WK, Nezhat F. Laparoscopic removal of dermoid cysts. Obstet Gynecol 73:278, 1989
24. Peterson HB, Hulka JF, Phillips JM. American Association of Gynecologic Laparoscopists 1988 membership survey on operative laparoscopy. J Reprod Med 35:587, 1990

25. Mage G, Canis M, Manhes H, Pouly JL, Wattiez A, Bruhat MA. Laparoscopic management of adnexal cystic masses. J Gynecol Surg 6:71, 1990
26. Lim-Tan Sk, Cajigas HE, Scully RE. Ovarian cystectomy for serous borderline tumors: a follow-up study of 35 cases. Obstet Gynecol 72:775, 1988
27. Trope C. The preoperative diagnosis of malignancy of ovarian cysts. Neoplasia 28:117, 1981
28. Barber HRK, Graber EA. The PMPO syndrome (post-menopausal palpable ovary syndrome). Obstet Gynecol Surv 28:357, 1973

CHAPTER 20

Torsion of the Ovary

Charles J. Dunton

Causes of acute abdominal pain unique to women include pelvic inflammatory disease, ectopic pregnancy, endometrioma, rupture or hemorrhage of a corpus luteum cyst, and torsion of adnexal structures.[1] Although uncommon, adnexal torsion is not rare and comprises approximately 3% of surgical emergencies in women.[2] Diagnosis of this condition is challenging. Prompt diagnosis may allow for preservation of the adnexal structures and fertility.

Causes

Torsion of the adnexa is caused by rotation of the ovary or adnexa about the ovarian pedicle, resulting in arterial, venous, or lymphatic obstruction (Fig. 20-1). Initially, the venous and lymphatic obstruction without arterial obstruction produces edema and enlargement of the ovary. If arterial obstruction occurs, the organs may become necrotic and gangrenous. This in turn may lead to peritonitis and intestinal obstruction. In some cases the twisted adnexa may be absorbed, leading to unilateral absence of the adnexa. Torsion of the fallopian tube alone is rare but has been associated with hydrosalpinx, neoplasms of the tube, and previous tubal ligation.[3]

Torsion of the adnexa may also accompany ovarian hyperstimulation syndrome caused by menotropin therapy for infertility.[4]

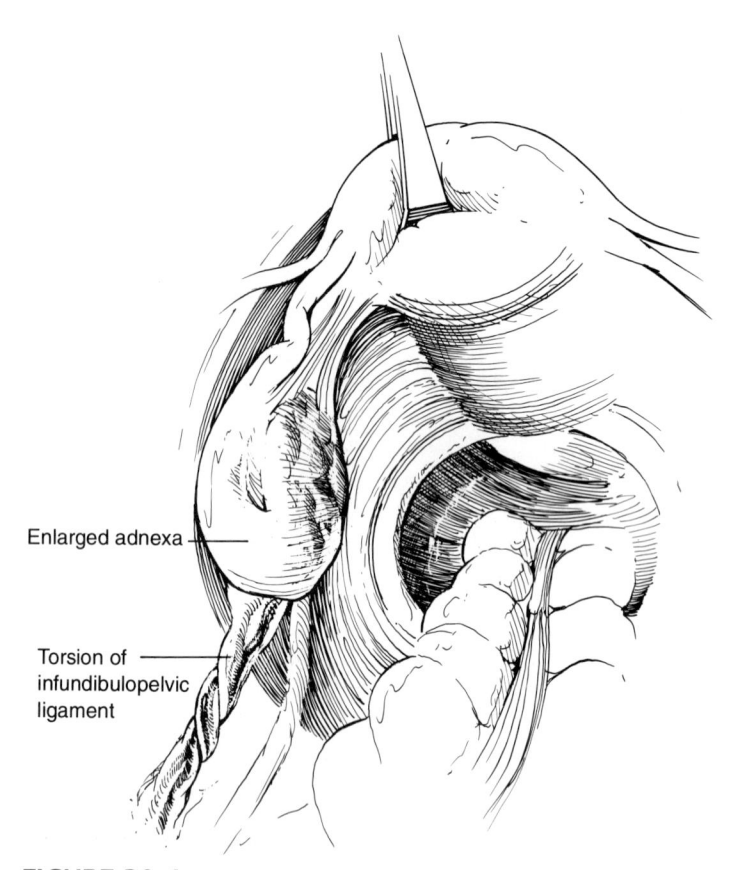

FIGURE 20–1.
Torsion of infundibulopelvic ligament.

Etiology

Torsion of the adnexa may involve the ovary, fallopian tube, or both structures together. In most cases, an ovarian neoplasm is involved. Nonetheless, in up to 18% of cases torsion may involve normal tubes and ovaries. In keeping with the age of the patient population, the neoplasms are usually benign (Table 20-1). Although the most common neoplasm is the dermoid cyst, paraovarian cysts have the highest relative risk of torsion.[2]

It is unusual for malignant neoplasm to present with symptoms of torsion. A review of 10 years' experience at the Women's Hospital, Los Angeles County, showed only two cases of malignant neoplasms undergoing torsion. In comparison, the relative risk for a benign neoplasm to undergo torsion was 12.9 (95% CI 10.2 to 15.9).[5] Torsion does occur in postmenopausal women. In Koonings and Grimes review of 301 tumors in postmenopausal women, 19 (6%) underwent torsion. Serous cystadenoma was the most common, and no malignant neoplasms underwent torsion.[6] In Lee's series, 17.5% of the neoplasms associated with torsion were malignant. This high number may be accounted for by the high percentage (27%) of postmenopausal women in this report.[7]

TABLE 20-1
Pathology of Torsed Adnexa*

Pathologic Diagnosis	Number
Dermoid cyst	38
Serous adenoma	12
Serous carcinoma	2
Mucinous adenoma	6
Fibroma/thecoma	4
Struma ovarii	1
Hemangioma	1
Paraovarian cyst	24
Corpus luteum	7
Serous cyst	6
Endometrioma	2
Total	101

*Modified from Hibbard LT. Adnexal torsion. Am J Obstet Gynecol 152: 456, 1985.

Torsion of a normal ovary may present as massive ovarian edema. This tumorlike condition presents with significant ovarian enlargement and pathologically shows only edema of a normal ovary.[8]

Clinical Features

The clinical diagnosis of adnexal torsion is often difficult. It occurs mainly in young women and less frequently in children and postmenopausal females. Pain, low-grade temperature; moderate leukocytosis; and nausea and vomiting are present in most cases. The pain may be acute in onset and may be associated with vigorous activity or a change in position.[2] The pain is described as colicky or constant and may be out of proportion to other findings. Later in the course if necrosis occurs, high fever and marked leukocytosis may be seen.[8]

In a review of 44 patients presenting with an acute abdomen and adnexal torsion, Lomano and colleagues described the following symptoms: pain (100%), nausea or vomiting (66%), abdominal fullness (16%), menstrual dysfunction (9%), diarrhea (7%), dysuria (7%), constipation (5%), rectal pressure (2%), and syncope (2%). The character of the pain was gradual in 26 patients and sudden in 16.[9]

Symptoms may be present for a number of days prior to the patient seeking medical attention, and physician delay prior to surgical treatment is not uncommon. Chronic pain associated with intermittent torsion may be seen in 10% of patients and is suggested by repeated attacks with asymptomatic intervals.[3]

Abdominal examination may show initial rigidity, spasm, tenderness, and unilateral pain on deep palpation. On pelvic examination, unilateral adnexal tenderness and a palpable mass are usually present. The torsion is more likely to involve the right adnexa (3:2), perhaps because of the proximity of the sigmoid colon to the left adnexa, resulting in less space for the torsion to occur.[2]

In most series the diagnostic accuracy for patients with demonstrated torsion is only approximately 70%.[2,10] If the patients with a preoperative diagnosis of torsion who proved to have other pathology are added to the total, the accuracy drops to about 40%. Incorrect preoperative diagnosis in patients subsequently having torsion included adnexal mass, appendicitis, myoma, ectopic pregnancy, abscess, and ruptured viscus.[2]

Torsion must be considered in the diagnosis of abdominal pain, especially when a palpable pelvic mass is present. If no palpable mass is present, ultrasonography may prove helpful in the diagnosis. Ultrasonography has been shown to demonstrate a mass in all patients with torsion. However, ultrasonic appearance of the masses was nonspecific. The use of Doppler evaluation of the ovarian vasculature may be helpful in the future but no data currently exist concerning this modality.[11]

Approximately 20% of patients with an adnexal torsion will have a concomitant intrauterine pregnancy. Ultrasound can demonstrate the location of the pregnancy and aid in differentiation of torsion with intrauterine pregnancy from an ectopic gestation.

Differential Diagnosis

The diagnosis of torsion of the adnexa must be considered in women with abdominal pain. The differential diagnosis includes ectopic pregnancy, appendicitis, pelvic inflammatory disease, adnexal mass without torsion, endometrioma, degeneration of a myoma, renal calculi, ruptured functional cyst.[1,3]

Ectopic pregnancy without an acute abdomen is diagnosed by serial beta-HCG testing along with appropriate use of ultrasound when quantitative beta-HCG level reaches a discrimination point. Although intrauterine pregnancy is associated with torsion of an adnexa, ultrasound and beta-HCG testing should be used to differentiate an intrauterine pregnancy with torsion from an ectopic gestation. In the event of an unstable patient, emergency laparotomy is indicated with either diagnosis.

In appendicitis, the symptoms of midline abdominal pain with migration to the right lower quadrant and negative pelvic findings other than tenderness on rectal examination differentiate this entity from torsion. In addition, the nausea and vomiting seen in torsion generally occur rapidly after the onset of pain, rather than gradually, as in acute appendicitis.

Pelvic inflammatory disease is usually characterized by bilateral pain and tenderness. Temperature elevation and leukocytosis may be more marked. Pertinent history—such as previous episodes of pelvic inflammatory disease, intrauterine device use, and multiple or new sexual partner—points to pelvic inflammatory disease.

Patients who have an adnexal mass without torsion generally present without pain. Those who have a ruptured functional cyst may present at the midpoint of the menstrual cycle (Mittleschmerz) or just prior to the next expected period. Symptoms of nausea and vomiting are less frequent. In cases where there is no hemorrhage, symptoms are less severe than those seen with adnexal torsion and resolve over 48 hours.

Renal calculi usually present with flank pain and hematuria. There is also lack of a palpable pelvic mass. Degeneration of a myoma, especially if pedunculated, may require laparoscopy to confirm the diagnosis. A history of chronic pelvic pain will usually accompany endometriosis. Fever, acute pain, and increased leukocyte count are not seen with endometriomas unless there is rupture. In cases of rupture, an acute abdomen may be seen, necessitating operative intervention.

In all cases of acute pain an empty bladder is necessary to ensure that urinary retention is not the cause of the pain. It will also allow for a more complete and accurate pelvic examination.

A high index of suspicion for torsion in cases of abdominal pain with a palpable or ultrasonically detected pelvic mass is necessary. Combined with laparoscopy in equivocal cases, early diagnosis and prompt treatment of this condition are possible.

Treatment

Treatment for torsion of the adnexa depends on the condition of the ovary at the time of surgery. In most series, treatment has consisted of removal of the affected adnexa because of fear of embolism from thrombosed ovarian veins or necrosis of the ovary and tube. In these cases it is wise to expose the ureter to determine its location prior to ligating the ovarian blood supply, as the tenting of the peritoneum by the torsion may cause the ureter to be in or adjacent to the twisted pedicle. It is also appropriate to ligate the ovarian vessels prior to untwisting to lessen the risk of embolism.[3]

If the ovary is not necrotic, it may be untwisted and stabilized by suturing to the posterior wall of the uterus or by shortening the ovarian ligament. Since torsion is usually associated with neoplasms of the ovary, the ovary should be carefully inspected and cystectomy carried out if necessary. If there is suspicion of a malignancy, unilateral adnexectomy should be performed. Appropriate surgical staging should be carried out if frozen section shows malignancy.[2,8]

Laparoscopic management of ovarian torsion has been reported. Mage and colleagues reported on 35 patients diagnosed with adnexal torsion at laparoscopy. All patients underwent untwisting of the pedicle and observation for 10 minutes. Conservative treatment was attempted in those who showed at least partial recovery of ischemic lesions. In addition to untwisting, laparoscopic oophoropexies were performed in two patients. Seventy-seven percent of these patients were managed with laparoscopy only. All had subsequent normal ovarian function. No complications were reported in these patients; however, one patient did develop a recurrence of the torsion 12 months later.[10]

Special Considerations

Torsion of the ovary is associated with ovarian hyperstimulation syndrome (OHSS) due to human menopausal gonadotropin (Pergonal) use for ovulation induction. This syndrome is characterized by high estrogen secretion, enlargement of the ovaries, abdominal discomfort, nausea, and vomiting. In severe cases clinical manifestations may include ascites, pleural effusions, electrolyte imbalance, oliguria, and shock. Torsion of the ovary was present in 7.4% of cases of OHSS in one series. It was more common (16%) in patients who were pregnant and had OHSS.[10] Recent reports of treatment of these patients by untwisting of the ovarian pedicle even when the ovary appears necrotic have demonstrated no complications. Normal subsequent ovarian function has been demonstrated by ultrasound in these patients. Continuation of pregnancy without problems was also shown. Although the number of patients treated in this manner is still small, this option should be considered for these patients in whom fertility is such an important issue. This method of treatment may not be applicable to patients who do not have OHSS.[10,12,13]

The diagnosis of ovarian torsion must be considered in children presenting with abdominal pain. In Lomano's series seven of the 44 patients were 9 years old or less.[9] This entity has been reported in the neonate as well.[14] In children the most common erroneous preoperative diagnosis was appendicitis. Up to 2% of children explored for appendicitis may have torsion of the adnexa.[15] In children the adnexal torsion may present as an abdominal mass.

Conclusions

Torsion of the adnexal structures must be considered in women of all ages presenting with abdominal pain. The incidence is highest in the reproductive-age group. A palpable or an ultrasonically detected pelvic mass along with pain should alert the clinician to consider this diagnosis. Because of the difficulty of clinical diagnosis, the more frequent use of laparoscopy may lead to early treatment and preservation of fertility.

REFERENCES

1. Silen W. Cope's Early Diagnosis of the Acute Abdomen, 15th ed, p 203. New York: Oxford Press, 1979
2. Hibbard LT. Adnexal torsion. Am J Obstet Gynecol 152:456, 1985
3. Nichols DH, Julian PJ. Torsion of the adnexa. Clin Obstet Gynecol 28:375, 1985
4. Mashiach S, Bider D, Moran O, Goldenberg M, Ben-Rafael Z. Adnexal torsion of hyperstimulated ovaries in pregnancies after gonadotropin therapy. Fertil Steril 53:76, 1990
5. Sommerville M, Grimes DA, Koonings PP, Campbell K. Ovarian neoplasms and the risk of adnexal torsion. Am J Obstet Gynecol 164:577, 1991
6. Koonings PP, Grimes DA. Adnexal torsion in postmenopausal women. Obstet Gynecol 73:11, 1989
7. Lee RA, Welch JS. Torsion of the uterine adnexa. Am J Obstet Gynecol 97:974, 1967
8. Burnett LS. Gynecologic causes of the acute abdomen. Surg Clin North Am 68:385, 1988
9. Lomano JM, Trelford JD, Ullery JC. Torsion of the uterine adnexa causing an acute abdomen. Obstet Gynecol 35:221, 1970
10. Mage G, Canis M, Manhes H, Pouly JL, Bruhat MA. Laparoscopic management of adnexal torsion. A review of 35 cases. J Reprod Med 34:520, 1989

11. Helvie MA, Silver TM. Ovarian torsion: sonographic evaluation. J Clin Ultrasound 17:327, 1989
12. Shalev J, Goldenberg M, Oelsner G et al. Treatment of twisted ischemic adnexa by simple detorsion. N Engl J Med 321:546, 1989
13. Bider D, Ben-Rafael Z, Goldenberg M, Shalev J, Mashiach S. Pregnancy outcome after unwinding of twisted ischaemic-haemorrhagic adnexa. Br J Obstet Gynaecol 96:428, 1989
14. Miller BM, Trocino AA, Gheewala A. Torsion of an ovarian cyst in a premature infant. NY State J Med 437, 1986
15. Schultz LR, Newton WA, Clatworthy HW. Torsion of previously normal tube and ovary in children. N Engl J Med 268:343, 1963

CHAPTER 21

Postoperative Emergencies

Gregory Sutton

This chapter discusses gynecologic emergencies typically occurring in the postoperative period. Although many of these emergencies are treated definitively by the gynecologic surgeon, because of the increasing pressure by third-party payors for expeditious hospital discharge, the emergency physician must be familiar with the recognition, diagnosis, and initial management of these complications. This chapter is divided into six sections, each dealing with a set of postoperative problems. They are (1) mechanical wound complications, (2) infectious complications, (3) thromboembolic complications, (4) gastrointestinal complications, (5) urinary tract sequelae, and (6) other postoperative emergencies.

Mechanical Wound Complications

Dehiscence

Dehiscence, or complete fascial disruption, is the most profound mechanical wound complication, occurring in up to 6% of general surgery cases and in from 0.3% to 0.7% of gynecologic surgical cases.[1,2] Associated mortality ranges from 10% to 35%. Risk factors for dehiscence include obesity, malnutrition, malignancy, previous surgical incision, infection, abdominal distention, bronchopulmonary disease, and corticosteroid therapy. Surgery following radiotherapy may also be complicated by fascial dehiscence.[3]

Dehiscence, also called "burst abdomen," generally reflects separation of all layers of the surgical wound, including skin, subcutaneous tissue, fascia, and peritoneum. This complication is usually, but not always, associated with evisceration, wherein the small bowel and other abdominal contents herniate through the incisional defect onto the abdominal wall (Fig. 21-1).

The choice of suture for wound closure may influence subsequent rates of dehiscence. Rapidly absorbed materials such as gut are associated with dehiscence rates as high as 14%.[4] Polyglactin (Vicryl) and polyglycolic acid (Dexon) are more durable but lose most of their tensile strength within 3 weeks of application. They are associated with higher failure rates than those observed with permanent sutures, such as stainless steel wire, nylon, polypropylene (Prolene), or polybutester (Novofil). Slowly absorbed synthetic sutures, such as polydioxanone (PDS) and polyglyconate (Maxon), maintain favorable characteristics for as long as 180 days,[5] which greatly exceeds the generally accepted 120-day period of fascial healing. The potential advantage of these materials is the absence of a foreign body that may lead to suture sinus formation or bowel entrapment.

Wound closure technique also influences outcome. Several studies have confirmed the superiority of mass closure techniques, such as that of Smead and Jones,[6] when compared to layered closure. More recently, continuous mass closure with permanent[7] or slowly absorbed materials, such as polyglyconate,[8] has been used with success approximating that of the Smead-Jones technique.

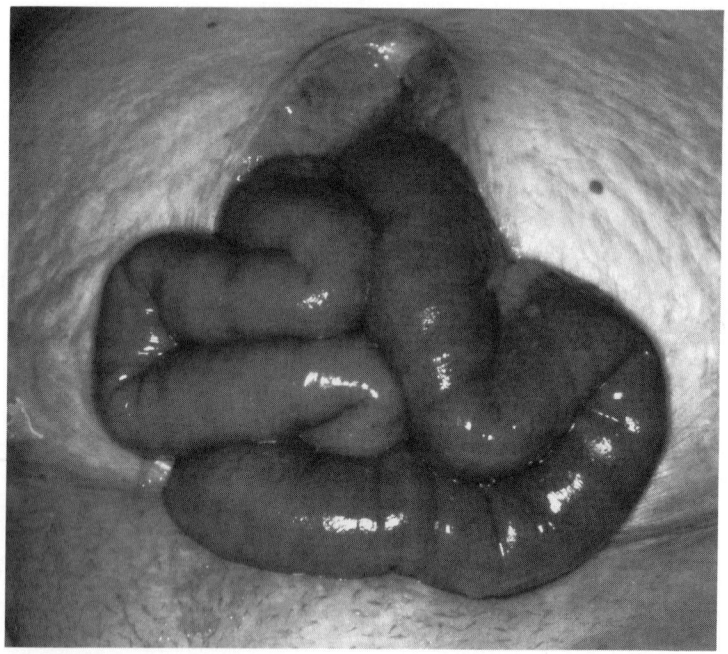

FIGURE 21-1
Herniation of abdominal contents through incisional defect.

Midline incisions are more commonly associated with dehiscence than paramedian, oblique, or transverse approaches, but the latter are not immune to this problem. This complication is often diagnosed by the patient, who describes a sudden rupture of the wound with straining, coughing, or a shift in position from supine to upright. The event may be heralded by a dramatic gush of fluid and small bowel loops, but just as often the skin remains intact.

Premonitory symptoms may be absent, however, and the most common finding is the presence of a serosanguineous discharge from the approximated skin edges of the wound. Such an occurrence always deserves evaluation. Even though dehiscence may occur from 5 to 15 days following surgery, the complication is much more safely managed in the inpatient setting. Gentle digital probing with a sterile gloved finger may reveal the fascial fault before catastrophe ensues. In the exceptional case where the skin has healed, ultrasound examination of the wound may identify actively peristalsing loops of small bowel subjacent to the skin with no evidence of intervening fascia or subcutaneous tissue. Superficial wound infection is associated with an increased risk of dehiscence and should not be regarded lightly. The fascia should be probed digitally during the initial evaluation of the superficial infection to ensure that it is not accompanied by a defect. Subcutaneous hematoma formation, although itself not a threat to fascial integrity, may indicate a hastily executed and faulty closure.

First treatment of wound dehiscence is the provision of a wide, moist, sterile dressing to protect the exposed viscera. The next concerns are intravenous access, gastrointestinal decompression, and urinary catheterization. Because dehiscence is often associated with sepsis or infection, central venous monitoring is beneficial, and right heart catheterization may be advisable if there is underlying pulmonary or cardiovascular disease.

Although surgical correction of the wound defect is of prime concern, hasty reoperation may jeopardize the condition of an unstable patient. Volume repletion must be accomplished before surgery, fluid and electrolyte disturbances must be corrected, and intravenous total peripheral nutrition should be considered, especially if there is a significant preexisting deficit. Broad-spectrum antibiotics should be employed but may be delayed until aerobic and anaerobic wound cultures can be obtained.

Once the patient's condition has been stabilized, the wound should be thoroughly evaluated under general anesthesia. Old suture material should be removed and the abdominal contents evaluated. If abscesses are present, drainage is imperative. The small bowel should be inspected from the ligament of Treitz to the ileocecal valve and nonviable areas should be resected and reanastomosed. The wound edges should then be generously debrided and the wound closed after voluminous irrigation of the peritoneal cavity. Fascial closure should employ a monofilament suture and should include all layers of the abdominal wall except the subcutaneous tissues and skin. Although the latter may be closed primarily, most surgeons prefer to leave the subcutaneous tissues open and allow healing by secondary intention. Delayed closure may be accomplished when granulation tissue is apparent throughout the wound. The use of drains should be discouraged unless an abscess is discovered.

Long-term sequelae of dehiscence may include an increased incidence of incisional hernias and cosmetic defects.

Vaginal Evisceration

Much rarer, but perhaps more dramatic than abdominal wound dehiscence, is vaginal evisceration. This uncommon complication has been reported most frequently following vaginal or abdominal hysterectomy but may also be seen as a result of spontaneous rupture of a large vaginal enterocele.[9] Additionally, iatrogenic evisceration may accompany inadvertent uterine perforation at the time of suction curettage. The latter condition is easily recognized at the time of surgery but may result in substantial injury to large segments of small bowel. Vaginal evisceration following hysterectomy or as the result of a large enterocele generally follows an episode of acutely increased intra-abdominal pressure. On recognition, the herniated bowel should be protected with moist, sterile towels or laparotomy packs and the patient should be kept in a supine position to prevent undue tension on the mesentery. Emergency laparotomy through a midline incision is imperative following stabilization and volume resuscitation. Antibiotics should be started prior to surgery and antiembolism precautions should be taken. At laparotomy, the entire gastrointestinal tract should be carefully inspected, with particular attention directed to the small bowel mesentery. Segmental resection is indicated if nonviable small bowel is identified. The vaginal vault should be securely closed. If the dehiscence is associated with a large enterocele, abdominal or vaginal repair may be undertaken unless the patient's condition warrants a delayed approach.

Mortality for vaginal evisceration may be as high as 10% and is usually associated with intestinal necrosis, peritonitis, or underlying medical illness. Such modern techniques as nutritional support, antibiotic therapy, and intensive monitoring should prevent fatalities.

Suture Sinuses

Chronic draining sinuses may occur when permanent suture is employed in the fascial or subcutaneous layer of abdominal wounds or in the vaginal or subvaginal tissues following vaginal procedures. Although the use of permanent sutures in the vagina is uncommon, this problem may arise when permanent materials are incorporated in procedures designed to suspend the vaginal wall or urethra. These sinuses first become apparent with erythema of the overlying skin or vaginal mucosa accompanied by pain or tenderness with or without fever. Over the course of a few days to weeks, the site opens and spontaneous drainage usually occurs. Skin flora may predominate in culture specimens, or the sinus may be sterile.

The only way to treat these annoying and rarely serious complications is by exploring the area under local anesthesia and removing the offending foreign body. In the case of abdominal wall sinuses, care must be taken to delay removal until fascial healing is complete.

Incisional Hernia

Most incisional hernias probably occur within 1 year of surgery. As the fascia and muscle separate, a sac of peritoneum bulges through the more superficial tissues and may be easily palpable through the skin. The patient may experience a tearing or shearing sensation upon straining or Valvalva's maneuver; the resulting hernia may or may not be appreciated by the patient.

Often the only symptom is a sense of abdominal discomfort or pulling, which is exacerbated by standing, walking, or straining.

The size of the hernia sac may bear no relationship to the defect in the fascia. Substantial omentum and bowel may slide through the hernia ring and occupy the extra-abdominal cavity. The smaller the fascial ring, the greater the risk for incarceration and strangulation. These dire complications are much rarer in incisional or ventral hernias than in inguinal or femoral defects. Nonetheless, care must be taken to demonstrate that the hernia can be manually reduced, usually with the patient in the supine position. If the suspicion of an incisional hernia is high, but the physical examination is inconclusive or the patient is obese, real-time ultrasound is a sensitive way to demonstrate the presence of omentum or the peristalsis of bowel above the level of the abdominal wall fascia.

Once the contents of the hernia sac are returned to the peritoneal cavity, it may be easier to assess the size of the fascial defect. Most incisional hernias may be repaired in a planned and deliberate manner. In elderly or ill patients, the relative advantages of repair and risks of surgical intervention must be carefully weighed. In those at high risk for surgery, an abdominal binder or corset may be sufficient to alleviate the symptoms of even a large defect. Surgical therapy may require the placement of synthetic mesh if the fascial defect is substantial.[10]

In the rare case of incarceration, the patient will present with symptoms of tenderness over the hernia and early peritoneal signs. If small or large intestine is present in the hernia, symptoms of obstruction will accompany the local findings. Strangulation may be associated with circulatory collapse, volume depletion, and sepsis. Stabilization and emergency surgery are indicated in such cases.

Vaginal Eversion

Total vaginal eversion, or vaginal prolapse, follows abdominal or vaginal hysterectomy in 2 to 4% of patients. Unless the patient has substantial obstructive pulmonary disease or an underlying connective tissue flaw, the prolapse usually results from failure to recognize and repair a defect in pelvic support at the time of hysterectomy or from neglecting to bolster the vagina following removal of the uterus.

Development of vaginal prolapse may have an insidious course, or, like other hernias, the onset may be abruptly symptomatic. The condition is seen more frequently in postmenopausal women, in those of high parity, and in those with a family history of support defects.[11] Urinary symptoms may be absent, but often the accompanying prolapse of the bladder leads to stress incontinence or, in more advanced stages, requires digital replacement of this organ before micturition. In addition to the bladder, the vaginal prolapse may contain sigmoid colon, rectum, and small bowel. Fecal retention may be present and a history of digital assistance with defecation may be elicited. Most authors feel that enterocele is nearly always present in the case of massive vaginal prolapse. As with other hernias, the associated symptoms may include a "dragging" or tractionlike abdominal discomfort that is exacerbated by long-term standing and relieved by lying down.

The complexity of genital eversion requires that corrective surgery be undertaken by an expert in the evaluation and repair of such defects. An abdominal procedure, such as sacral colpopexy, may be the more durable repair, but vaginal approaches such as the sacrospinous repair permit rapid postoperative recovery and are ideally suited for elderly or medically unstable patients.

Almost without exception, vaginal prolapse can be reduced with gentle sustained pressure with the patient in the supine position, and it thus rarely requires emergency surgical intervention. Once the prolapsed small bowel and pelvic viscera have been repositioned, a pessary may be placed and worn until appropriate surgical evaluation can be carried out. In this regard, a medium or large donut or inflatable balloon pessary may be best, since the smaller ring, cube, and stem pessaries may not be large enough to support the redundant mucosa of a complete eversion.

Infectious Complications

Superficial Wound Infections

In patients who have not received prophylactic antibiotics, the incidence of wound infection following abdominal hysterectomy for benign indications is about 5%.[12] However, this number may be significantly higher in some populations. The infection rate for cesarean section may be as high as 10%. The risk of infection may be reduced significantly by administering preoperative antibiotics. Abdominal hysterectomy and cesarean section are, by definition, "clean-contaminated" operations, since the genitourinary tract is entered.

Wound infection rates are affected by the size of bacterial inoculum, the virulence of the responsible organism, the presence of foreign bodies, the experience of the primary surgeon, and host factors. The latter include nutritional status, diabetes, liver disease, age, and immunosuppression.

Superficial surgical infections typically become apparent 5 to 7 days postoperatively, when serosanguineous or seropurulent drainage from the incision line is noticed. Frequently, the patient has been been discharged; thus the diagnosis is made on emergency room visit. Fever and leukocytosis frequently accompany this finding, but systemic toxicity is mild unless the wound is neglected. These infections are typically due to *Staphylococcus aureus* contamination or arise from enteric or vaginal flora. In diabetic or obese patients the subcutaneous infection may be quite extensive despite apparently normal surrounding skin (Fig. 21-2). The skin and subcutaneous layers of superficially infected wounds should be opened completely even if partial skin healing has occurred. This facilitates evaluation and subsequent care of the entire incision. If the fascial and muscular layers are intact, the wound can be successfully treated without systemic antibiotic therapy. Following gentle initial debridement, four-times-daily irrigation with dilute hydrogen peroxide or Dakin's solution (sodium hypochlorite), and packing with dry, nonfilled fine gauze such as Kerlix promotes rapid development of granulation tissue and a healthy wound bed. Delayed closure can be safely performed once the surface of the wound is completely covered with granulation tissue. Gram stain and culture of such superficial infections is of little clinical value but may provide important information to the hospital infection control committee.

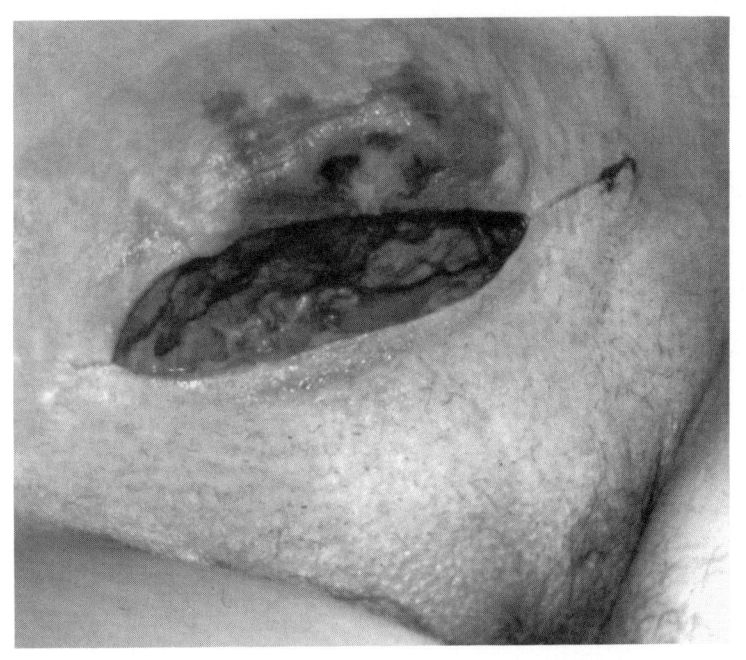

FIGURE 21–2
Subcutaneous infection secondary to *Staphylococcus aureus*.

Infections with group A beta-hemolytic *Streptococcus* induce high fevers within 24 to 48 hours after surgery and are characterized by rapidly spreading erythema of the wound edge. Lymphangitic spread and regional adenopathy are characteristic. Toxicity may be striking, and drainage from the incision may be limited to a small amount of thin, watery fluid. The rash of scarlet fever may accompany the infection.

Antibiotic therapy without mechanical wound disruption will normally control an uncomplicated streptococcal infection. Parenteral penicillin is the antibiotic of choice, although it may be desirable to use a more broad-spectrum antibiotic if the etiology of the infection is uncertain.

Necrotizing Fasciitis

Although necrotizing fasciitis, a devastating infection, may arise from a trivial insult, approximately 50% of cases are associated with a surgical incision. This infection was initially described by Meleney, who differentiated it from clostridial or gas gangrene.[13] He was the first author to advocate early diagnosis and prompt, aggressive surgical resection of the involved tissues. Although the term *necrotizing fasciitis* was introduced by Wilson in 1951,[14] Fisher first enumerated the following six criteria for the diagnosis[15]:

1. Extensive necrosis of the superficial fascia with widespread undermining of skin
2. Moderate to severe systemic toxic reaction
3. Absence of muscle involvement

4. No demonstration of *Clostridia* in wound and blood cultures
5. Absence of major vascular occlusion
6. Intensive leukocytic infiltration, necrosis of subcutaneous tissue, and microvascular thrombosis on pathologic examination of debrided tissue.

This condition has been most commonly described in the lower extremity. When it is not seen in association with an abdominal incision, it occurs, in order of frequency, in the perineum or groin, upper extremity, and back or buttocks. Not only is diabetes an important risk factor for the development of necrotizing fasciitis, but patients with diabetes have a much worse prognosis than those without this condition.[16] The cause of necrotizing fasciitis is unknown, but it has been attributed to both hemolytic streptococci and staphylococci. Recent bacteriologic studies suggest that mixed infections predominate and that the anaerobes are frequently involved.[17]

In addition to diabetes, other risk factors include advanced age, peripheral vascular disease, malnutrition, debilitating illness, malignancy, radiation therapy, morbid obesity, hypertension, and renal insufficiency.

Early symptoms include subcutaneous edema and induration of the area around the surgical incision.[18] The skin may become dusky or erythematous. Although tenderness may be pronounced, it is not uncommon for hypesthesia to develop in the central area of infection as cutaneous nerves become ischemic in transversing the subcutaneous tissue in the area of infection. Crepitation may occasionally be elicited. Perhaps the most striking feature is systemic toxicity far in excess of the apparent infection. Although fever and leukocytosis may be pronounced, they may not be as severe as the hypotension, tachycardia, and lethargy that accompany this infection.

As this infection spreads peripherally, cutaneous bullae may develop and the skin may appear necrotic. It is not uncommon for incision and drainage to be performed at this point in the clinical course, for necrotizing fasciitis is rarely diagnosed before the third to fifth day of the infection. With incision, the subcutaneous tissues appear necrotic. A grayish watery "dirty dishwater" exudate may emanate from the wound. The deep fascia may be black or gray and necrotic (Fig. 21-3), and the infectious process may travel along the planes of the deep fascia, undermining normal-appearing skin and giving little clue to the extensive nature of the disease.

Subcutaneous necrosis is the hallmark of this infection and may be demonstrated by passing a finger or blunt instrument through the fatty tissue with little or no resistance.

Early in the clinical course, necrotizing fasciitis becomes a multiorgan process. Intravascular depletion may be extreme, secondary to local tissue edema and increased vascular permeability. Hemoconcentration is a common finding and must be corrected before operative intervention is undertaken. Similarly, saponification of subcutaneous fat is associated with pronounced and often unexpected hypocalcemia. Hemolysis, hyperbilirubinemia, and hepatic, renal, and pulmonary insufficiency are not uncommon.

The most important aspects of treatment in necrotizing fasciitis are early diagnosis and subsequent wide surgical debridement to healthy skin, subcutaneous, and fascial margins. Such supportive measures as central venous monitoring, total peripheral nutrition, very-broad-spectrum antibiotic therapy, and aggressive replacement of fluids, colloids, and calcium are also of great importance. The critical role

Obstruction of the Large Intestine

Obstruction of the large intestine is a rare postoperative problem. Most common are sigmoid and cecal volvuluses. The former usually occurs when the sigmoid is overlong or redundant, but it may be the result of tethering adhesions. The latter only occurs when the cecum is attached by a mesentery, rather than being secured in its usual retroperitoneal position. Large bowel obstruction most commonly presents with the symptoms of obstipation and abdominal distention. Only if the ileocecal valve is incompetent does the small bowel also become dilated.

Large bowel obstruction may result in intestinal perforation, peritonitis, and death. The cecum is the most common site of perforation owing to the greater diameter of this organ and resulting in higher stress per unit wall area. Radiographic examination shows air-filled dilated colon up to the point of obstruction. Clinically, patients with large bowel blockage may not manifest the signs of volume depletion or severe nausea and vomiting observed in small bowel obstruction.

The management of large bowel obstruction is operative. Volvulus or adhesions must be corrected or reduced surgically. Preoperative colonoscopy not only is important to determine the level and the severity of obstruction, but also may facilitate the management of early sigmoid volvulus.

Gastrointestinal Fistulas

Enterocutaneous fistulas are rare following surgery for benign gynecologic conditions. When widespread endometriosis is present, the small bowel may be inadvertently injured and, usually after a protracted postoperative course, enterocutaneous fistula may develop. Another cause of postoperative enterocutaneous fistulas is the accidental inclusion of a loop of small bowel in the abdominal closure. Again, the typical postoperative course is one of fever, partial small bowel obstruction, wound infection, and finally, recognition of the fistula. Enterovaginal fistulas are less common than enterocutaneous fistulas.

Enterocutaneous fistulas are much more common after surgery upon the small bowel during oncologic procedures and following radiotherapy for cervical cancer. After small bowel surgery, an anastomotic leak may be heralded by symptoms of diffuse or localized peritonitis, abscess formation, and drainage of small bowel contents through the incision or another point on the abdominal wall.

Treatment of postoperative small bowel fistula depends upon the presence of associated abscess or obstruction. In the absence of radiotherapy, abscess, and distal obstruction, the leak may be successfully managed in over 70% of cases by gastrointestinal tube decompression, total peripheral nutrition, and somatostatin. Fistulas associated with radiotherapy, obstruction, or abscess frequently require operative correction.

Initial therapy for enterocutaneous fistulas should include protection of the skin from the proteolytic enzymes present in small bowel fluid by isolating the drainage into an ileal or colostomy drainage bag. Karya paste or a wafer may be fitted to protect the skin. Volume depletion should be corrected, and arrangements for semipermanent central access made. It is important to demonstrate that the colon is patent if surgical intervention is anticipated.

Colovaginal or rectovaginal fistulas may complicate deep or fourth-degree episiotomies, overzealous culdotomy, difficult posterior cul-de-sac dissections associated with endometriosis, or the condition of patients who have had radiotherapy. Low rectovaginal fistulas that occur in the postpartum period may be repaired without diverting the large bowel. Early sigmoid-vaginal fistulas following abdominal hysterectomy may resolve spontaneously if they are small, recognized early, and unassociated with abscess formation. An elemental diet must be employed to reduce the fecal stream to a negligible amount.

Larger leaks must be treated with a diverting colostomy and surgical repair. In the case of large bowel/vaginal fistulas following radiotherapy or associated with recurrent malignancy, colostomy is the best method of palliation, although these problems may be managed with elemental diets in patients either not desiring or unable to undergo major surgery.

Laparoscopic Bowel Injury

Transmural small or large bowel injuries recognized at the time of laparoscopy require repair. Small bowel injuries and minor large bowel injuries may be repaired by way of the laparoscope if the surgeon is capable of this type of procedure. Puncture wounds incurred by the Verres needle may be successfully managed with antibiotics and tube decompression. Larger injuries, especially those of unprepared colon, should be treated by laparotomy and repair or diversion.

Half of all bowel burns that occur at the time of laparoscopy are recognized at the time of surgery, and most can be handled conservatively. In complicated cases, signs of peritonitis are recognized between 2 and 7 days from surgery and indicate the need for surgical intervention and resection of the damaged segment.

More serious are laparoscopic injuries that go unrecognized until the patient develops an acute abdomen, usually within 24 to 72 hours following the procedure. In such cases, emergency laparotomy is indicated after stabilization and initiation of broad-spectrum antibiotic coverage. Important in the diagnosis of a bowel injury at the time of laparoscopy is the presence of free air under the diaphragm on upright films of the abdomen. At the time of laparotomy, large bowel injuries should be repaired and the fecal stream diverted. Small bowel injuries may require resection and reanastomosis if the bowel is irreparably damaged. Minor injuries may be oversewn.

Genitourinary Injuries Resulting in Postoperative Emergencies

The most common urologic complications following gynecologic surgery are ureteral obstruction, ureterovaginal fistula, and vesicovaginal fistula. The majority of ureteral injuries are ligations, angulations, or transections unrecognized at the time of abdominal hysterectomy.[22] Approximately three quarters of all ureterovaginal fistulas in the United States are the result of abdominal hysterectomy.

Postoperative ureteral obstruction remains silent more often than not. Usually the obstructed ureter is only recognized months or years later at the time of evaluation for unrelated diagnoses. Unfortunately, at such an interval, the renal cortex is generally thin and residual function in the involved kidney is poor. Asymptomatic obstructed kidneys are best left alone unless nuclear scanning demonstrates significant function. Symptomatic obstruction results in flank pain, colicky discomfort occasionally referred to the ipsilateral groin or labium majus, and fever and chills if there is obstructed pyelonephritis. Symptomatic obstruction is usually recognized early and can be treated.

If intravenous pyelography and retrograde studies demonstrate a low-grade obstruction, stents may be placed across the narrowed segment by cystoscopy, and the urinary system can be restudied 3 to 4 months later for improvement. If the injury is severe or the bladder too edematous to allow visualization of the ureteric orifices, percutaneous nephrostomy should be performed. If the injured segment can be stented in antegrade fashion using a double-J or pigtail catheter, the nephrostomy may be capped and the blockage managed expectantly. Occasionally, if the narrowed segment is recognized early, dilatation using a Grunzig balloon catheter may be possible.

If stenting is ineffective, then surgical reconstruction of the ureter is necessary. For low injuries, psoas hitch ureteroneocystostomy is the procedure of choice. For middle-one-third lesions, interposition of small bowel may be possible, and for higher lesions, ureteroureterostomy may be indicated.

Ureterovaginal fistulas are handled in much the same way as ureteral obstruction. These injuries may be most common following radical hysterectomy and very frequently respond to stenting with a multiperforate "fistula" stent. Adequate radiographic evaluation is critical to exclude a concomitant vesicovaginal communication.

Patients with both vesicovaginal and ureterovaginal fistulas commonly present with continuous urinary incontinence following surgery. Occasionally, the urinary leakage may be positional and may actually improve at night when the patient is in the supine position. Careful history and vaginal examination may demonstrate the vaginal site of urinary leakage. A small point of granulation tissue commonly marks the fistula tract, and both vesico- and ureterovaginal fistulas are most common at the vaginal apex. If the fistula cannot be visualized with the patient in the supine position, it is often helpful to repeat the examination in the knee-chest position. The weight of the intra-abdominal contents expands the vagina and facilitates inspection of the entire cylinder.

Other techniques useful in demonstrating urinary fistulas include tampon or cotton ball tests. These indicators are placed in the vagina and the urine is dyed using methylene blue or indigo carmine instilled by way of an indwelling Foley catheter. The catheter is clamped and the patient is allowed to ambulate for 15 minutes. After this time the marker is removed from the vagina and inspected for stain. A similar technique useful in demonstrating ureterovaginal leakage involves the administration of 400 mg pyridium by mouth about 30 minutes before the vaginal markers are placed. Orange discoloration of the marker in the presence of a negative methylene blue test indicates the presence of a ureterovaginal communication.

Once the leak is identified, intravenous pyelography, cystoscopy, and retrograde studies complete the evaluation and help lay the groundwork for repair. Early postoperative ureterovaginal fistulas may respond very well to stenting. Early vesicovaginal fistulas that are limited in size may heal if a suprapubic catheter is placed. Large, complicated, or late fistulas require surgical intervention.

Urinary Retention

Although this problem occurs most commonly within the first day or two following gynecologic surgery, usually after removal of an indwelling urethral catheter, patients who have undergone radical hysterectomy or retropubic urethropexy may experience voiding difficulty several weeks or even months following surgery. As in other cases of urinary retention, the diagnosis and treatment of this problem is catheter drainage. Whereas women who have had urinary suspension become symptomatic at relatively low bladder volumes, those who have had radical hysterectomy are quite often unable to appreciate bladder filling and may present with vague lower abdominal pain, suprapubic mass, and history of oliguria. These women may require instruction in intermittent self-catheterization to be performed two to three times daily until the bladder tone and function return.

Other Postoperative Emergencies

Venous Thrombosis

Injury to pelvic venous plexuses is not uncommon during gynecologic or oncologic surgery, if to this is added some degree of immobilization in the immediate perioperative period, and the diagnosis of a gynecologic malignancy, Virchow's triad of stasis, vascular injury, and hypercoagulability is met and the stage is set for deep venous thrombosis. Patients who do not have a malignancy may have obesity or diabetes or a hereditary hypercoagulability; thus many patients undergoing gynecologic surgery are at risk for clot formation.

Although the presence of a hot, tender, swollen lower extremity raises the suspicion of deep venous thrombosis, clinical diagnosis of this condition is often inaccurate. Homans' sign, or resistance to forced dorsiflexion of the foot, is just as unreliable in the diagnosis of thrombosis. Contrast venography, the gold standard for the diagnosis of lower-extremity clots, has been replaced to a large extent by impedance plethysmography and color-flow Doppler venography, and compression ultrasonography in the detection of lower-extremity clot.

Superficial thrombophlebitis may occur in the veins of the calf or along the distribution of the greater saphenous vein. Physical findings are limited to erythema and tenderness in the distribution of these venous systems, and therapy consists of extremity elevation, aspirin, and heat. Most superficial clots will respond to such conservative therapy.

Deep venous thrombosis requires inpatient heparinization and immobilization of the extremity until anticoagulation is achieved. After 7 to 10 days of heparin therapy, Coumadin is started and maintained for 3 to 6 months, depending upon the extent of the clot and the relative risk of the patient for recurrence. The three most common sequelae of deep venous thrombosis—recurrence, pulmonary embolus, and postphlebitic syndrome—should be minimized if aggressive anticoagulation is utilized.

Pulmonary Embolus

Although it is a very common cause of death among hospitalized patients, the increased risk of pulmonary embolus follows the patient home after discharge. The risk of postoperative pulmonary embolism ranges from 0.1% in patients undergoing uncomplicated gynecologic surgery to 5% in those with the diagnosis of malignancy undergoing extensive pelvic operations.

Although prophylaxis with low-dose subcutaneous heparin or external pneumatic extremity compression garments has reduced the risk of postoperative thromboembolic disease, pulmonary embolism should always be considered in the differential diagnosis of postoperative pulmonary complaints.

Signs of thromboembolism may be very mild or massive. They may be as unimpressive as tachycardia or tachypnea in a patient with mild breathlessness. Many patients with pulmonary embolism develop signs and symptoms of pulmonary infarction, including fever, pleuritic chest pain, cough, and hemoptysis. Those with massive emboli may simply experience cardiovascular collapse, respiratory failure, coma, and death. Most patients who die of pulmonary emboli do so within 2 hours of the event.

Physical findings associated with pulmonary embolism are nonspecific and may be confused with those of other pulmonary processes. The presence of a pleural friction rub in the setting of dyspnea and tachycardia should be considered highly suspicious, however. Radiographic studies are no more specific. Infiltrates, pleural effusions, or volume loss may be associated with a variety of pulmonary diseases.

Perfusion scanning is very helpful. A normal lung perfusion study effectively excludes the diagnosis of pulmonary embolism. Perfusion defects unassociated with ventilation abnormalities suggest pulmonary emboli and, if these defects are large, very often indicate the presence of blood clot. Matching ventilation/perfusion abnormalities may be caused by primary pulmonary processes, such as mucus plugs or bronchitis. Indeterminate scans require evaluation by pulmonary angiography.

Although pulmonary arteriography is not risk-free, selective studies with small volumes of contrast are relatively safe and probably associated with less morbidity than long-term anticoagulation. Another approach to the patient with abnormal perfusion scans is lower-extremity color Doppler or compression ultrasound evaluation. If a deep venous thrombosis is identified in the proximal lower extremity, anticoagulation must be employed, regardless of the ventilation/perfusion scan results.[23] Serial impedance plethysmography has been used similarly to exclude the presence of lower-extremity clot.

Continuous heparin should be administered in doses that produce an activated partial thromboplastin time (APTT) of 1.5 to 2.0 times control. Oral anticoagulation may be initiated at the same time heparin is started. Heparin can then be discontinued after 5 days of therapy, provided a 1.5 to 2.0 times prolongation of prothrombin time has been achieved.

Coumadin should be maintained for 3 months in patients with uncomplicated thrombosis or embolism but should be continued for a year in those patients with recurrent thromboembolic problems.

The role of thrombolytic therapy is uncertain, but intravenous streptokinase therapy should be considered in patients with acute life-threatening pulmonary emboli.

Inadvertent Residual Foreign Bodies

Despite perioperative sponge, needle, and instrument counts, surgical equipment is occasionally left behind in the abdomen or pelvis. Such situations require prompt, judicious diagnosis and treatment, so that such an error is not compounded by secondary mismanagement.

Perhaps the most common misplaced item is the surgical sponge or laparotomy tape that is not removed from the vagina following minor vaginal surgery or obstetric repairs. Although such an object may reside in the vagina innocuously for several days, overgrowth of bacterial flora eventually produces olfactory clues that lead to professional consultation. Vaginal sponges may cause local necrosis if they are placed tightly or if impregnated with an astringent such as ether or ferrous subsulfate.

After removal of the sponge or tape, the vagina should be carefully inspected for epithelial injury and residual fragments or fibers.

Intra-abdominal laparotomy pads, sponges, or tapes occasionally remain asymptomatic for long periods of time, particularly if the object is small and the patient in good general health.[24] More commonly, vague abdominal symptoms such as fullness, cramping, obstipation, or localized discomfort are present. If infection occurs, symptoms mimic those of postoperative abscess.

Localized peritoneal signs may lead to generalized peritonitis. Since most surgical sponges contain a radio-opaque marker strip, the diagnosis of a foreign body can generally be made with abdominal plain films, although an upright or lateral view may aid in the differential diagnosis of acute abdomen. Air trapped between the fibers of the pad may produce a "whorled" appearance, which is characteristic of these foreign bodies. Computerized tomography scanning with gastrointestinal contrast may aid in the preoperative localization of sponges and may indicate whether the object requires retrieval by laparotomy or whether laparoscopy may suffice. All such bodies must be removed, even if the patient is asymptomatic at the time of diagnosis.

Surgical instruments such as clamps and scissors are rarely lost in the wound. When this unfortunate event occurs, the patient may complain of abdominal pains that are accentuated by extremes of posture, such as bending, lifting, or stretching. Infection is rare, but the danger of perforation or true "mechanical" bowel obstruction demands removal of these objects.

Surgical needles may occasionally be lost intraoperatively. Small needles rarely cause problems, but larger needles may migrate and cause bowel injury or localized peritonitis. Reexploration is probably not indicated in cases where needles are discovered late, although otherwise unexplained bowel symptoms should prompt a thorough radiographic evaluation.

REFERENCES

1. Greenburg AG, Saik RP, Peskin GW. Wound dehiscence. Arch Surg 114:143, 1979
2. Baggish MS, Lee WK. Abdominal wound disruption. Obstet Gynecol 46:530, 1975
3. Madden JW. Wound healing: biologic and clinical features. In: Sabiston DC, ed. Textbook of Surgery, 10th ed. Philadelphia: WB Saunders, 1972
4. Goligher JC, Irvin TT, Johnston D et al. A controlled clinical trial of three methods of closure of laparotomy wounds. Br J Surg 62:823, 1975
5. Stone IK. Suture materials. Clin Obstet Gynecol 31:712, 1988
6. Jones TE, Newell ET, Brubaker RE. The use of alloy steel wire in the closure of abdominal wounds. Surg Gynecol Obstet 72:1056, 1941
7. Gallup DG, Talledo OE, King LA. Primary mass closure of midline incisions with a continuous running monofilament suture in gynecologic patients. Obstet Gynecol 73:675, 1989
8. Gallup DG, Nolan TE, Smith RP. Primary mass closure of midline incisions with a continuous polyglyconate monofilament absorbable suture. Obstet Gynecol 76:872, 1990
9. Fox WP. Vaginal evisceration. Obstet Gynecol 50:223, 1977
10. George CD, Ellis H. The results of incisional hernia repair: a twelve-year review. Ann R Coll Surg Engl 68:185, 1986
11. Nichols DH. Eversion of the vagina. In: Nichols DH (ed): Reoperative Gynecologic Surgery. St Louis: CV Mosby, 1991
12. Ohm MJ, Galask RP. The effect of antibiotic prophylaxis on patients undergoing total abdominal hysterectomy. Am J Obstet Gynecol 125:442, 1976
13. Brewer GE, Meleney FL. Progressive gangrenous infection of the skin and subcutaneous tissues following operation for acute perforative appendicitis. Ann Surg 84:438, 1926
14. Wilson BL. Necrotizing fasciitis. Am J Surg 18:416, 1952
15. Fisher JR, Conway MJ, Takeshita et al. Necrotizing fasciitis. Importance of roentgenographic studies for soft-tissue gas. JAMA 241:803, 1979
16. Addison WA, Livengood CH, Hill GB et al. Necrotizing fasciitis of vulvar origin in diabetic patients. Obstet Gynecol 63:473, 1984
17. Golde S, Ledger WJ. Necrotizing fasciitis in postpartum patients. Obstet Gynecol 50:670, 1977
18. Sutton GP, Smirz LR, Clark DH, Bennett JE. Group B streptococcal necrotizing fasciitis arising from an episiotomy. Obstet Gynecol 66:733, 1985
19. Stone HH, Martin JD. Synergistic necrotizing fasciitis. Ann Surg 175:702, 1972
20. Cohen MB, Pernoll ML, Gevirtz CM et al. Septic pelvic thrombophlebitis: an update. Obstet Gynecol 62:83, 1983
21. Beutler B, Cerami A. Cachectin: more than a tumor necrosis factor. N Engl J Med 316:379, 1987
22. Symmonds RE. Urologic injuries: ureter. Clin Obstet Gynecol 19:623, 1976
23. Hull RD, Raskob GE. Pulmonary thromboembolism. In: Kelly WN (ed): Textbook of Internal Medicine. Philadelphia: JB Lippincott, 1992:1776
24. Jones S. The foreign body problems after laparotomy. Am J Surg 122:785, 1971

CHAPTER 22

Oncologic Emergencies

Guy I. Benrubi, Robert C. Nuss, and Ann Harwood-Nuss

Obstetric and Gynecologic Emergencies, edited by Guy I. Benrubi. J.B. Lippincott Company, Philadelphia © 1994.

Approximately 71,500 new invasive cancers of the female reproductive tract are diagnosed annually in the United States.[1] These cancers eventually result in approximately 24,400 annual deaths.[1] The yearly incidence of these diseases is increasing. As the baby boom cohort in the population ages, more ovarian, vulvar, and endometrial cancers will develop. An increased prevalence of human papillomavirus infection will result in an increase in cervical dysplasia and, possibly, cervical cancer, particularly if cytologic surveillance is not aggressively encouraged.[2]

With the advent of cytologic screening and the consequent decrease in invasive cervical cancer, the most frequently diagnosed cancer of the female reproductive tract is now endometrial.[1] This condition is followed in incidence by ovarian, cervical, and vulvar cancer and, less frequently, by gestational trophoblastic neoplasia, and tubal and vaginal cancer. Although the most frequent cause of emergencies in this population is ovarian cancer, emergency department physicians probably see patients primarily with cervical cancer. These patients typically belong to lower socioeconomic groups and are more likely to seek help in emergency department settings than with their primary physicians. This chapter discusses gynecologic cancer emergencies according to their most frequent clinical presentations, rather than according to the primary malignancies that cause these presentations.

Vaginal Bleeding

Patients who present with vaginal bleeding secondary to a gynecologic malignancy probably have either cervical or endometrial cancer.[3] Occasionally, other corpus malignancies, such as sarcomas and gestational trophoblastic disease, are the cause. Rarely, the cause is advanced vulvar cancer.

Women who present with vaginal bleeding owing to cervical cancer have a mean age of between 40 and 45 years.[4] This mean age has recently decreased because younger women have been contracting cervical cancer secondary to an increased incidence of human papillomavirus infection.[5] Essential points in the history of patients who present with vaginal bleeding owing to cervical cancer include the following: painless vaginal bleeding, exacerbated or caused by coitus; lack of previous cytologic screening, or a history of prior abnormality; findings on cytologic screening; lower socioeconomic status; multiple sexual partners.

Though physical examination should assess extra-pelvic spread of disease, such as supraclavicular or inguinal adenopathy, the main focus of the examination should be the pelvis. In a patient whose cancer is so advanced that vaginal bleeding is the presenting complaint, the lesion should be visible on speculum examination. The speculum should be inserted gently to avoid trauma to the bleeding site. The vulva, vagina, and cervical os should be carefully inspected. If there is no visible lesion on the cervix and the bleeding is coming through the cervical os, then cervical cancer is an unlikely cause of bleeding. Bimanual examination as well as a rectovaginal examination should be performed to assess possible involvement of the parametrial tissues. Laboratory studies should include a pregnancy test and a complete blood count. Measures that are effective in control of vaginal bleeding include packing the vagina, after insertion of a Foley catheter; use of Monsel's solution; and application of Oxycel. When all else fails, the packing material can be impregnated with a solution of epinephrine (1:500,000). If the bleeding is unremitting, the patient may need to be admitted for hypogastric artery ligation, embolization, or high-dose radiation therapy.[6]

In vaginal bleeding caused by endometrial or other corpus cancers the bleeding is usually not as severe as that caused by cervical cancer. Patients tend to be in an older age group. The mean age for patients with this disease is 60.[7] In approximately 5% of cases endometrial cancers occur in women under age 40.[3] Essential points in the history of the older patient include obesity and use of unopposed exogenous estrogens. In younger women obesity, nulliparity, and infertility may be predisposing factors. Although vaginal bleeding is the most common presenting complaint for this disease, it is seldom of such magnitude as to cause an emergency visit. In women who present with postmenopausal vaginal bleeding the diagnosis should be endometrial cancer until proved otherwise.

Careful examination should be performed to assess the size of the uterus and the presence of extrauterine tumor. On speculum examination the bleeding will be from the cervical os. Occasionally, endometrial cancer presents with a visible lesion on the cervix. The bleeding is seldom life-threatening.

Vaginal bleeding caused by gestational trophoblastic neoplasia occurs in women in either early or late reproductive age. With increasing numbers of immigrants from the Far East this may become an increasingly common cause of vaginal bleeding. Gestational trophoblastic neoplasia occurs in 1 out of 1200 pregnancies in the United States, but it is much more common in Asia.[8] In addition, as the pregnancy rate among inner-city teens burgeons, physicians will see a steadily increasing incidence of this disease. Vaginal bleeding is the most common presentation for gestational trophoblastic neoplasia.[8] Salient points in the history include uterine enlargement greater than expected for gestational age, absence of fetal movements, repeated visits to medical facilities for bleeding (often the diagnosis is threatened abortion), and hypertension in early pregnancy.

Physical examination reveals a large-for-gestational-age fundal height; speculum examination shows bleeding coming from the os. Vesicular material also may be seen extruding through the os. The definitive diagnosis is made by ultrasonography, which shows a distinctive multiechogenic pattern. Bleeding caused by vulvar cancer is unusual.[9] Women who present with this entity usually have an advanced lesion. Most are over age 60 and have other signs of neglect. Because of the possibility of either self- or institutional neglect, it is advisable to admit women who present with large, bleeding vulvar cancer lesions. Therapy can then be instituted promptly.

Bowel Emergencies

Bowel emergencies in patients with gynecologic malignancies are divided into two major subheadings: those that occur in nonradiated bowel and those with complications secondary to radiated bowel.

In the nonradiated bowel group the most common bowel emergencies are bowel obstruction, colostomy problems, fistula formation, and perforation.

Bowel Obstruction

Small-bowel obstruction that is not in the perioperative period is usually due to internal adhesions secondary to a previous surgical procedure or to gynecologic malignancy. In ovarian cancer approximately 5% of patients have small-bowel obstruction as the presenting complaint.[7] Ovarian cancer spreads on the serosal surfaces of the bowel and can cause either adhesive or bulk obstruction. The presentation of small-bowel obstruction secondary to ovarian cancer is similar to that of bowel obstruction caused by nongynecologic causes. Two important points are unique to gynecologic cancer: (1) in elderly patients with no history of prior abdominal surgery small-bowel obstruction is a harbinger of ovarian cancer and (2) in patients with prior history of pelvic malignancy small-bowel obstruction may be the first sign of recurrence. Frequently, patients with obstruction secondary to long-standing ovarian cancer should not have surgical intervention immediately on presentation. They should be managed conservatively.

Large-bowel obstruction can occur by direct extension of a cervical malignancy that blocks the rectum. It is also seen when a large tumor in the omentum causes compression at either the splenic or hepatic flexure. The evaluation of the patient with large-bowel obstruction secondary to gynecologic malignancy is the same as that in any other patient. The most critical aspect of the evaluation is to rule out overdistention of the cecum. If the obstruction is in excess of 10 cm in diameter, prompt surgical decompression is necessary.[10]

Colostomy

Colostomy complications occur in approximately 30% of patients. These complications include stenosis of the stroma, peristomal hernia, wound infection, and prolapse.[11] Most problems can be managed by a stomal therapist. However, some stomal complications require prompt surgical correction. Mucosal prolapse of the stoma can be reduced by gentle digital pressure, but it should be done expeditiously to prevent infection and stomal damage.

Fistula Formation

Bowel fistulas in patients with gynecologic malignancies are usually enterocutaneous, enterovaginal, or rectovaginal. Rarely, these fistulas are the presenting sign of a gynecologic malignancy. More often they occur secondary to therapy.

Complications of Radiated Bowel

The role of radiation therapy in gynecologic malignancies is constantly changing. Radiation therapy is currently most frequently used for the primary treatment of advanced cervical cancer or cervical cancer in patients who are not operative candidates. It is also used with increasing frequency as adjuvant therapy for endometrial cancer and as adjuvant or consolidation therapy in ovarian cancer. Two stages of complications result from radiation therapy: early and late. An early bowel complication is radiation enteritis with diarrhea. This injury can be seen during therapy (resulting in therapy interruption) or shortly after the completion of therapy. Patients with severe diarrhea secondary to radiation enteritis or proctitis can usually be treated conservatively and seldom need to be admitted. The diarrhea can be managed with diphenoxylate (Lomotil). Fluid resuscitation may be necessary secondary to severe diarrhea.

Late complications of radiation injury to the bowel are caused by endarteritis and progressive sclerosis of the smaller vessels.[12] This leads to several complications, including ulceration, infarction, entero-entero fistulas, necrosis, and stenosis.[13] Usually the patient presents with either intestinal obstruction or severe intractable abdominal pain.

Another common emergency presentation is rectal bleeding owing to radiation proctitis. If the bleeding is minimal, the patient can be treated with Cort enemas (hydrocortisone) and a low-residue diet. When the bleeding is severe or symptoms of shock exist, fluid resuscitation and transfusion are indicated. When medical management fails, intervention may include angiographic embolization and colostomy.

Urologic Emergencies

Patients with genital tract cancer may present with urologic emergencies secondary to surgery, radiation therapy, or the malignancy itself.

Ureteral Obstruction

Ureteral obstruction may result from any of the preceding three factors. Ureteral obstruction most often presents as nonspecific flank pain, occasionally radiating to the pelvis and groin. Urinary infection is common and may result in urosepsis. In rare cases where there is bilateral obstruction, anemia and azotemia may result. Ureteral obstruction can occur at any time after surgery or radiation therapy, but it is usually seen during the first posttreatment year. It may be the first presenting sign of late recurrence of genital malignancy. It can also be an initial sign of cervical cancer. The diagnosis is made on intravenous pyelography, computed tomography, renal nuclear scanning, or renal ultrasonography. Management depends on the severity of the obstruction. In patients with urosepsis, hospitalization should be arranged and antibiotics started after specimens for blood and urine cultures have been obtained. In patients who are stable and have insidious signs of ureteral obstruction, arrangements need to be made for continuing follow-up.

Urologic Fistulas

Urinary fistulas occur because of extensive primary disease or secondary to radical hysterectomy for cervical or endometrial cancer. Surgical fistulas occur from 7 to 21 days after surgery.[13] Occasionally, fistulas occur secondary to radiation therapy and are diagnosed 6 to 12 months after completion of treatment. The incidence of fistula formation after radical hysterectomy is approximately 1%.[14] There is a three- to fourfold increase in this rate when radiation is given in conjunction with surgery. Fistulas that occur in patients after radical surgery are usually diagnosed by the patient's surgeon and seldom present to the emergency department. However, in inner-city situations, it is possible that the presenting sign of the malignancy may be vesicovaginal fistula secondary to spread of the disease into the trigone of the bladder.

Fistulas can be diagnosed either by direct observation of urine in the vagina or by injection of indigo carmine intravenously and placement of a tampon in the vagina.

Hemorrhagic Cystitis

Hemorrhagic cystitis can be due to either radiation therapy or chemotherapy. Hemorrhagic cystitis may be secondary to cyclophosphamide or ifosfamide chemotherapy. Hemorrhagic cystitis is not uncommon after radiation, and the pathophysiology is similar to that of radiated bowel. Management includes a three-way catheter, irrigation, and possibly a hydrocortisone-containing solution. Once clots are removed and if the bleeding is not severe, the patient may be discharged with follow-up. In severe hemorrhage the patient will need to be admitted and managed either with cautery by way of cystoscopy or by instillation of a sclerosing agent such as formalin.

Urinary Conduit Complications

Urinary conduits are either ileal or transverse colon conduits. Complications include blockage of the ureteroconduit anastomotic site with ureteral obstruction and possibly urosepsis, conduit necrosis, stomal necrosis secondary to avascularity, stomal problems as described under the section on colostomy, and electrolyte imbalance owing to absorption of chloride in an overly long conduit, resulting in hyperchloremic acidosis.[15] Intravenous pyelography or ultrasonography usually defines the problem. If urinary obstruction has resulted in urosepsis, emergency percutaneous nephrostomy is necessary.[16]

Postoperative Complications

Interval postoperative complications usually involve (1) bowel obstruction secondary to surgery, (2) urologic fistula secondary to surgery, and (3) postoperative infection. The first two were discussed earlier.

In the vast majority of cases postoperative infections are diagnosed while the patient is still in the hospital. This is particularly the case with ovarian cancer, in which the first course of chemotherapy is initiated in the hospital in the absence of postoperative infection. The postoperative infections most likely to be seen at an interval postdischarge are wound infection, wound dehiscence, and wound evisceration. Wound dehiscence occurs 5 to 7 days after surgery; in some situations it may occur after discharge. The patient can usually be managed with debridement and dressing changes. In situations where home care is inadequate, the patient may need to be admitted. If signs of necrotizing fasciitis (skin discoloration, skin necrosis, and crepitus) are present, the patient needs to be admitted for surgical debridement.[17] If there is fascial separation (evisceration), the wound should be covered with sterile, moist towels and arrangements should be made for the patient to be taken to the operating room for fascial closure.

The other common postoperative infections in patients with gynecologic malignancies are vaginal cuff cellulitis and cuff abscess.[17] Vaginal cuff cellulitis occurs in 8% of those who receive antibiotic prophylaxis before a hysterectomy. The most common cause is a mixed infection of anaerobes endogenous to the vagina. Occasionally gram-negative aerobic bacteria may be involved. When this diagnosis is made, the patient should be admitted and broad-spectrum antibiotic coverage should be started. If the diagnosis is certain, the antibiotics can be started in the emergency department. Appropriate drugs for anaerobic bacteria are metronidazole, ampicillin-sulbactam, and ticarcillin-clavulanate. If an abscess is identified, arrangements should be made for drainage in the operating room.

Complications secondary to outpatient therapy such as colposcopy, conization, and laser therapy most commonly involve postoperative cervical bleeding. This can usually be managed by the application of Monsels solution or packing the vagina with phenylephrine Neosynephrine hydrochloride (-) or epinephrine-impregnated pack. Occasionally, the cervix needs to be sutured. If the patient is not bleeding severely and the bleeding is controlled with the procedures outlined earlier, the patient may be sent home and told to avoid intercourse and to follow up promptly.

Complications of Chemotherapy

Chemotherapy is used primarily in ovarian cancer and gestational trophoblastic disease and is an adjuvant in endometrial cancer. The most commonly used drugs in gynecologic oncology are cisplatin and carboplatinum. Complications caused by cisplatin are nausea and vomiting, which may be unremitting. In gynecologic oncology cisplatin is given as a bolus medication. Most of the nausea and vomiting can be severe enough that the patient may seek emergency care the day after chemotherapy instillation. Once fluid and electrolyte status are assured, the patient often can be managed by intravenous antiemetic medication as well as metoclopramide (Reglan). If nausea and vomiting are unremitting, the patient needs to be admitted for hydration. Elderly patients tend to have less nausea and vomiting on cisplatin.[18] Other drugs that are commonly used in gynecologic oncology are cyclophosphamide, methotrexate, flouro-uracil, doxorubicin, dactinomycin, vinblastine, etoposide, ifosfamide, and paclitaxel (Taxol). The most common complication with these medications is bone marrow suppression. If the patient presents with a neutropenia of less than 500 granulocytes and fever, she should be admitted for antibiotic therapy. Rarely, the patient presents with a very low platelet count. If the platelet count is less than 20,000 and there is spontaneous bleeding, the patient needs to be admitted for transfusion as well as platelet therapy. Bleomycin, another commonly used drug, may cause pulmonary fibrosis. The patient may present with dyspnea, cough, and bibasilar rales. A chest radiograph usually shows basilar infiltrates. The patient needs to be admitted, particularly if there is an upper respiratory tract infection in addition to the bleomycin toxicity.

Complications of Total Parenteral Nutrition

In the past, patients seldom had emergency complications secondary to total parenteral nutrition (TPN). However, as home infusion services have increased, it is now more common to see extramural complications of TPN. The most likely complications secondary to home infusion TPN are infection and metabolic derangements.[19] The patient with signs and symptoms of sepsis should be managed aggressively and admitted promptly. Metabolic complications include acid/base and electrolyte abnormalities and abnormalities in glucose metabolism as well as hypokalemia, hypomagnesemia, hypophosphatemia, and hypocalcemia. Patients may present with muscle weakness, hyporeflexia or hyperflexia, lethargy, and mental status change.

Organ Failure

Patients with gynecologic malignancies may experience organ failure because of either the primary disease or therapy. As discussed, renal failure can occur from ureteral obstruction, conduit anastomosis problems, or urosepsis. It may represent a primary presentation of cervical cancer with bilateral ureterovesical junction obstruction. Liver failure is most frequently due to metastasis from ovarian cancer and less frequently from gestational trophoblastic neoplasia and endometrial, vulvar, or cervical cancer. Pulmonary metastasis is seen most frequently with endometrial cancer or cervical cancer; parenchymal pulmonary metastasis is seen somewhat less frequently with ovarian cancer.[20] It is not infrequent, however, to see pleural effusions secondary to ovarian cancer in association with ascites. Brain metastasis is rare in gynecologic malignancies except for gestational trophoblastic neoplasia. In the presence of gestational trophoblastic neoplasia, complaints of headache, seizure, visual disturbance, or mental status change should be evaluated with a computed tomographic scan of the head.[21]

REFERENCES

1. Boring C, Squires T, Tong T. Cancer Statistics 1993. CA 43:7, 1993
2. Guijon F. Sexually transmitted disease and cervical neoplasia. Curr Opin OB/GYN 2:857, 1990
3. DiSaia P, Creasman W. Clinical Gynecologic Oncology, 4th ed. St Louis: CV Mosby, 1993
4. Hoskins W, Perez C, Young R. Principles and Practices of Gynecologic Oncology. Philadelphia: JB Lippincott, 1992
5. Barnes W, Delgado G, Kurman R et al. Possible prognostic significance of human papilloma virus type in cervical cancer. Gynecol Oncol 29:267, 1988
6. Dehaeck C. Transcatheter embolization of pelvic vessels to stop intractable hemorrhage. Gynecol Oncol 24:9, 1986
7. Berek J, Hacker N. Practical Gynecologic Oncology, Baltimore: Williams & Wilkins, 1989
8. Droegemueller W, Berbst A, Mishell D, Stenchever M. Comprehensive Gynecology. St Louis: CV Mosby, 1987
9. Morley G. Cancer of the vulva: a review. Cancer 48:597, 1981
10. Schwartz S, Shires G, Spencer F. Principles of Surgery, 5th ed. New York: McGraw-Hill, 1989
11. Kretschmer P. The Intestinal Stoma. Philadelphia: WB Saunders, 1978
12. Beer W, Fan A, Halsted C. Clinical and nutritional implications of radiation enteritis. Am J Clin Nutr 41:85, 1985
13. Delgado G, Smith J. Management of Complications in Gynecologic Oncology. New York: John Wiley, 1982
14. Chamberlain D, Hopkins M, Roberts J et al. The effects of early removal of indwelling urinary catheter after radical hysterectomy. Gynecol Oncol 43:98, 1991
15. Hancock K, Copeland L, Gershenson D. Urinary conduits in gynecologic oncology. Obstet Gynecol 67:680, 1986
16. Dudley B, Gershenson D, Kavanaugh J et al. Percutaneous nephrostomy catheter use in gynecologic malignancy: an MD Anderson Hospital experience. Gynecol Oncol 24:273, 1986

17. Nichols D. Reoperative Gynecologic Surgery. St Louis: CV Mosby, 1991
18. Benrubi G, Norvell M, Nuss R, Robinson H. The use of methylprednisolone and metoclopramide in control of emesis in patients receiving cis-platinum. Gynecol Oncol 21:306, 1985
19. Rayburn W, Walk R, Roberts J. Parenteral nutrition in obstetrics and gynecology. Obstet Gynecol Surv 41:200, 1986
20. Peeples W, Inalsingh C, Tapon A et al. The occurrence of metastasis outside the abdomen and retroperitoneal space in invasive carcinoma of the cervix. Gynecol Oncol 4:307, 1976
21. DuBeshter B, Berkowitz R, Goldstein D et al. Metastatic gestational trophoblastic disease: experience at the New England Trophoblastic Disease Center 1965–1985. Obstet Gynecol 69:390, 1987

CHAPTER 23

Gynecologic Emergencies in Childhood and Adolescence

Kristi Morgan Mulchahey

Children and adolescents do not present frequently to the emergency department with gynecologic problems; however, this age group may have a number of unique medical and surgical problems and special psychosocial needs that require sensitive and skillful care. The purpose of this chapter is both to familiarize the reader with the special gynecologic needs of these young patients and to review some of the common problems that may be encountered in the emergency department setting. The emergency department may be a frightening place for a child or teenager; care of the "whole patient" requires that both medical and individual developmental needs be considered.

Anatomy and Physiology of the Developing Child

At birth the newborn is hormonally very similar to her mother. Estradiol and gonadotropin levels are elevated at birth and are responsible for a mucoid vaginal discharge, a small amount of breast development, and a blood-tinged vaginal discharge that may occur within the first few days of life. The endocrinology of infancy is marked by a gradual decline in gonadotropins along with a fall in estradiol levels as the negative feedback of the hypothalamic pituitary axis develops. By late infancy or early childhood, the child is hypoestrogenic and will remain so until the onset of puberty.[1]

The prepubertal child obviously differs from the adult in the absence of secondary sexual characteristics. There are also other, less obvious differences that may influence the development or presentation of gynecologic disorders. The labia majora and mons have less fatty tissue than those in an adult. The labia minora are thin and slitlike, and the distance between the vaginal and anal openings may be relatively smaller than that found after puberty. The vaginal epithelium of the prepubertal child resembles that of a postmenopausal woman, a thin epithelium with parabasal cells. The wet prep in a prepubertal child will reveal smaller epithelial cells with a larger nuclear to cytoplasmic ratio, as found in a postmenopausal unestrogenized woman. The cervix and uterus of a prepubertal child are quite small, with the cervix making up a relatively larger proportion of the total uterus than will be encountered later. The portio of the cervix is covered with a thin squamous epithelium. Endocervical glands are present but are high in the canal of the cervix, unlike the adolescent, where columnar epithelium is often found on the ectocervix.

In this hypoestrogenic state, normal vaginal flora is different. After the initial period of infancy, where vaginal flora resembles that of normal maternal vaginal flora, *S. epidermidis* and diphtheroids are the predominant normal flora in the vagina of a child. In contrast, lactobacillus is one of the predominant organisms after puberty. Gram-negative rods are also commonly encountered in the vagina of a child, particularly in the diaper age group (Table 23-1). The absence of lactobacillus to metabolize glycogen and produce lactic acid creates the alkaline vaginal pH found in childhood. Because of these physiologic differences in the prepubertal child, children may develop vaginitis with organisms that would not be considered pathogens in adults. In addition, such organisms as *Neisseria gonorrhoeae* and *Chlamydia trachomatis*, which traditionally cause endocervicitis and ascending genital tract disease in adults, will cause vaginitis in a child but rarely upper genital tract infection. The alkaline pH of the vagina may make the child more resistant to infections such as trichomoniasis. The thin vaginal epithelium also explains the frequent association of vaginal bleeding with vaginal infection in prepubertal children.

Normal hymeneal anatomy has received greater attention in recent studies. The hymen of the prepubertal child is generally described as crescentic, annular, or fim-

TABLE 23-1
Normal Vaginal Flora of the Prepubertal Child

Diphtheroids
Staphylococcus epidermidis
Nonhemolytic streptococci
Alpha-hemolytic streptococci
Group D streptococci
Escherichia coli
Klebsiella
Staphylococcus aureus
Haemophilus influenzae
Pseudomonas aseruginosa

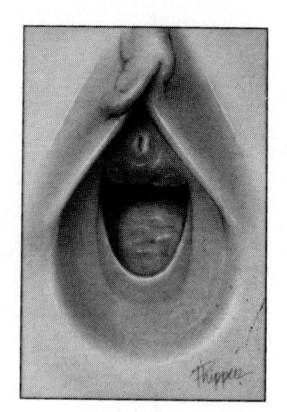

FIGURE 23-1
Normal hymenal anatomy—crescentic. (From Pokorny S. Pediatric vulvovaginitis. In: Kaufman RH, et al, eds. Benign Diseases of the Vulva and Vagina. Chicago: Year Book Medical Publishers, 1989. Used with permission.)

briated, with crescentic being the most commonly encountered. Figures 23-1 through 23-3 illustrate the common appearances of the normal hymen in prepubertal children. Although some authors state that the transverse diameter of the hymen should be no more than 4 to 5 mm in a healthy prepubertal child, other studies of normal children suggest that the hymeneal diameter may vary with age. Although hymeneal diameter is not the only factor in assessing hymeneal anatomy, a general "rule of thumb" may be helpful. For children over 4 to 5 years of age, one may allow 4 to 5 mm plus 1 mm for each year of age as upper limits of normal for transverse diameter. It is important to remember that this diameter also will vary in an individual child, according the state of relaxation.

As the child grows, secondary sexual characteristics will begin to appear. The onset of puberty is generally marked by a rapid growth spurt, followed by thelarche. Eight years is the lower limit of normal for the onset of adrenarche or thelarche, and 10 years is the lower limit for menarche. The timing of adrenarche relative to thelarche may vary somewhat from child to child, as this is an adrenally mediated event under a separate control mechanism. Most children will experience menarche 2 years after the onset of breast development. The absence of secondary sexual characteristics by 14 years of age or absence of menarche at 16 should be carefully evaluated. In some cases, earlier evaluation may be warranted.[2]

The early bleeding pattern of the young adolescent is frequently irregular be-

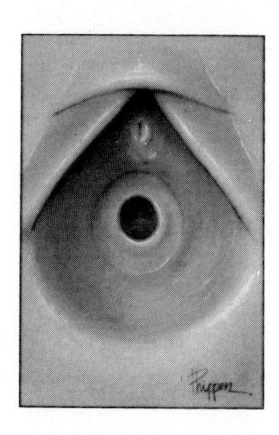

FIGURE 23-2
Normal hymenal anatomy—annular. (From Pokorny S. Pediatric vulvovaginitis. In: Kaufman RH, et al, eds. Benign Diseases of the Vulva and Vagina. Chicago: Year Book Medical Publishers, 1989. Used with permission.)

FIGURE 23-3
Normal hymenal anatomy—fimbriated. (From Pokorny S. Pediatric vulvovaginitis. In: Kaufman RH, et al, eds. Benign Diseases of the Vulva and Vagina. Chicago: Year Book Medical Publishers, 1989. Used with permission.

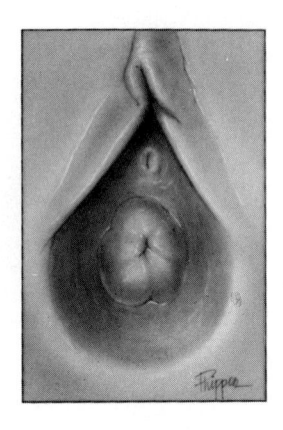

cause of anovulatory cycles. The hypothalamic pituitary ovarian positive feedback mechanism responsible for ovulation may not mature until 1 to 5 years after menarche, with 1 to 2 years being most common. During this time, fluctuating estradiol levels will provide stimulus to the endometrium to proliferate. Bleeding episodes are generally in response to fluctuations in estradiol levels and often irregular. This bleeding pattern may occasionally result in heavy or prolonged pubertal bleeding that may require evaluation and intervention.

The adolescent experiences differential growth in the body of the uterus, so the fundus comprises approximately two thirds of the entire uterus. Changes in the transformation zone of the cervix result in the ectropion with columnar epithelium so often seen on the speculum examination during the adolescent years. This columnar epithelium is particularly susceptible to infection with *N. gonorrhoeae* and *C. trachomatis*. Figures 23-4 and 23-5 illustrate the normal progression of pubertal development as described by Tanner and colleagues.

Examination of the Adolescent and Young Child

For a health care provider accustomed to dealing primarily with adults, the appearance of a mother and a child in an emergency setting brings two individuals, each with unique concerns and worries. Obtaining a careful medical history from the mother is essential. However, there may be times when obtaining a history from the child independently can be critical. Particularly in situations where child abuse is in the differential diagnosis, it may be imperative to interview the child alone in a comfortable, nonthreatening setting. Often the use of allied health personnel may be helpful in this regard. In addition to the usual items covered in an adult history, special concern must be paid to developmental issues in the child.

Accomplishing a productive and atraumatic genital examination in a prepubertal child requires a patient, skillful examiner who is also creative and flexible. The physical examination of the child should always begin with a general physical examination. In addition to screening for other medical problems, this allows the child to be comfortable with the touch of the physician and will improve cooperation during

GYNECOLOGIC EMERGENCIES IN CHILDHOOD AND ADOLESCENCE ♦ 319

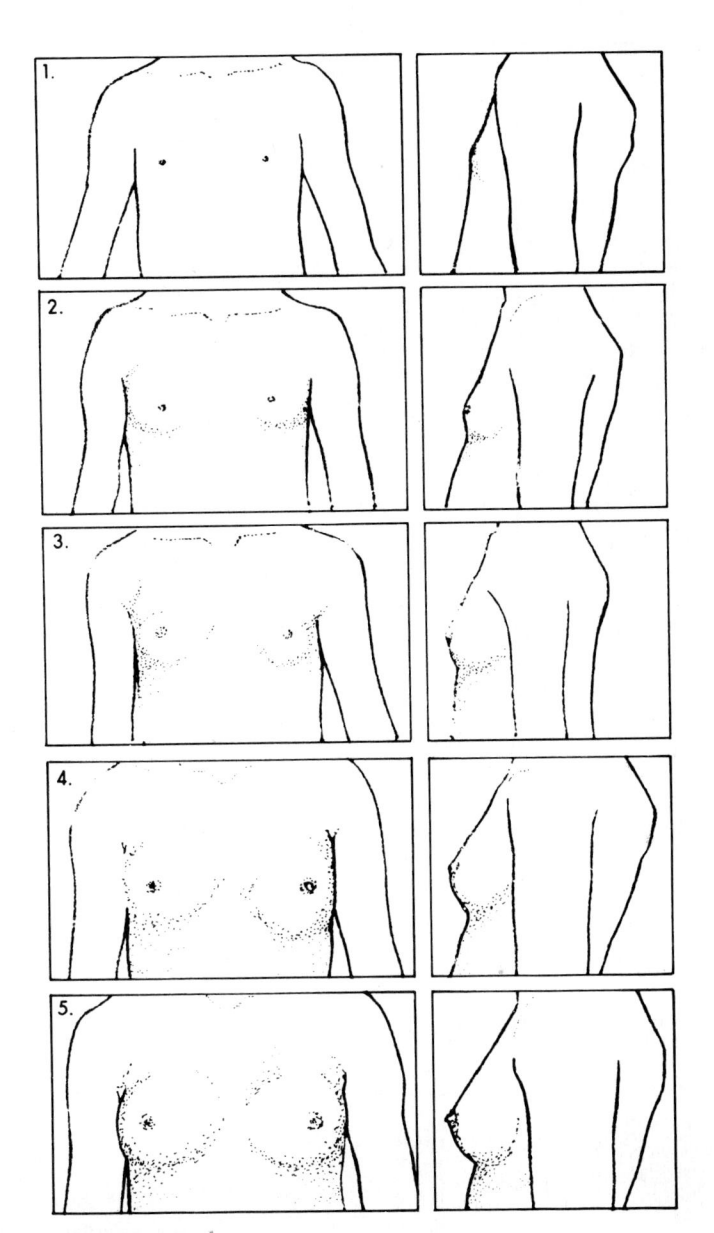

FIGURE 23-4
Tanner staging for breast development. (From Coupey S, Saunders DS. Physical maturation. In: Laveny JP, Sanfilippo JS (eds): Pediatric and Adolescent Obstetrics and Gynecology. New York: Springer-Verlag, 1985. Used by permission.)

FIGURE 23–5
Tanner staging for pubic hair development. (From Coupey S, Saunders DS. Physical maturation. In: Laveny JP, Sanfilippo JS (eds): Pediatric and Adolescent Obstetrics and Gynecology. New York: Springer-Verlag, 1985. Used by permission.)

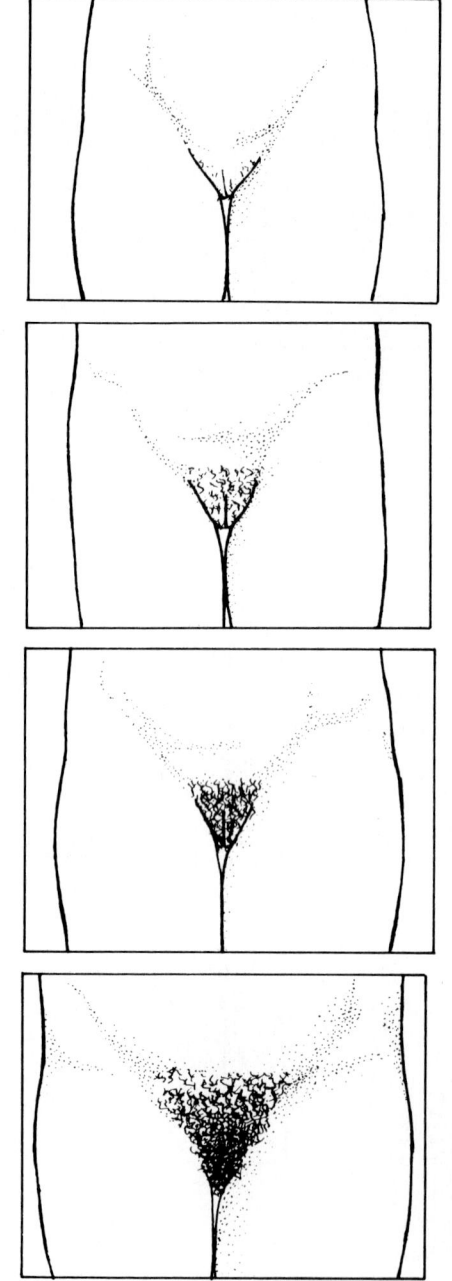

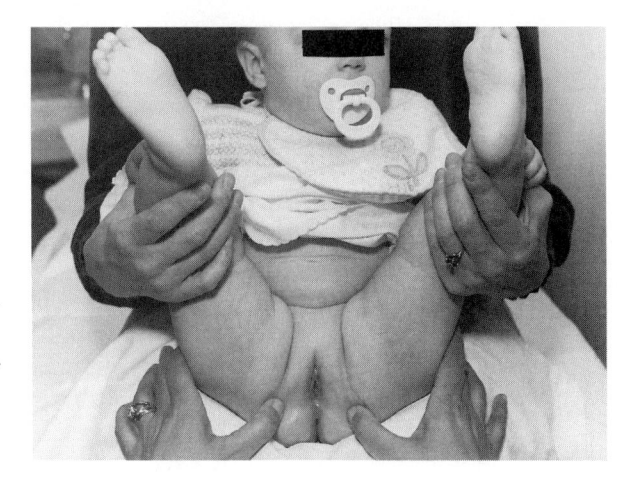

FIGURE 23–6
Examining the small child in the frog-leg position. (From Gidwani GP. Approach to evaluation of the premenarchal child with a gynecologic problem. Clin Obstet Gynecol 30:643, 1987. Used with permission.)

the genital examination. A variety of positions for accomplishing a genital examination in children have been described. In the infant, toddler, and preschooler, examining the child in her mother's lap in a frog-leg position is very helpful. The child sits in the mother's lap while she supports the legs in a flexed position. This allows excellent exposure of the genitalia for visual inspection and is excellent for obtaining cultures. A catheterized urine specimen is also easily obtained in this position when necessary. This position also allows the young child to watch the examiner; attempts to examine a child behind a drape sheet are generally futile and nonproductive (Fig. 23-6). Older children may be able to tolerate the standard dorsolithotomy position, especially if the head of the examining table is raised. For children who are too frightened for this position, placing the mother, fully clothed, in the dorsolithotomy position with the child lying in a prone position on her lap may also be helpful (Fig. 23-7).[3]

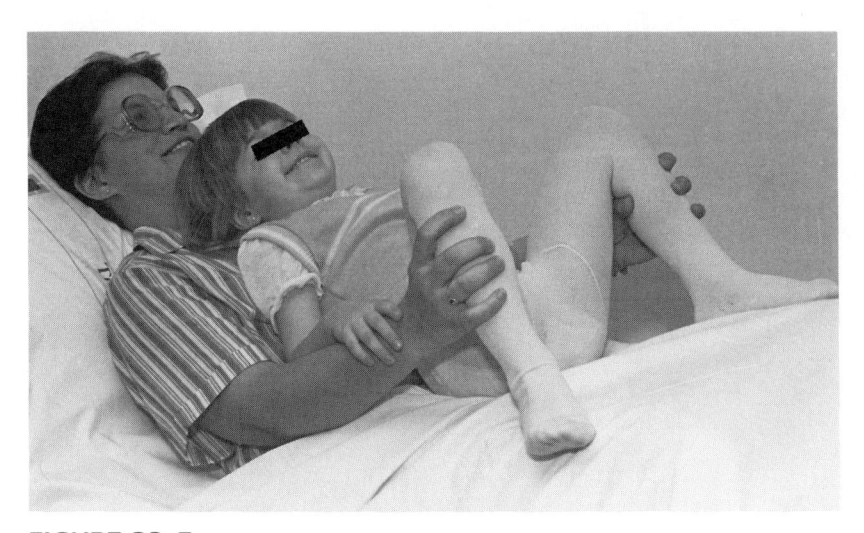

FIGURE 23–7
Examination of the child in the dorsolithotomy position. (From Gidwani GP: Approach to evaluation of the premenarchal child with a gynecologic problem. Clin Obstet Gynecol 30:643, 1987. Used with permission.)

322 ♦ OBSTETRIC AND GYNECOLOGIC EMERGENCIES

Examination of children in the knee-chest position can be quite helpful, particularly for assessment of the lower portion of the vaginal canal (Fig. 23-8). Air enters the vagina with lordosis of the back, and at least the lower half of the vagina may be visualized with either the naked eye or the use of a hand-held otoscope without the ear speculum. The "cannonball" position may be helpful in children for assessing the perianal area. The vulva can usually be visualized best with general outward and lateral traction on the labia majora. This places the hymeneal ring in a slight amount of stretch and is tolerated well by most children. It also allows careful assessment of the hymen and good visualization of the periurethral area (Fig. 23-9).

The use of the "pediatric speculum" in the unanesthetized child is inhumane and nonproductive. Visualization of the cervix is rarely necessary, since most gynecologic pathology in children is located on the vulva or the lower portion of the vagina. When visualization of the cervix is necessary, a vaginal examination under anesthesia with a pediatric vaginoscope or cystoscope is required. The traditional bimanual examination is not feasible in a small child; however, a rectal examination with abdominal palpation may reveal useful information about the pelvis. On rectal examination in the prepubertal child, a midline uterus is easily palpated, with the cervix being most prominent. In most children, this has the size and consistency of a pencil eraser. The pelvis in the child is shallow, and pelvic masses originating in the adnexa quickly rise out of the pelvis. For this reason a careful abdominal examination is always included with the genital examination in a prepubertal child.

Very little equipment, aside from a good light source, is required to accomplish a genital examination in children. Often a quiet room, a supportive mother, and a

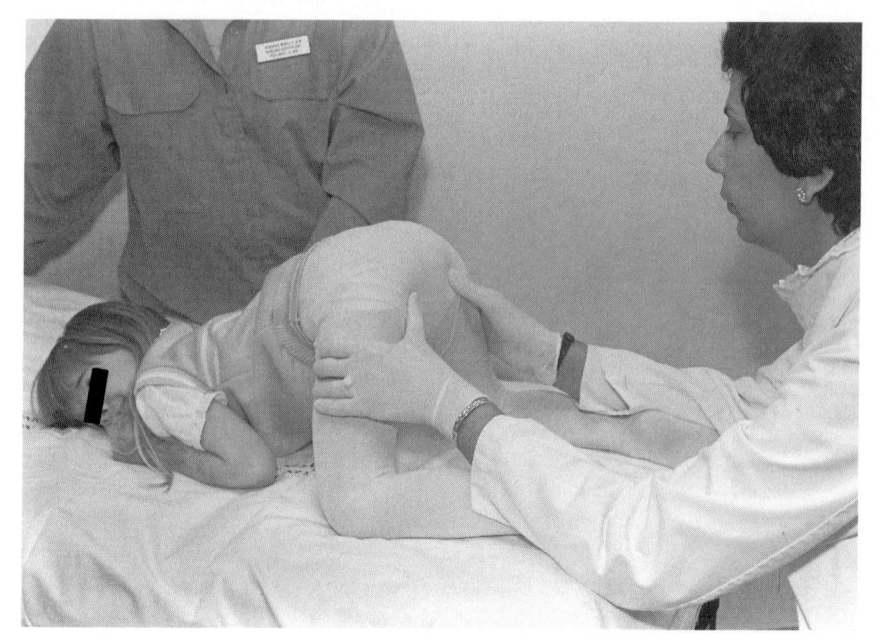

FIGURE 23-8
Examination of the child in the knee-chest position. (From Gidwani GP. Approach to evaluation of the premenarchal child with a gynecologic problem. Clin Obstet Gynecol 30:643, 1987. Used with permission.)

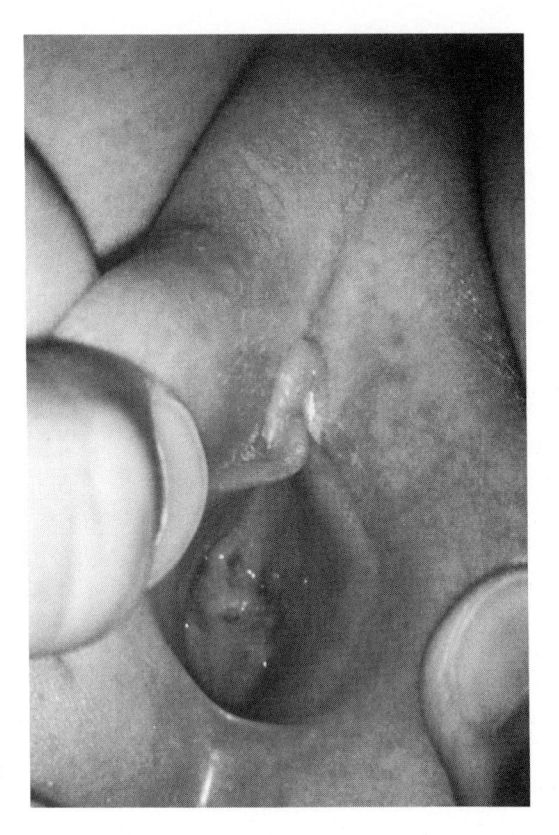

FIGURE 23-9
Separation technique for examination of the vulva.

well-relaxed child are all the ingredients required. If it is necessary to collect specimens for culture, it is important to remember that a dry cotton-tipped applicator in the vagina of a child may be painful. A small swab, such as a Calgis swab, moistened with nonbacteriostatic saline greatly facilitates obtaining specimens in prepubertal children with minimal discomfort (Fig. 23-10). Other authors have also described the use of a small pediatric feeding tube or plastic IV catheter attached to a syringe for obtaining specimens (Fig. 23-11).[4]

In the adolescent patient, issues of patient confidentiality become more crucial. The young adolescent may be reluctant to disclose history related to sexual activity to a strange emergency department physician. This is again a situation where the use of other supportive medical personnel may be helpful. Although parents need to be involved for certain portions of the medical history, it is essential that the adolescent also be interviewed alone and be reassured of the confidentiality of information related to sexual activity, possible pregnancy, or sexually transmitted diseases. In addition to the usual components of a medical and gynecologic history, particular attention to developmental issues is important.

A pelvic examination for an adolescent is often a frightening experience. In situations where it is warranted, a thorough explanation and preparation by the physician or nurse are helpful. Positioning the patient with her head elevated in the dorsolithotomy position and the drape sheet adjusted so that good eye contact may be maintained between the patient and examiner decreases anxiety. The presence of the mother or a nurse as a support person may also be helpful. Teenagers can

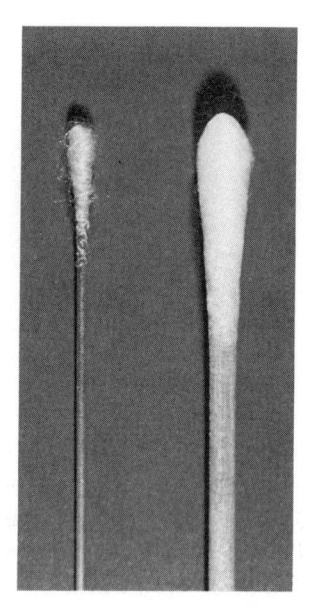

FIGURE 23-10
Size comparison of swab types.

often tolerate the use of a speculum prior to the onset of sexual activity if a narrow Pederson-type speculum is used, such as a Huffman speculum. This speculum is much like the traditional medium Pederson speculum but has narrower blades, approximately 0.5 inch in diameter. In a young adolescent unable to tolerate a vaginal bimanual examination, a rectal bimanual examination may provide essentially the same information.

Sedation in Children

Most children who present to the emergency department with a gynecologic problem may be adequately evaluated in an awake state. A patient examiner, armed with the examination techniques that were discussed earlier, will nearly always be able to accomplish a complete examination. In certain situations, however, sedation may be required. Sedation may be required in a child who has been injured in order to

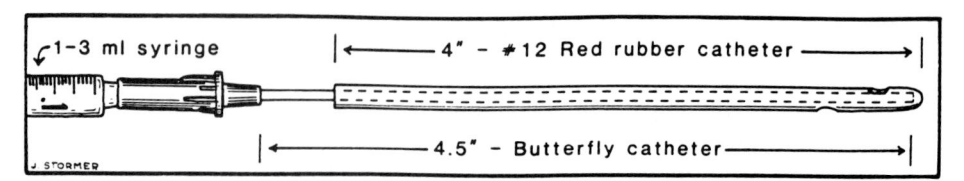

FIGURE 23-11
Collection technique for pediatric vaginal specimens. (From Pokorny SF, Stormer J. Atraumatic removal of secretions from prepubertal vagina. Am J Obstet Gynecol 156:581, 1987. Used with permission.)

determine the extent of the injuries. Occasionally, suturing may be safely done with sedation. However, if evaluation of the vagina and cervix is required, this will need to be accomplished in the operating room with careful airway control by an anesthesiologist. The level of sedation required to suppress a reflex in the perineal body and allow for vaginoscopy will also leave the child's airway unprotected.

Lesser degrees of sedation may be achieved by individuals who are experienced at sedation of children and in settings where children may be adequately monitored. Sedation should be used in a setting where a protocol for conscious awake sedation has been established. In this setting, oral Versed has been successfully used in a dose of 0.3 mg/kg. Intravenous Demerol may also be given in a dose of 0.05 mg/kg in incremental doses up to a maximum of 0.3 to 0.5 mg/kg. Older regimens using chloral hydrate at 25 to 100 mg/kg per dose orally or Demerol, Phenergan, and Thorazine are less predictable and frequently provide less adequate sedation (Table 23-2).[5] Sedation should be provided only in clinical settings where the airway and respiratory status of the child can be carefully monitored. Most protocols for conscious awake sedation include the use of supplemental oxygen, monitoring with a pulse oximeter, and a specifically designated individual whose only responsibility is to monitor the child.

Vaginal Bleeding in Children

Vaginal bleeding is one of the most common problems that bring a child to the emergency department for evaluation. Vaginal bleeding can be caused by a host of problems, as listed in Table 23-3.[6] Some of these problems may require a more detailed evaluation; others may be easily diagnosed and treated in the emergency department. The presentation of a child with vaginal bleeding should *always* be taken seriously. It is not appropriate to delay a work-up to "see if it happens again."

Vaginitis

Vaginitis is one of the most common causes of vaginal bleeding in children. The hypoestrogenic vagina of the child is susceptible to infection with organisms that would not be pathogenic to the well-estrogenized adult female (Table 23-4). Girls

TABLE 23–2
Pediatric Sedation

1.	Meperidine (Demerol)	2 mg/kg IM
	Promethazine (Phenergan)	1 mg/kg IM
	Chlorpromazine (Thorazine)	1 mg/kg IM
2.	Chloral hydrate	25 to 100 mg/kg per dose orally (maximum dose 2 g)
3.	Midazolam (Versed)	0.008 to 0.15 mg/kg per dose IM or IV 0.3 mg/kg PO

TABLE 23-3
Causes of Prepubertal Vaginal Bleeding

Vaginitis
Vaginal foreign body
Genital trauma
Hematuria
Urethral prolapse
Lichen sclerosis
Genital condyloma
Physiologic neonatal bleeding
Estrogen withdrawal bleed
Precocious puberty
Vaginal neoplasm

with group B streptococcus may frequently present with frank vaginal bleeding. Other organisms may cause a blood-tinged vaginal discharge. The presence of a foreign body often causes a severe vaginitis with a profuse, foul-smelling vaginal discharge that may be blood-tinged. Examination of the child in the knee-chest position may be helpful in evaluating the child for the possibility of a foreign body.

Obtaining cultures to identify the causative agent in pediatric vulvovaginitis may be helpful. These cultures should be obtained in atraumatic fashion with a small swab moistened with nonbacteriostatic saline or with a syringe aspiration system described earlier. It is important to communicate to the laboratory personnel that the

TABLE 23-4
Causes of Pediatric Vaginitis

Nonspecific vaginitis (e.g., local irritants)
Vaginal foreign body
Respiratory pathogens
   Group A B. streptococcus
   Streptococcus pneumoniae
   Neisseria meningitis
   Staphylococcus aureus
   Haemophilus influenzae
Enteric pathogens
   Candida
   E. coli
   Klebsiella
   Shigella
   Yersinia
Sexually transmissible pathogens
   Neisseria gonorrhoeae
   Chlamydia trachomatis
   Trichomonas vaginalis
   Herpes simplex

specimen is coming from a prepubertal child, so that each organism present may be identified. Otherwise, a report of "normal flora" may be obtained that is not helpful in dictating management of the child.

The diagnosis of a potentially sexually transmissible agent in a child should alert the clinician to the possibility of sexual abuse. *C. trachomatis*, *N. gonorrhoeae*, and trichomonads may be sexually transmitted in the child; however, the possibility of perinatal transmission in a younger child must also be considered. The involvement of support staff from social services is essential in this setting. Each clinician is responsible for appropriate reporting of suspected child abuse to the local Child Protective Services.

The treatment of the child with nontraumatic vaginal bleeding usually is not instituted in the emergency setting. When vaginitis is responsible, culture results are necessary to determine the need for antibiotics and the exact sensitivity of the organism. However, in the event that empiric therapy is felt to be warranted, oral amoxicillin or Bactrim may be helpful. The broad range of potential organisms responsible for the infection must be considered in choosing an antibiotic. Treatment usually may be delayed until culture results are obtained and the child symptomatically treated with sitz baths.

Careful follow-up of the child presenting with vaginal bleeding thought to be due to vaginitis is essential. Culture results need to be reviewed and antibiotics instituted as indicated. Children with vaginal bleeding whose obvious source cannot be identified on physical examination should undergo examination under anesthesia to rule out vaginal lesions.

Genital Trauma in Children

Vaginal bleeding is commonly a presenting complaint of children who have sustained a straddle injury or nonaccidental injury to the genitalia through sexual abuse. Because children may be reluctant to disclose to a parent or caretaker that such an injury has occurred, finding blood on the child's clothing may be the first clue to the caretaker that the child needs attention. In this setting a careful interview of the child is necessary to help determine the source of the injury. The initial disclosure of sexual abuse may often occur weeks or months after the event, and children who have been abused may simply state that they have fallen or in some way injured themselves. Interviewing the child alone, as well as interviewing playmates or adults who had witnessed the injury, may be helpful in assessing the source of the injury. Assistance from social service workers may be a valuable asset.

A careful physical examination is essential when a child has sustained genital trauma. A general physical examination looking for other evidence of trauma is the first priority. A careful abdominal examination looking for signs of abdominal trauma or possibly indirect peritoneal injury through the vagina or the rectum is essential. The reader is referred to the earlier section describing a variety of different positions for examining children. Sedation may be necessary in a child who is frightened. Irrigation of the injured area with warm sterile water and inspection with a good light are other helpful tools.

Certain clinical features can help determine if the injury was accidental or intentional. In general, straddle injuries (Fig. 23-12) present with the most severe injury occurring in the area that sustained the major impact from the fall. More external areas, such as the mons, labia majora, and buttocks, as well as the inner thighs, are more often injured in a straddle injury. If bruising is present it is important to note its color and extent. Small lacerations of the labia minora are not infrequently seen and may occasionally bleed briskly. Periurethral injuries may also bleed relatively briskly.[7]

Although it is not possible to determine the source of the injury simply based on physical examination, injuries due to sexual assault (Fig. 23-13) are more likely to involve the hymenal area, with less severe injuries on the periphery. Any evidence of an acute hymenal injury or blood coming from the vagina or rectum of the traumatized child warrants prompt evaluation by a pediatric gynecologist with an examination under anesthesia. The small unestrogenized vagina of the child does not have rugae as in adults, and penetrating injuries to the hymen may cause significant injuries to the vaginal wall and may perforate into the peritoneal cavity. The same is true for injuries that may involve the anal canal in children.

Management of pediatric vulvar injuries may sometimes take place in the emergency setting. Any hematomas present should be watched very carefully for evidence of rapid expansion that may indicate a small vessel that is bleeding and may require operative ligation. The majority of small hemostatic injuries heal well with minimal cosmetic effect and can be conservatively managed. A pressure dressing with an ice pack frequently accomplishes hemostasis in the small injuries. Application of topical thrombin or similar material may be helpful. In the older cooperative child or the child who can be adequately and safely sedated, some repair of small injuries may be accomplished. However, further trauma to the child should be avoided in situations where cooperation cannot be obtained or the child cannot be adequately and safely sedated. The topical use of TAC for local anesthesia is not recommended on mucosal surfaces because of the potential for enhanced systemic absorption. However, the

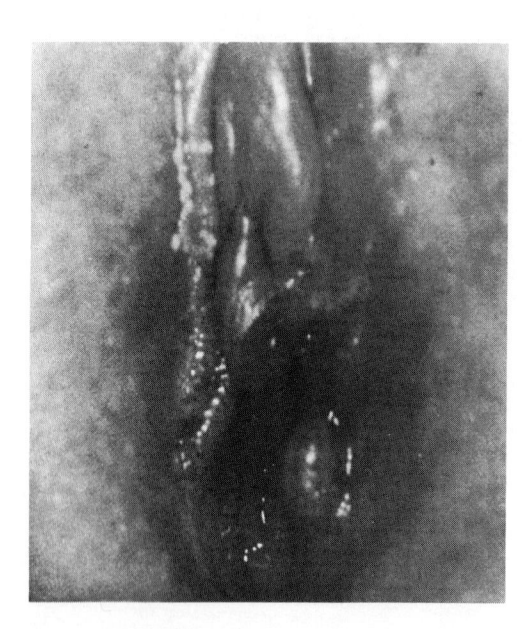

FIGURE 23–12
Straddle injury. (From Chadwick DL, et al. Color Atlas of Child Sexual Abuse. Chicago. Year Book Medical Publishers, 1989:62. Used with permission.)

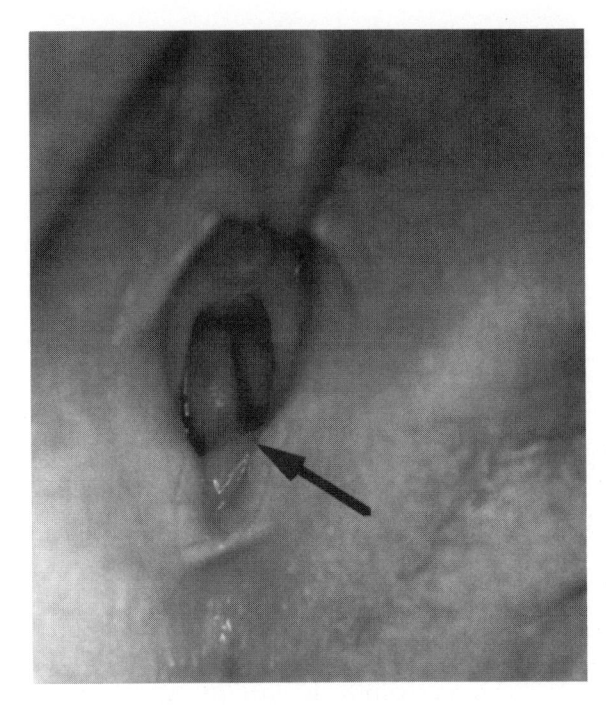

FIGURE 23–13
Hymenal and vaginal laceration from sexual assault. (From Muram D. Child sexual abuse. *Obstet Gynecol Clin North Am* 19 (1):199, 1992. Used with permission.)

addition of the small amount of sodium bicarbonate to 1% Lidocaine will buffer the solution and diminish discomfort associated with its use. A very fine 28- or 30-gauge needle may also be helpful in infiltration. The use of a delayed absorbable suture such as Vicryl or Dexon is recommended. Permanent suture that must be removed at a later date adds to the trauma of the experience for the child. Human bites should be allowed to heal by secondary intent and covered by broad-spectrum antibiotics.

For more severe injuries, liberal use of available consultants is important. An abdominal x-ray should be obtained if there is any concern about abdominal trauma or bony injury. A rectal examination may detect occult pelvic injuries. Observation for urinary retention is important. Admission to the hospital for observation may be indicated.

The clinician in the emergency department may not be able to determine the exact etiology of the injuries of the child in the acute care setting. As with the diagnosis of a sexually transmissible disease in a child, practitioners in the emergency department must be familiar with the local reporting laws for suspected child abuse. In children where sexual assault has occurred within 72 hours, the completion of a forensic evaluation with the use of a "rape kit" is also indicated. This kit varies from state to state but is generally designed for use with adult rape victims. It is important to remember that collecting cervical specimens from the unanesthetized child will be traumatic and unnecessary. Careful follow-up of children who have sustained genital injuries is essential. Referral for both medical and social services follow-up is recommended. Simple care at home with warm sitz baths is helpful. Estrogen cream to speed the healing of genital injuries in children has also been recommended. Tetanus toxoid immunization should be up-to-date.

Urologic Causes of Vaginal Bleeding in Children

As is often demonstrated on voiding cystourethrogram, urine frequently pools in the vagina when a child urinates. A small amount of urine may sometimes be seen coming from the vagina of the child if she is examined immediately after urination. This phenomenon has been called "vaginal voiding." For this reason the child with hematuria may appear to have vaginal bleeding. In the case of a simple urinary tract infection, bloody urine may sometimes be seen coming from the vagina. In cases of severe hemorrhagic cystitis or upper urinary tract lesions, such as Wilms' tumor, gross hematuria and frank blood may occasionally be seen from the vagina. If hematuria is suspected, a catheterized urine specimen will differentiate the source of the bleeding.

Children may occasionally present with a large hemorrhagic, spongy-appearing mass in the periurethral area due to urethral prolapse (Fig. 23-14). Urethral prolapse often occurs in prepubertal girls following straining with vomiting, coughing, or constipation. Minor degrees of urethral prolapse may present with friable redundant tissue in the periurethral area. At times the tissue involved in the prolapse may become very edematous and quite large. It may sometimes be difficult to determine whether this mass of tissue is coming from the vagina or from the urethra. Observing the child voiding on a bedpan and seeing a stream of urine come from this mass may be very helpful in the differential diagnosis.

In children with hematuria, screening for urinary tract infection should be performed and the antibiotics begun if indicated. Proper referral for more detailed evaluation and treatment is important, especially if infection is not identified and the cause of the hematuria is undetermined. Urethral prolapse can be very success-

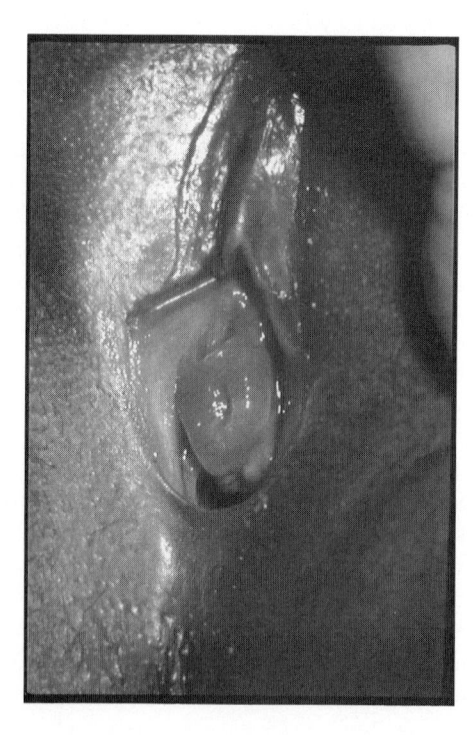

FIGURE 23-14
Urethral prolapse. (Photographs courtesy of S. Jean Emans, Children's Hospital, Boston, MA).

fully treated with simple conservative measures of sitz baths and the application of topical estrogen cream. Several surgical techniques for excision of the redundant and swollen urethral tissue have been described. However, more recent reviews have suggested that this be limited to situations where hemodynamically significant bleeding is occurring. Even quite large areas of urethral prolapse usually respond promptly and nicely to medical treatment.

Dermatologic Lesions Presenting as Vaginal Bleeding in Children

Small breaks in the skin may occur fairly frequently in children with pediatric vulvar seborrhea or psoriasis. Although it is rare for these to be associated with large amounts of bleeding, visual diagnosis is usually fairly straightforward. However, the diagnosis of pediatric lichen sclerosus (Fig. 23-15) should also be considered in the differential. Lichen sclerosus occurs in the prepubertal and postmenopausal woman, both states of hypoestrogenism. The classic findings of lichen sclerosus in children will include a figure of eight depigmented area around the vulva and the anal area. With even minor degrees of trauma, such as might occur from riding a tricycle, hemorrhagic bullae may develop in these areas. To an examiner who is unfamiliar with this condition, this may appear as severe bruising from a straddle injury or sexual abuse. Although generally precipitated by only very minor degrees of trauma, this dermatologic condition has been mistakenly reported as sexual abuse in children.

The child with genital human papilloma virus infection may often present with vaginal bleeding. Condyloma (Fig. 23-16) in children tend to be less cornified than those seen in adults. The warty lesions, especially in moist mucosal areas, may be friable and bleed easily. Condylomata may appear in the periurethral and perianal areas as well as in the area immediately surrounding the hymen.

Definitive treatment of these dermatologic conditions requires referral to a pediatric gynecologist or a dermatologist. For the acute treatment of lichen sclerosus, sitz baths and application of 1% hydrocortisone may give symptomatic relief. Sitz baths and careful attention to hygiene can often relieve significant symptoms in children with genital condyloma. The bleeding accompanying these lesions usually responds promptly to the application of gentle pressure. Again, because human papilloma virus is a sexually transmissible agent, involvement of colleagues and social services is essential.

Other Causes of Vaginal Bleeding in Children

On occasion, a well, asymptomatic child may present to the emergency department with vaginal bleeding and be found to have an entirely normal physical examination. One possible cause of this is a mild vaginitis that spontaneously resolves, leaving no etiologic organism to identify on culture. In the absence of frank precocious puberty, the prepubertal girl may occasionally develop a small functional ovarian cyst that will produce estradiol and thicken the endometrial lining. When this cyst resolves, an estrogen withdrawal bleed may occur. Although frank precocious pu-

332 ◆ OBSTETRIC AND GYNECOLOGIC EMERGENCIES

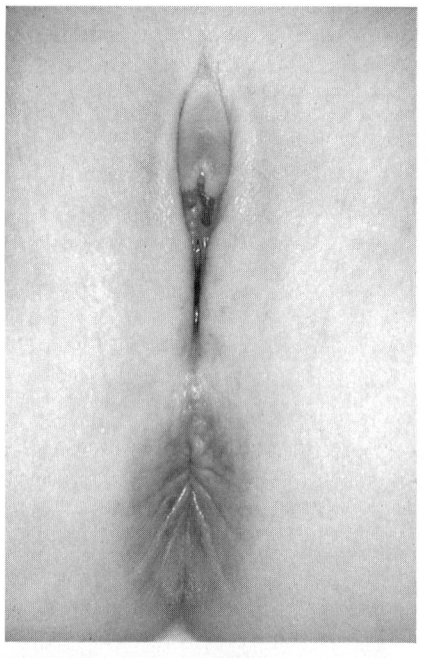

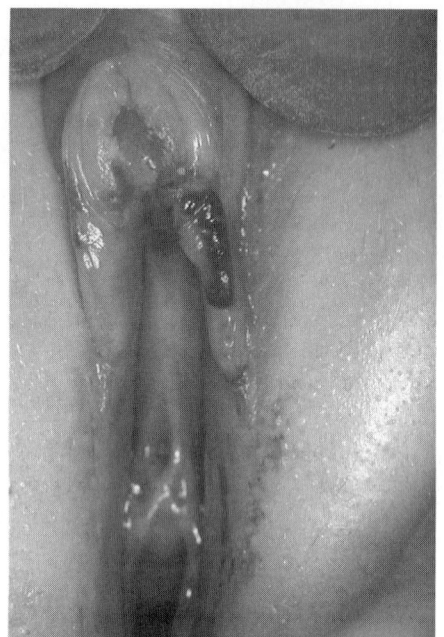

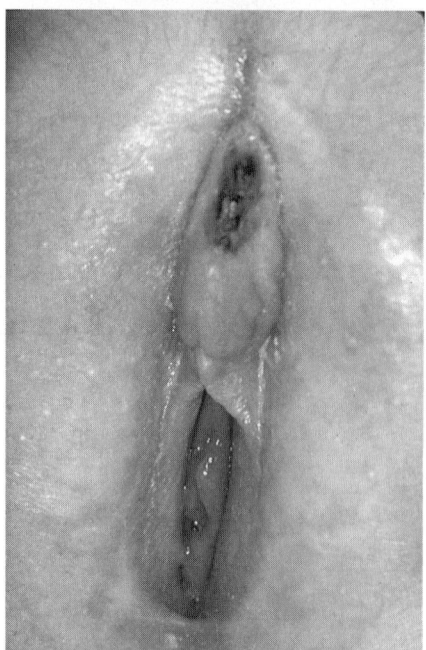

FIGURE 23-15
Vulvas of three girls with lichen sclerosus. (Photographs courtesy of S. Jean Emans, Children's Hospital, Boston, MA).

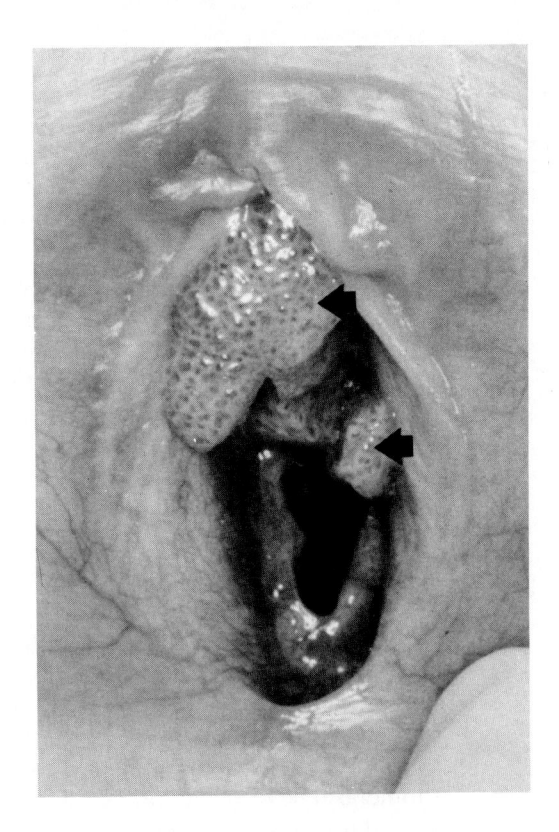

FIGURE 23-16
Genital condyloma. (From Pokorny SF. Pediatric vulvovaginitis. In: Kaufman RH, Friedrich EG, JR., Gardner HL, eds. Benign Diseases of the Vulva and Vagina, 3rd ed. Chicago: Year Book Medical Publishers, 1989:62. Used by permission.)

berty with the development of secondary sexual characteristics is not a difficult visual clinical diagnosis, reports of isolated premature menarche also have been noted. In these prepubertal girls, cyclic vaginal bleeding may occur, in the absence of secondary sexual characteristics. Clearly, these are diagnoses beyond the scope of evaluation in the emergency setting, and appropriate subspecialty referral is essential.

Fortunately, the incidence of malignant neoplasms in the genital tract is low, accounting for less than 1% of vaginal bleeding in most series. Tumors such as rhabdomyosarcoma, vaginal clear cell adenocarcinoma, and endodermal sinus tumors have been reported. Because of this possibility an examination under anesthesia is warranted in all children with unexplained vaginal bleeding.

Gynecologic Emergencies in the Adolescent Years

Pubertal Bleeding

Irregular menses during the first 1 to 2 years after menarche are quite common. Young adolescents frequently have anovulatory cycles and will experience estrogen withdrawal bleeding that may occur at irregular intervals. In general, this bleeding will not be sufficiently heavy or long-lasting to result in anemia. On occasion a young adolescent may present to the emergency department with unusually heavy bleeding associated with her first menses or with heavy bleeding resulting in anemia that may require intervention. In young adolescents who experience hemodynamically significant bleeding at menarche, clotting disorders may be found in up to 50%. Primary coagulation disorders are responsible for 19% of cases of acute menorrhagia in adolescents.[8]

When a teenager presents to the emergency department for vaginal bleeding, it is important to obtain the date of menarche and a specific history regarding the interval, duration, and amount of menstrual bleeding. It is not sufficient to ask a teenager if her menses have been "normal," for the teenager with heavy bleeding may have no basis of comparison. An accurate sexual history should also be obtained from the young woman to assess her risk of pregnancy. She should be questioned as to a history of other manifestations of a coagulopathy, such as nosebleeds, or easy bruising. A careful past medical history is also important, along with a family history specifically asking for bleeding disorders. She should be asked about the use of oral contraceptives, since some young women will not make the association between pill use and breakthrough bleeding.

The physical examination should assess for volume status with orthostatic vital signs. A general physical examination looking for evidence of systemic illness should be performed. As discussed earlier, many adolescents will tolerate a pelvic examination if a Huffman adolescent speculum is used, and a rectal examination may often be adequately substituted. The history and physical examination of the patient should also be directed toward ruling out other causes of vaginal bleeding, such as genital tract trauma, infection, or genital lesions.

Laboratory studies should include a complete blood count with platelet count and differential and a serum pregnancy test. Especially in the setting where there is concern regarding coagulopathy, clotting studies and bleeding time may be helpful. Since von Willebrand's disease is one of the most common causes of clotting disorders in young women, the bleeding time is essential. A more detailed endocrine work-up, including thyroid studies, may be necessary; ultimately, however, this may be deferred for a more thorough follow-up evaluation.

The adolescent with mild to moderate irregular uterine bleeding and a stable hematocrit without anemia will generally require no emergency treatment. Follow-up with a pediatrician or gynecologist is nevertheless important for these girls to ensure that their bleeding pattern does normalize. With significant bleeding or a falling hematocrit, more acute treatment may be indicated. For the stable patient who can be managed as an outpatient, using tapering doses of a low dose oral contraceptive may be helpful. The adolescent may be treated with a 35-mcg monophasic pill three times day, gradually tapering down to a daily dose. A schedule of one pill three times a day for 3 days, followed by one pill twice a day for 3 days, followed by one pill daily is usually successful. Most anovulatory bleeding that requires treatment will respond to this regimen. In certain clinical situations, particularly in settings where an atrophic endometrium is anticipated, oral estrogen may be required. If oral progestins are used, it is important to remember that a second withdrawal bleed will occur when the medicine is discontinued. The patient's hematocrit must be able to tolerate this second withdrawal bleed if this regimen is to be used. With higher doses of tapering oral contraceptives, nausea is a common side-effect. It may be prudent to provide an antiemetic for the patient to use at home.[9]

On occasion, significantly heavy vaginal bleeding may require inpatient management, with administration of intravenous conjugated estrogens. Premarin 25 mg IV every 6 hours for two to three doses may control heavy bleeding. Antiemetics should be provided, as severe nausea is very common with this regimen. This should be followed by oral progestins to stabilize the endometrium. In teenagers the likelihood of the structural abnormality of the uterus, such as leiomyoma or a polyp, is not high. With the possible exception of the very obese adolescent, who may have a very thick endometrium, a dilatation and curettage is rarely required. If contemplated, a transvaginal ultrasound to assess endometrial thickness and detect structural abnormalities may be helpful preoperatively.

A coagulopathy will be found in 50% of girls with very heavy bleeding at menarche. Among coagulopathies, von Willebrand's is most commonly encountered. The possibility of a myeloproliferative disorder, immune thrombocytopenia, or other hematologic conditions should be considered. In this setting, identification of the coagulopathy and correction of the specific defect will bring the most prompt relief to the bleeding. Particularly in the teenager with a chronic medical illness who may be bleeding from uremia or a myeloproliferative disorder, the hormonal manipulations discussed earlier may be helpful until the underlying disorder can be corrected. In adolescents who are undergoing chemotherapy, hormonal manipulation often may be necessary in an acute setting.

When a pregnancy is diagnosed in the young adolescent, the possibility of threatened spontaneous abortion, incomplete spontaneous abortion, or ectopic pregnancy should be considered. In this setting the differential diagnosis, diagnostic studies, and management are very much like those for an adult.

Again, the importance of careful follow-up after the emergency department visits must be emphasized. Although anovulatory bleeding is quite common in the young adolescent, a more detailed endocrine work-up may be indicated in selected situations.

Abdominal and Pelvic Pain in the Adolescent

Abdominal pain in the teenager is a relatively common problem. Occasionally, the pain may be sufficiently severe that the teenager and her family may present for emergency care. The differential diagnosis is very similar to that found in an adult. Acute or chronic GI processes, pelvic inflammatory disease, adnexal pathology, and pregnancy complications must be considered. Constipation seems to be an especially common problem in teenagers, especially with a presenting complaint of left lower quadrant pain.

In the teenager with abdominal and pelvic pain, a careful history should be obtained regarding the nature, duration, and location of the discomfort. A history of sexual activity is also important to evaluate. Questions screening for gastrointestinal and genitourinary diseases should also be asked.

A general physical examination, careful abdominal examination, and pelvic examination are also important, as is screening for sexually transmitted diseases, such as *N. gonorrhoeae* and *C. trachomatis*. In the teenager with abdominal or pelvic pain, the examiner may wish to screen for these sexually transmitted diseases regardless of the history provided about sexual activity. A complete blood count and sedimentation rate may be helpful in screening for infection. A pelvic ultrasound to assess for adnexal pathology, especially in the young adolescent where the adnexa may be difficult to evaluate, can offer additional information. A serum pregnancy test should be obtained. Urinalysis, urine culture, and testing for occult fecal blood are other clinically indicated studies.

Especially in the teenager where pelvic inflammatory disease is suspected, serious consideration should be given to hospitalization for parenteral antibiotics. Teenagers may be poorly compliant with outpatient oral antibiotics and often may have difficulty in making follow-up appointments. There is also some evidence to suggest that teenagers with pelvic inflammatory disease tend to present for care later than adults. The incidence of unsuspected tubo-ovarian abscess in adolescents with pelvic inflammatory disease appears to be greater than that for an adult. If outpatient treatment is contemplated, it is important that testing for both *N. gonorrhoeae* and *C. trachomatis* be obtained prior to therapy being instituted. Reevaluation by an experienced examiner within 12 to 24 hours is very important to ensure response to treatment. The adolescent who is febrile and has leukocytosis and significant abdominal tenderness, especially with peritoneal signs or any suggestion of a mass, should definitely be considered a candidate for hospitalization. Moreover, if the likelihood of compliance with medication or close follow-up is in doubt, hospitalization should be considered. Because of the disastrous consequences of an episode of pelvic inflammatory disease for the fertility of a young woman, hospitalization for all adolescents with suspected pelvic inflammatory disease should be strongly considered.[10]

For the teenager with more acute abdominal pain, consultation with a gynecologist and general surgeon in the emergency department may be necessary. Diagnostic laparoscopy can be used to differentiate between appendicitis and pelvic infection.

Psychosocial and Developmental Issues in The Emergency Care of Children

A visit to the emergency department is a stressful experience for both the child and her parents. Children may have specific age-related developmental needs that affect the way a child reacts to the illness or injury and the routines of the emergency department setting. A thorough understanding of these issues will enable the health care provider to minimize the trauma to the child and also obtain more thorough evaluation from a more cooperative child.

For the very young infant and toddler, separation from the parent is the child's main fear. Toddlers also quite commonly are afraid of the dark and of being left alone. As the child ages, he or she may continue to fear separation from the parent but also develop a greater fear of injury to the body by invasive procedures. Preschoolers may also engage in magical thinking and somehow feel that they are responsible for their illness or injury. Fear of bodily injury or harm is quite common during the school-age years. As children grow and mature, they become more concerned about the effects that an illness or injury may have on them in the eyes of their peers. Loss of control, either in their reaction to pain or through general anesthesia, is a concern in school-age children. In the adolescent years issues of control and autonomy are particularly important in interacting with parents. Concerns about bodily function and appearance are crucial during these years. There is a strong need to identify and to be similar to one's peers.

The developmental issues discussed earlier are very important to remember when dealing with children of different ages. In the youngest patients, having a parent present during examination or procedures can be very reassuring. It is important to assess the emotional status of the parent, however, and to encourage the anxious or distraught parent to provide as much support for the child as possible. Careful explanations to the parents may enable them to handle their own anxiety and fears in a more productive fashion. The presence of a security blanket or other familiar object can be reassuring to a young child. Restraints should be avoided in children of all ages. The vast majority of examinations and procedures can be accomplished without the use of restraints, or at the most, using a parent to help hold the child. The use of appropriate and safe sedation is preferable over the use of forcible restraint. Older children will respond well to a simple explanation of an examination or procedure. If a procedure will be uncomfortable, such as an injection, it is best to be straightforward with the child and prepare her for this. Explanations should be given in age-appropriate language that the child will understand. It is important always to be honest and truthful with a child. Especially in the adolescent, clear explanations of procedures and expectations will be most helpful. The teenager should be allowed to participate in the decision-making process and informed-consent process as much as possible. Especially in the teenage years, respect for the young woman's privacy and right to confidentiality regarding matters of sexual activity, sexually transmitted diseases, and contraception is very important.[11]

The emergency department experience for children or adolescents may be remembered throughout their lives. The way in which they are treated and how they perceive their experience will color their future interactions with the health care system. For this reason it is of the utmost importance that careful consideration be given to the child's psychosocial as well as physical needs.

REFERENCES

1. Emans SJ. Vulvovaginitis in the child and adolescent. Pediatr Rev 8:12, 1986
2. Coupey S, Saunders DS. Physical maturation. In: Laveny JP, Sanfilippo JS (eds): Pediatric and Adolescent Obstetrics and Gynecology. New York: Springer-Verlag, 1985
3. Gidwani GP. Approach to evaluation of the premenarcheal child with a gynecologic problem. In: McDonough PG (ed): Pediatric Gynecology. Clin Obstet Gynecol 30:643, 1987
4. Pokorny SF, Stromer, J. Atraumatic removal of secretions from prepubertal vagina. Am Obstet Gynecol 156:581, 1987
5. Greene MG (ed). The Harriet Lane Handbook, 12th Ed. St Louis: CV Mosby Year Book, 1991

6. Muram D, Massouda D. Vaginal bleeding in children. Contemp Obstet Gynecol 26:41, 1985
7. Muram D. Genital tract injuries in the prepubertal child. Pediatr Ann 15:616, 1986
8. Claessens EA, Cowell CA. Acute adolescent menorrhagia. Am J Obstet Gynecol 139:277, 1981
9. Gidwani GP. Vaginal bleeding in adolescents. J Reprod Med 29:417, 1984
10. Washington AE, Sweet RL, Shafer MB. Pelvic inflammatory disease and its sequelae in adolescents. J Adolesc Health Care 6:298, 1985
11. Thompson SW. Emotional and psychological support of the child and family. In: Thompson SW (ed): Emergency Care of Children. Boston: Jones and Bartlett, 1990

Obstetric and Gynecologic Emergencies, edited by Guy I. Benrubi. J.B. Lippincott Company, Philadelphia © 1994.

CHAPTER 24

Emergency Evaluation and Treatment of the Sexual Assault Victim

James L. Jones and Jay M. Whitworth

Sexual assault or rape is a common violent crime in the United States. The Federal Bureau of Investigation statistics show that in 1990 there were 120,000 reported cases of rape in adults (over 18 years of age).[1] Accurate statistics are difficult to obtain because rape is often not reported to authorities. Bureau of Justice statistics[2] found in a survey of a representative sample of the U.S. adult population that only 54% of all victims report the crime. A study of college-aged women showed that 37% of the respondents reported a history of sexual abuse but that only 4% had reported the crime or sought professional help.[3] Other sources estimate that the actual number of rapes reported to police is between 4 and 25%.[3-5]

Since the 1970s, rape crisis centers have been developed in larger urban areas of the United States to deal with the particular problems of the sexual assault victims. Rape crisis centers provide training for physicians and nurses in performing sexual assault examinations. These centers also provide continuity of care and counseling that is difficult to obtain in many other settings. The multidisciplinary approach used by many centers underscores the importance of the psychological aspects of sexual assault. In addition to meeting the acute medical needs of the patient, the medical staff is responsible for seeing to the immediate and long-term emotional needs of the victim as well.

Ninety-five percent of adult assault victims are women. It is important to realize that the male victim will require the same consideration and support as the female victim.

Many physicians are uncomfortable performing sexual assault examinations. Unless the victim is seriously injured, she may not require the presence of a physician. Sexual assault examinations are performed by nurse examiners in many states.[6] The most important considerations in determining who should perform a sexual assault examination are experience and interest. The forensic aspects of the examination require strict attention to detail and experience in performing sexual assault examinations. The psychological aspects of sexual assault demand that the examiner be compassionate, patient, and understanding. A list of the responsibilities of the examiner in caring for a victim, as described by Kobernick and colleagues, follows.[7]

1. Prompt treatment of physical injuries
2. Collection of legal evidence
3. Careful physical examination
4. Documentation of pertinent history
5. Prevention of pregnancy
6. Prevention of venereal disease
7. Psychological support and arrangements for follow-up counseling

The physician or examiner should be familiar with all these aspects of care of sexual assault victims.

Triage

Upon arrival in the emergency department the victim should not wait in a public area but should be quickly and discretely escorted to a private examination area. An assessment should be made on admission as to the extent of the victim's injuries. Critically injured victims should be treated without delay in an urgent care area. The forensic examination should be performed only after the victim is stabilized. If the victim has to be taken to the operating room, specimens can often be safely collected during an operative procedure. Fortunately, sexual assault victims are not usually severely injured. A review of 100 consecutive assaults reported to the Sexual Assault Center at University Medical Center, Jacksonville, Florida, found that only two patients required hospitalization for injuries sustained during an assault. One patient was bleeding heavily from a labial laceration and required an examination under anesthesia; the other was a victim of a severe beating. A study by Hicks of rape victims presenting to a Miami emergency room also found that less than 1% of all victims require hospitalization.[8]

The victim should be instructed not to wash, use the toilet, or eat and drink until the examination is completed. If friends or family members are present, they may remain with the victim if she wishes. If the victim is alone, a nurse or rape crisis counselor should stay with her. Do not leave the victim alone.

Control is an important psychological factor in rape; it is important to help the victim reestablish control over her surroundings. It is important that the victim be reassured as to her safety. The examiner should carefully explain the procedures that will be performed. At the Sexual Assault Center at University Medical Center,

Jacksonville, Florida, the victim is given a folder containing information about each step of the examination. A list of tests that have been ordered is included, along with the expected completion date. The victim should be informed that she may refuse any part of the examination. Consents for the examination and release of the information to the police should be reviewed carefully and signed. Whether the victim intends to report the crime should be immaterial; she is still entitled to medical care.

Forensic Medicine

Many physicians find the medicolegal aspects of sexual assault intimidating. It is important that the physician be familiar with the specific guidelines issued by the prosecuting attorney for sexual assault examination. Prepackaged rape kits are also available that should fulfill a particular state's guidelines for collecting evidence. Common medical practices, such as using the newer rapid DNA probe technologies for detection of *Neisseria gonorrhoeae* and *Chlamydia trachomatis* are not admissible in some courts. As newer technologies are introduced, state guidelines change, and the hospital's protocol should be updated.

The most important aspect of a forensic examination is adequate and careful documentation. Notes must be legible. One may be called to testify years after the assault, and the physician must be able to rely solely on notes taken during the examination. It is equally important that the physician not make remarks that may be misinterpreted at a later date or in court. This can be avoided if the physician realizes that his or her role is not to determine if the victim has been raped, but to determine if the examination is consistent with sexual assault. Avoid conclusive statements that are not supported by facts or the experience of the physician. Remarks concerning the victim's behavior should not be entered into the record unless they are purely descriptive. Coping mechanisms produce a wide spectrum of response to rape; thus the physician may encounter behavior that seems inappropriate to a history of assault. Statements, for example, that the victim's behavior was inconsistent with sexual assault are inappropriate. The patient's affect can be described instead.

The physician should also understand the concept of "chain of custody." Courts will not consider evidence admissible if a direct line of custody cannot be established between the examiner and the court. As the evidence is gathered, it is placed into separate envelopes, sealed, and initialed. All specimens must be clearly labeled with the victim's name, the date, the examiner's name, and the source of the specimen. Clothing is placed in paper bags. Glass slides should be placed in carriers with rigid sides. The bags, envelopes, and carriers should be sealed with plastic tape and the examiner's initials written across the tape or seal. This should be done in such a fashion that if the container is opened, the tampering would be obvious. The evidence should then be placed into a large paper bag or envelope and sealed. The evidence is then either handed directly to a police officer or placed in a locked cabinet. A receipt should be obtained for the evidence when it is transferred to the police. Breaking the chain of custody, by faulty handling or record keeping, may make the entire examination inadmissible in court.

Obtaining a Medical History

The purpose of obtaining a history in a sexual assault case is to record as soon as possible the events that have occurred and to guide the physician during the examination. If the patient is an adult and a good historian, one may eliminate some parts of the exam and tests, such as obtaining rectal or oral cultures when only vaginal penetration has occurred. In the absence of an adequate history the physician should perform an encompassing physical examination. If the physician records remarks made directly by the victim, these should be placed in quotations; otherwise the remarks are assumed to be paraphrased.

The history should include the following:

1. *Medical and surgical history.* This should include allergies and medications.
2. *Gynecologic history.* The examiner should emphasis menstrual history, current method of contraception, history of venereal disease, history of pelvic inflammatory disease, last coitus, tampon use, and douching practices.
3. *Obstetric history.* Methods of delivery, gravidity, and parity.
4. *Location, date, and time of assault.*
5. *Description of assault.* The victim would be asked to describe the assault in her own words. The examiner should ask the victim to include the number of assailants, whether force was used, the presence of weapons, what type of assault occurred. If the patient does not volunteer enough information it would be appropriate to ask, for example, "Did he put his penis in your vagina?"

The Physical Examination of the Adult

It is particularly important to inform the patient again as to exactly what the examination involves and to reassure her that the examination will not be painful.

The examiner should collect as much of the victim's clothing as feasible, particularly the panties. The victim should remove the clothing herself, preferably over a clean paper or cloth sheet to catch any debris. If it is necessary to cut the victim's clothing in order to remove it, torn or stained areas should be avoided.

The victim should then be carefully examined with close attention to lacerations, bruises, and foreign material (Fig. 24-1). Any foreign material should be carefully removed and placed in an envelope and identified as to location. Bruises, bite marks, and lacerations should be carefully described and diagramed. Lacerations should be inspected carefully, particularly if a sharp object was used in the assault, to rule out a deep, penetrating injury. Photographs may be helpful if they effectively demonstrate an injury but should be taken by a police or medical photographer. Photographs can actually harm a case if they do not add significant graphic detail. The photograph should be labeled with an indelible marker or by other permanent means of identification.

Any suspicious stains or deposits on the skin should be collected by scraping with a tongue blade or with a moist, cotton-tipped applicator. Since semen fluoresces a bright yellow-green, deposits can be identified with a Woods light. The head hair

EMERGENCY EVALUATION AND TREATMENT OF THE SEXUAL ASSAULT VICTIM ◆ 343

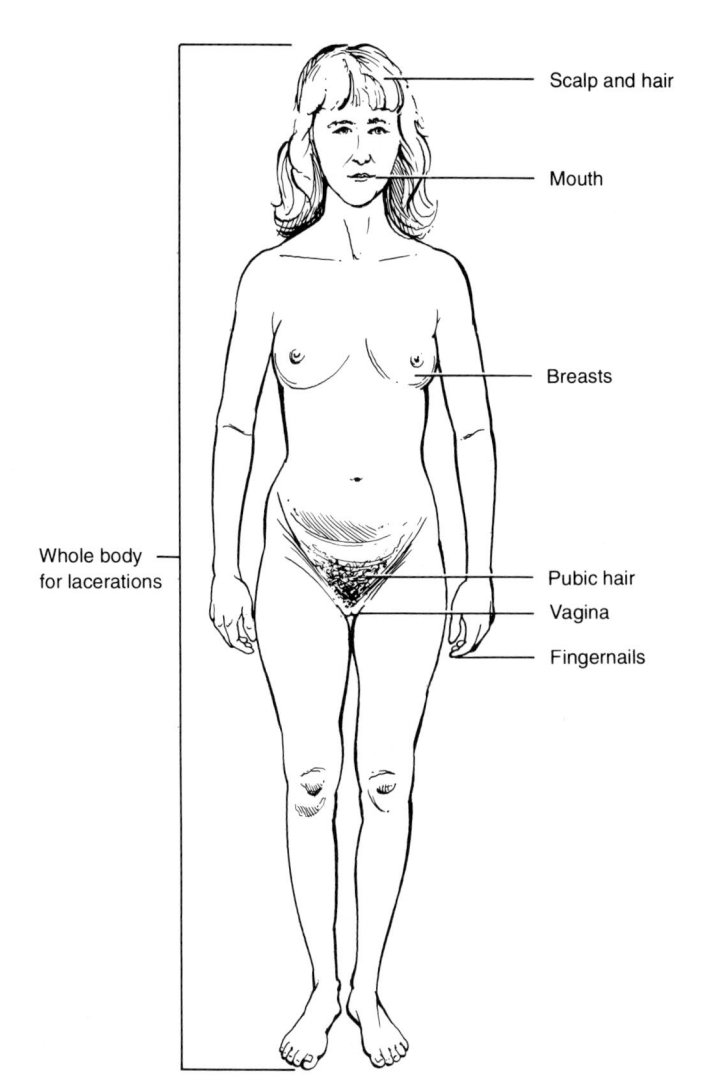

FIGURE 24–1
Examination of the sexual assault victim.

should be combed with a new comb over a paper towel, carefully collecting foreign material. Hair standards should be obtained by plucking, so as to include the roots if possible. The pubic hair should be examined in a similar fashion.

The oral cavity should be carefully examined with a tongue blade. Victims will often bite themselves during a sexual assault, producing small abrasions in the buccal mucosa. Fellatio may also cause small submucosal hemorrhages, which are usually seen at the junction of the hard and soft palate (Fig. 24-2).[9] If there is a history of fellatio, the oral cavity, especially the areas between the gum and lips, should be swabbed with a cotton-tipped applicator and glass slides should be prepared. When obtaining specimens for determination of the presence of sperm, two slides should be made. One goes directly to the forensic laboratory; the other is used immediately

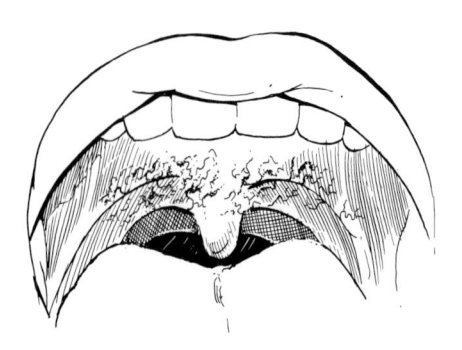

FIGURE 24–2
Fellatio syndrome: echymoses of palate.

as a wet mount. The specimens should be made with several swabs. After the slides are prepared, the swabs are allowed to air-dry before placing them in an envelope. The presence of sperm as noted by the examiner should be recorded in the chart, and a separate notation should be made as to whether the sperm are motile. Pharyngeal cultures should be taken for *N. gonorrhoeae*. A saliva specimen is obtained from the victim for blood antigen determination. A small square of filter paper is placed in the victim's mouth, and the victim is encouraged to saturate it with saliva. It is important that no one handle the filter paper except the victim. If there is a history of fellatio, the victim should rinse her mouth out with water and wait 5 minutes before preparing the specimen.

The fingernails should be inspected for foreign material under the nails. If any foreign material is present, including dirt, it should be collected over a paper towel with a blunt wooden probe. Scrapings from each hand should be submitted separately.

The victim is then asked to lie on the examination table in the dorsal lithotomy position, so that a pelvic examination can be performed. The labia, posterior fourchette, and vestibule are carefully inspected under adequate lighting. Bruises, lacerations, and tender areas are carefully explored, diagramed, and photographed, if necessary. The Woods light should again be employed to highlight semen deposits. In younger victims the posterior fourchette is very susceptible to injury, which appears as fine lacerations. In cases of chronic sexual abuse, the examiner should look for scarring in posterior fourchette and posterior vestibule.

Physical findings suggestive of vaginal penetration are present in approximately 50% of sexual assault victims, but only 2% have clinical evidence of significant genital trauma.[10] Injuries are typically minor and appear as small abrasions and lacerations. The examiner should describe any visible lesions and diagram their location. The most commonly injured sites are the posterior aspect of the introitus, hymen, and posterior fourchette (Fig. 24-3).[9] In the absence of gross lacerations, two techniques can be employed to highlight microlacerations: colposcopy and toluidine blue staining. The colposcope is a medium-powered binocular with an internal light source that is commonly used to visualize the cervix. In a study of 18 volunteers examined within 6 hours after coitus, Norvell and colleagues showed that microlaceration of the introitus and vagina could be identified in 61%.[11] Toluidine blue staining can also be used in the absence of gross lesions to highlight microlacerations.[12] The stain should be applied directly to the perineum and then carefully wiped off using lubricating jelly on a gauze. Toluidine blue is a nuclear

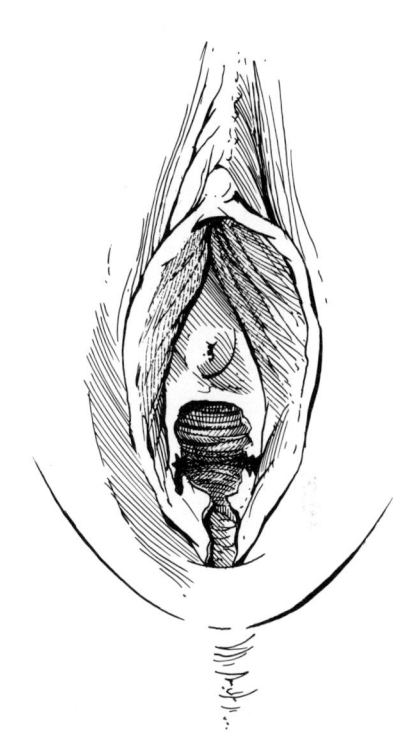

FIGURE 24-3
Laceration of hymenal ring and posterior fourchette.

stain, so normal keratinized skin will not stain. Microlacerations show up as finely stained blue lines.

The buttocks are then gently separated and the anus is inspected for evidence of small fissures, lacerations, and scarring. Hemocult should be obtained for evidence of occult rectal bleeding. If there is a history of anal penetration, the physician should look for evidence of rectal bleeding. Unexplained rectal bleeding should alert the physician to the possibility of bowel perforation. Proctoscopy or flexible sigmoidoscopy would then be indicated to rule out bowel perforation.

Anal swabs should be taken and glass slides prepared. Sperm may be recovered from the rectum, but the yield is usually significantly lower than that from the vagina or cervix.[13] Cultures should also be obtained from the rectum.

A speculum moistened with warm water (do not use lubricant) can now be gently inserted in the vagina. The cervix is visualized for any evidence of trauma. Microlacerations on the cervix resulting from sexual trauma can be visualized with the aid of the colposcope.[10] A specimen should be taken from the external os, and two glass slides should be prepared. Samples are also taken from the vaginal pool. It should be noted if the sperm are motile. Sperm may remain motile in the vaginal pool for 12 hours.[14] Sperm survival in the cervical os is considerably longer; motile sperm can be recovered from the cervix for up to 7 days.[14]

Cultures for gonorrhea and chlamydia should be taken. As noted earlier, most courts will not accept direct antigen tests for determination of gonorrhea. The rapid antigen tests, such as the chemiluminescent Gen-probe, offer a significant improvement over the traditional culture. The assay is highly sensitive and specific, and the results can be ready in as little as 2 hours. At University Medical Center in Jacksonville, Florida, the sensitivity and specificity of the Gen-probe assay is 93.3 and 99% for *N. gonorrhoeae* and 93.9 and 99.1% for *C. trachomatis,* respectively.

Two vaginal swabs are obtained for antigen determination. Blood group antigens are secreted into body fluids by approximately 80% of the population.[15] Although unable to identify a specific assailant, the technique is useful nonetheless to exclude or include someone from a list of suspects.

Vaginal swabs are also obtained for the analysis of prostatic antigen, p30, and acid phosphatase. The finding of these seminal factors can be used to establish penile penetration in absence of sperm.

Additional swabs, usually six to eight, also can be obtained from the vaginal pool for DNA fingerprint analysis. This technique is rapidly gaining acceptance in U.S. courts. DNA fingerprint analysis uses restrictive enzyme analysis and can yield a unique map from a single sperm. This technique is a tremendous advance, since it can be used to identify an assailant, much as the classic fingerprint does. Again it is extremely important that the examiner not cross-contaminate the specimen.

The vaginal walls are then inspected for lacerations. This is most easily accomplished while slowly withdrawing the speculum. In very young or postmenopausal patients who have poorly estrogenized vaginal mucosa, lacerations of the vaginal sidewalls are more common. Laceration of the cul-de-sac or the posterior vaginal fornix can also be seen, particularly if a foreign object is inserted into the vagina. Injury from insertion of a foreign object can also cause perforation of the cul-de-sac and bowel injury. If a penetrating injury is suspected, a laparotomy should be performed to rule out injury to the bowel.

Many courts request pubic hair samples. The victim should again be informed that hair samples are going to be taken. Samples should be taken by pulling the hair out by the roots. Head hair samples should also be obtained for comparison purposes. Twenty individual hairs should constitute an adequate sample. Since this procedure is uncomfortable, it is often prudent to perform it at the end of the examination.

Examination of the Child

A discussion of sexual abuse in children must begin with the physician's legal requirement for reporting of cases. In all states a physician having a reason to suspect child sexual abuse must report to a designated agency. Agencies that receive reports vary in different states and localities, and it is essential that the physician inform himself of these requirements before any examination is done. The services of a multidisciplinary assessment team, if available, can be of extreme assistance in evaluation of the child and the total family situation.

Examinations for alleged sexual abuse in children usually do not result from allegations of acute rape.[16] More commonly, the allegation is of incest, fondling, molestation, or exploitation. In the unusual situation where there may be forensic collection considerations, a protocol for specimens should be used similar to that in adult patients. Chronic or recurrent sexual abuse in children is usually manifest by subtle physical signs and is likely to be accompanied by behavioral or developmental signs or symptoms. For this reason the child sexual assault examination must be carried out in the context of a total pediatric health assessment and by an examiner skilled in assessing for the specific manifestations of child sexual abuse.[17] After a history has been taken by the examiner or by a trained interviewer, the examiner should decide the extent of the examinations necessary, decide the cultures and specimens to be collected, and incorporate an explanation for each into an age-appropriate explanation to the child. The child should always have the option of a trusted adult being present during the examination and should know that the examination is not painful or more intrusive than necessary. The examiner should be understanding and patient but should not play games with the child to gain cooperation. This is a common ploy of abusers.

Children should never be examined against their will. If the examination is absolutely necessary for medical or legal reasons, the examination should be performed under anesthesia. Genital examinations in children should be carried out in the modified dorsal lithotomy (frog-leg) and/or knee-chest positions. Children are often uncomfortable in the knee-chest position, but it may offer visualization up to the cervix without instrumentation. Uncooperative or frightened children often do quite well in their mother's lap on an examining table (Fig. 24-4). Stirrups may be used in older children but are usually unnecessary and frightening in younger children. The use of a colposcope in the examination offers a light source, magnification, and photographic documentation and greatly simplifies evaluation and documentation.[18]

Findings associated with child sexual abuse have been more clearly documented in recent years.[19–21] In addition, there is a greatly enhanced understanding of normal anatomic variations based on recent studies.[22,23] Most of the physical findings seen

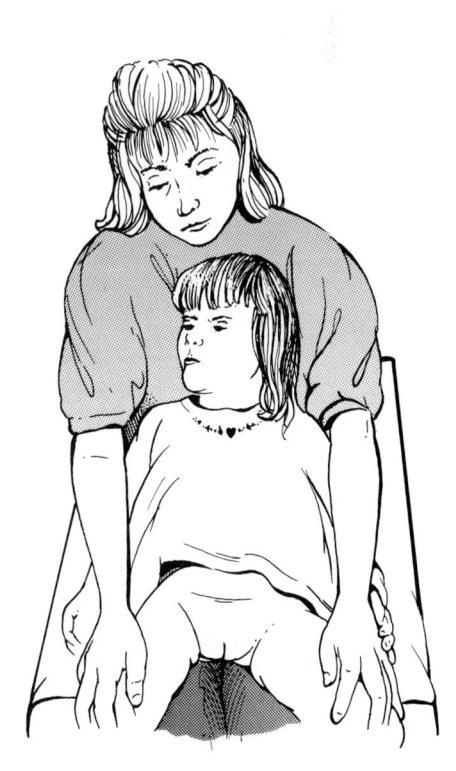

FIGURE 24–4
Position of child on mother's legs for examination (See also Fig. 23-7).

with sexual abuse are indicators of genital trauma and must be coupled with the history to raise a serious question of abuse. Some findings or combinations of findings, however, are so compelling as to be reasonably diagnostic of abuse. In our experience with a highly selected referral population, 65% of examinations result in no findings, 30% have findings consistent with sexual abuse, and 5% have findings considered diagnostic of sexual abuse. It is useful to remember that a normal examination is expected if the allegation is of fondling or oral sex. Many times the offender has confessed to specific sexual acts and there are no physical findings. Therefore a physical examination can never rule out the possibility of sexual abuse.[24,25]

The genital examination is best performed by using labial traction, in which the labia majora are grasped between the thumbs and index fingers and gently lifted laterally and toward the examiner, or labial separation, where the thumbs of the examiner are placed on the labia majora and mild lateral pressure is applied. The latter is more comfortable, whereas the former usually offers better direct visualization of the edges of the hymen. Digital or speculum examinations are rarely advisable or necessary except in sexually active older children.

Many of the findings associated with genital trauma focus on changes in the hymen. A clear understanding of normal variants is essential. The hymen can normally be circular (annular), semilunar (crescentic with attachments at about 2 o'clock and 10 o'clock), cribriform, or septate. In unusual circumstances, the hymen may be imperforate, which has medical implications but no implications for sexual abuse. Congenital absence of the hymen has never been reported.[26] In the first few months of life the hymen is still estrogenized from maternal influences and becomes estrogenized again in early puberty. Estrogenization produces an appearance of hypertrophy, redundancy, and a white, pearllike mucosa. It often is more difficult to assess for scars with these changes.

Any of the following findings may occur in sexually abused children:

- Bruises, scars, or bleeding of the genitalia, perineum, or perianal structures
- Chafing, abrasions, or bruising of inner thighs or genitalia
- Scarring, tears, or severe distortion of the hymen
- Hymenal measurements that exceed currently accepted norms
- Torn, stained, or bloody underclothing
- Sexually transmitted disease
- Sperm on body, clothes; lax rectal tone
- Reflex anal dilatation
- Rectal lacerations

Documentation issues are even more important in children than in adults, as the time between the examination and possible testimony is even longer. Photographs are the method of choice, but detailed diagrams of body findings and specific genital findings may suffice. Laboratory support may be very useful in supporting the diagnosis of child sexual abuse. Cultures for *N. gonorrhoeae* should routinely be done in all cases where genital contact by the abuser is possible. Since positive cultures are common from sites other than the primary contact, cultures should be obtained from vaginal, rectal, and oropharyngeal sites. A positive result from culture makes sexual contact a certainty if the patient is not a newborn. Cultures for *C. trachomatis* and herpes, types 1 and 2, may be indicated under certain clinical conditions. The presence of genital warts on gross inspection or *Trichomonas vaginalis* in wet preparations is usually considered a strong indicator of sexual abuse in children. HIV antibody testing and serologic test for syphilis are not routinely done unless more specific indicators are present.[17,27]

Treatment of Sexual Assault Victims

Most physical injuries sustained during rape or sexual assault are minor. Minor cuts, abrasions, and bruises on the external genitalia will respond to cold compresses and sitz baths. Vaginal sidewall lacerations often do not require repair unless they are deep. Deep lacerations are best repaired under anesthesia, where the extent of the lesion can be more fully appreciated. As noted earlier, penetrating injuries to the cul-de-sac also require examination under anesthesia and possible exploratory laparotomy. Patients assaulted with foreign objects should also receive tetanus prophylaxis.

Prevention of Venereal Disease

The risks of acquiring a sexually transmitted disease from a single act of sexual assault are difficult to determine. The risks depend on the prevalence of the disease in the local community and on the nature of the assault. Infections detected within 24 hours of the assault most likely represent a preexisting condition.[28] In a small study of 109 sexual assault victims who returned for follow-up, Jenny and coworkers found that the risks of *N. gonorrhoeae* and *C. trachomatis* were 4% and 2%, respectively.[29] The prevalence of these infections in assault victims is higher—6% for gonorrhea and 10% for chlamydia. The prevalence of syphilis in rape victims has been reported in several studies to be less than 3%.[28,29]

Lack of adequate follow-up is a significant problem in treating sexual assault victims. The experience of the Sexual Assault Center at University Medical Center, Jacksonville, Florida, is that only 20% of victims return for follow-up counseling or testing. In Jenny's study, cited previously, the follow-up was accomplished in only 53%. Because of poor follow-up many centers use prophylactic antibiotics. The treatment regimen should cover the most common pathogens, gonorrhea, chlamydia, and incubating syphilis. The Centers for Disease Control recommends Ceftriaxone 250 mg IM for coverage of gonorrhea and incubating syphilis.[27] Penicillin-allergic patients should be given spectinomycin 2 g IM. This should be followed by oral doxycycline 100 mg bid for 7 days. Pregnant women and young children should not be given tetracycline and should be treated with erythromycin 500 mg QID for 7 days. Selection of prophylaxis should also be determined by local sensitivity studies. A new therapy for chlamydia is azythromycin (Zithromax) 1 g (four tablets of 250 mg) as a single oral dose. It has the advantage of completing therapy at a single dose.

The risk to young children of acquiring *N. gonorrhoeae* or chlamydia from sexual assault is low. Prophylaxis is not recommended unless the assailant is known to be infected and treatment with antibiotics is withheld until diagnostic tests are completed. Treatment of *N. gonorrhoeae* and *C. trachomatis* in children is adjusted to body weight and is given in Table 24-1.[30]

The risks of acquiring sexually transmitted viral infections such as HPV, HIV, hepatitis, and herpes simplex is not known. Since there is a prolonged latency period, testing rape victims for viral infections is controversial. This is particularity true for testing for HIV. Except for possible medicolegal implications, there is no rationale for drawing baseline HIV titers at the initial examination. However, it would be appropriate to offer the victim HIV testing at subsequent visits, particularly if the assailant is a known carrier of the virus.

If the assailant was known, attempts should be made to determine if he is a carrier of hepatitis B. If the victim requests, she should be offered prophylaxis with hepatitis B immunoglobin.

Prevention of Pregnancy

The risk of pregnancy after a single unprotected act of intercourse is anywhere from 0 to 26%, depending on the victim's cycle. If the victim is at risk for pregnancy and the assault has occurred within 72 hours, postcoital hormonal birth control should be offered. A sensitive pregnancy test should be obtained before any medications are given. The most commonly prescribed regime uses a combination oral contraceptive containing 50 mcg of ethinyl estradiol and 0.5 mg of dl-norgestrel, sold in the United States as Ovral. Two tablets are given by mouth, and this is repeated 12 hours later. The most common side-effect is nausea, which can be treated with an antiemetic. The pregnancy rate with this regime is approximately 1.6%.[31]

Insertion of a copper-bearing intrauterine device (IUD) within 5 days of conception is also an effective means of preventing implantation.[32] The potential for devel-

TABLE 24–1
Treatment of N. gonorrhea and Chlamydia trachomatis in Children (by weight of patient)

	N. gonorrhea	Chlamydia trachomatis
< 45 Kg	Amoxicillin 50 mg/kg po with probenecid 25 mg/kg	Erythromycin 40 mg/kg/day QID for 7 days
	Ceftriaxone 125 mg im	
	Spectinomycin 40 mg/kg im	
≥ 45 Kg	Amoxicillin 3.0 gm po with probenecid 1.0 gm po	Erythromycin 500 mg po QID for 7 days
	Ceftriaxone 250 mg im	Doxycycline 100 mg po QID for 7 days
	Spectinomycin 2.0 gm im	Tetracycline 500 mg po QID for 7 days

opment of pelvic inflammatory disease in rape victims may preclude the use of an IUD, since the presence of the IUD can potentiate the infection. It should be remembered that postcoital hormonal or IUD birth control is considered by some religious groups to be a form of abortion. The mechanism of action of these techniques should be carefully explained to the victim.

Psychological Support and Counseling

The most significant medical problem that the rape victim presents is a psychological one. The rape trauma syndrome was initially described by Burgess and Holmstrom in 1974.[33] The syndrome is composed of two phases, an acute phase and a long-term reorganization phase.

The response to sexual assault as seen in the acute phase is described as either controlled or expressive. Expressive behaviors, demonstrated by 75% of victims, include anger, grief, and anxiety. Twenty-five percent of victims respond in a controlled fashion and internalize their emotions. Such controlled behavior has led some examiners to conclude that the victim has not been assaulted because her behavior is different from what is expected.

Somatization is a common feature of the acute phase. Victims may complain of a wide variety of somatic manifestations of the sexual assault, including sleep disturbances, muscle tension, headaches, and gastrointestinal problems. The acute phase typically lasts from 3 to 6 months.[34]

The long-term reorganization phase may last for years. The clinical signs include depression, sexual dysfunction, substance abuse, and low self-esteem.[34] Felitti found a significant increase in morbid obesity in victims of child abuse.[35] Chronic pelvic pain is also strongly associated with a history of sexual abuse. When dealing with patients who present with complaints of depression, sexual dysfunction, or chronic pain, one should rule out sexual abuse as an underlying factor. Physicians commonly treat sexual assault victims, but they are not always aware of it.

Sexual assault is a major social and medical problem in the United States. Treatment of sexual assault victims presents a unique challenge to the physician. The examination should only be performed by professionals who have both the technical skills to perform and interpret the physical examination and the compassion and understanding to deliver medical care to victims.

REFERENCES

1. Uniform Crime Reports for the United States. Federal Bureau of Investigation, US Department of Justice, Washington, DC, 1990
2. US Department of Justice. Female Victims of Violent Crime. Publication No. NCJ-126826, January 1991
3. Koss M. The scope of rape: implications for the clinical treatment of victims. Clin Psychologist. 88, 1983

4. Kilpatrick D. Rape victims: detection, assessment and treatment. Clin Psychologist 92, 1983
5. Binder R. Why women don't report sexual assault. J Clin Psychiatr 42:437, 1981
6. Antognoli-Toland P. Comprehensive program for examination of sexual assault victims by nurses: a hospital-based project in Texas. J Emerg Nurs 11(3):132, 1985
7. Kobernick ME, Seiferts S, Sanders AB et al. Emergency department management of the sexual assault victim. J Emerg Med 2:205, 1985
8. Hicks DJ. Rape: sexual assault. Am J Obstet Gynecol 137(8):931, 1980
9. Geist RF. Sexually related trauma. Emerg Med Clin North Am 6(3):439, 1988
10. Slaughter L, Brown C. Cervical findings in rape victims. J Obstet Gynecol 164(2):528, 1991
11. Norvell MK, Benrubi GI, Thompson RJ. Investigation of microtrauma after sexual intercourse. J Reprod Med 29(4), 1984
12. Lauber AA, Souma ML. Use of toluidine blue for documentation of traumatic intercourse. Obstet Gynecol 60(5):644, 1982
13. Tucker S, Claire E, Ledray LE et al. Sexual assault evidence collection. Wis Med J. 89(7):407, 1990
14. Soules MR, Pollard AA, Brown KM et al. The forensic laboratory evaluation of evidence in alleged rape. Am J Obstet Gynecol 130(2):142, 1978
15. Cabaniss ML, Scott SE, Copeland L. Gathering evidence for rape cases. Contemp Obstet Gynecol 25(3):160, 1985
16. American Academy of Pediatrics, Committee on Adolescence. Rape and the adolescent. Pediatrics 81:595, 1988
17. American Academy of Pediatrics, Committee on Child Abuse and Neglect, Guidelines for the evaluation of sexual abuse of children. Pediatrics 87:254, 1991
18. McCann J. The use of culposcope in childhood sexual abuse examinations, Pediatr Clin North Am 37(4):863, 1990
19. Heger A, Emans SJ. Introital diameter as the criterion for sexual abuse. Pediatrics 85:222, 1990
20. Hobbs CJ, Wynne JM. Sexual abuse of English boys and girls: the importance of anal examination. Child Abuse Negl 13:195, 1989
21. Chadwick DL, Berkowitz CA, Kerns DA et al. Color Atlas of Child Sexual Abuse. Chicago: Year Book, 1989
22. McCann J, Voris J, Simon M, Wells R. Perianal findings in prepubertal children selected for non-abuse: a descriptive study. Child Abuse Negl 13:179, 1989
23. McCann J, Voris J, Simon M, Wells R. Comparison of genital examination techniques in prepubertal girls. Pediatrics 85:182, 1990
24. Muram D. Child sexual abuse: relationship between sexual acts and genital findings. Child Abuse Negl 13:211, 1989
25. DeJong A, Rose M. Legal proof of child sexual abuse in the absence of physical evidence. Pediatrics 88(3):506, 1991
26. Jenny C, Kuhns ML, Arakawa F et al. Hymens in female infants. Pediatrics 80(3):399, 1987
27. Centers for Disease Control. 1989 Sexually transmitted diseases treatment guidelines. MMWR 38(September 1, suppl S-8):1, 1989
28. Schwarcz SK, Whittington, WL. Sexual assault and sexually transmitted diseases: detection and management in adults and children. Rev Infect Dis 12(suppl 6), 1990
29. Jenny C, Hooten TM, Bowers A et al. Sexually transmitted diseases in victims of rape. N Engl J Med 322(11):713, 1990
30. Paradise JE. The medical evaluation of the sexually abused child. Pediatr Clin North Am 37(4):839, 1990

31. Yuzpe A, Smith P, Rademakeer A. A multi-center clinical investigation employing ethinyl estradiol combined with dl norgestrel as a postcoital contraceptive agent. Fertil Steril 37(509):508, 1982
32. Lippes J, Tatum HJ, Maulik D. Postcoital copper IUDs. Adv Planned Parenthood 14:87, 1979
33. Burgess AW, Holmstrom LL. Rape trauma syndrome. Am J Psychiatry 131(9):981, 1974
34. Gise LH, Paddison P. Rape, sexual abuse, and its victims. Psychiatr Clin North Am 11(4):629, 1988
35. Felitti VJ. Long term medical consequences of incest, rape and molestation. South Med J 84(3):328, 1991

CHAPTER 25

Gynecologic Trauma

Tracey Abner

Gynecologic trauma can result from a variety of situations. Included in this discussion will be trauma that is sexually related, that is associated with women's sports or leisure activities, and that occurs from pelvic fractures.

Sexually Related Trauma

A substantial body of literature addressing trauma from rape as well as trauma occurring during consensual coitus exists.[1-10] Interestingly, the major forms of sexually related trauma dealt with in recent literature have resulted from unexpected trauma occurring between consenting adults. Though sexual abuse and its related trauma may be seen in emergency departments, abused women without life-threatening injuries or hemorrhage are generally evaluated in a well-controlled setting established for rape victims.[1-3] Nevertheless, the gynecologic injuries that can occur during consensual and forced coitus are similar.

Women presenting for emergency evaluation due to sexually related trauma not only will be in pain but will harbor feelings of embarrassment and anguish. In such a setting, compassion is as important as diagnostic acumen, if not more so.

Trauma secondary to oral-genital sex can present in many ways. One finding seen in the oral cavity is referred to as the fellatio syndrome. Erythema, petechia, purpura, and ecchymoses of the soft palate are seen.[4] These are due to hemorrhage, possibly from repetitive negative pressure in the oral cavity combined with the action of the tensor and levator veli palatini muscles, or solely from thrusting against the highly vascular soft palate.[4] The lesions are painless, nonulcerative and nonblanching.[4] A history of fellatio can deter an extensive diagnostic work-up, but a differential diagnosis includes paroxysmal coughing, sneezing, vomiting, infection, tumors, blood dyscrasias, and capillary fragility.[4] Cunnilingus syndrome results from oral-genital sex in which the tongue is used on the partner's genital areas.[4] The findings are pain of the ventral surfaces of the tongue and throat with abrasions and ulcerations of the lingual frenulum.[4] Chronic irritation can result in a traumatic fibroma on the frenulum.[4]

Two possible, but rare, occurrences can be seen in the female recipient of oral-genital sex. One is a pneumoperitoneum. This can result after air is blown into the vagina, traverses the cervical canal and endometrial cavity, and enters the abdomen through the fallopian tubes.[4] Cases have been reported in patients with their uterus in situ.[4] Posthysterectomy cases have also been encountered with the supposition that the air entered through a small dehiscence in the vaginal cuff.[4,5] These patients generally present with lower abdominal pain, upper quadrant pain, or shoulder pain.[4] Peritoneal signs tend to be absent, allowing for conservative management.[5] The clinical course is benign, with the air gradually absorbed spontaneously. Cuff defects should be repaired when encountered.[4,5]

Air embolism is the second complication seen in the female recipient of oral-genital sex. It is uniformly fatal.[4] Death occurs rapidly, and resuscitative measures are usually too late. This complication has been reported in seven gravid women, all more than 20 weeks of gestation.[4] Whether or not oral-genital-related air embolism can occur in nonpregnant women is not known.

Another possible, though rarely written about, complication of oral-genital sex is a vulvar hematoma from a human bite. One case report exists in the literature.[11] Finally, oral-genital sex can lead to lesions of the oral cavity caused by sexually transmitted diseases. This should be kept in mind by the practitioner, so that information can be elicited from the patient (Fig. 25-1).

Trauma with coitus can range from hymenal tearing during initial intercourse to evisceration with hemorrhage. Small tears of the hymen are usually associated with minimal discomfort, but occasionally profuse bleeding can occur that requires repair.[4]

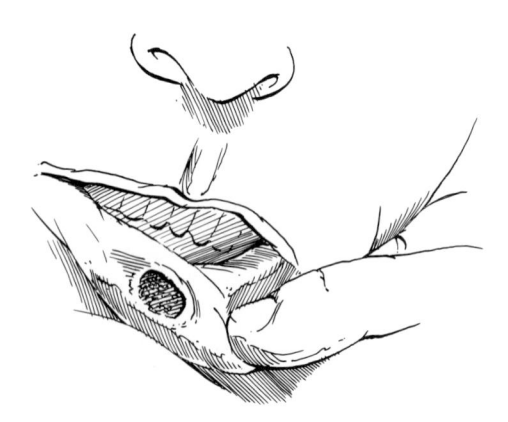

FIGURE 25-1
Chancre behind lip.

Vaginal lacerations and ruptures are rare, but when they are seen, they usually occur in women of reproductive age who had been having consensual intercourse.[4,6,9] Metsala and Nieminen found that approximately 88% of vaginal ruptures occurred during penile coital activity, with most of the remaining due to other direct mechanical effects.[9] The exact cause of the rupture often cannot be determined. Many predisposing factors have been suggested.[4,7,9] In 1965, Purnell reported several cases of apparently spontaneous rupture of the vaginal vault.[9] All these cases were in postmenopausal women with vaginal atrophy. They occurred with sudden increases in intra-abdominal pressure during lifting, coughing, falling, or defecation. Purnell's theory was that the sudden intra-abdominal pressure acted through the pouch of Douglas on a weakened posterior fornix to bring about a rupture. Women in both these situations generally presented with vaginal bleeding. Exsanguination has been reported.[4,6,7] Sometimes a history of sharp vaginal pain during intercourse is obtained.[6,7] Surrounding structures may also be injured, and evisceration of abdominal contents has been seen (Fig. 25-2).[4,8]

Management starts with controlling the bleeding and treating shock if present. If the bleeding is heavy, a moist vaginal packing can be placed to tamponade the bleeders, while the history and physical is completed with particular emphasis on other signs of trauma. When the bleeding has slowed, the vagina can be examined to determine the extent of the laceration. Most lacerations are in the posterior and right lateral fornix (Fig. 25-3).[6,7,9] Often the examination has to take place in the operating room under general anesthesia for patient comfort. If evisceration has occurred and the penetration is known to be either a penis, finger, or other blunt object, one may attempt to replace the eviscerated organs, usually bowel, back into

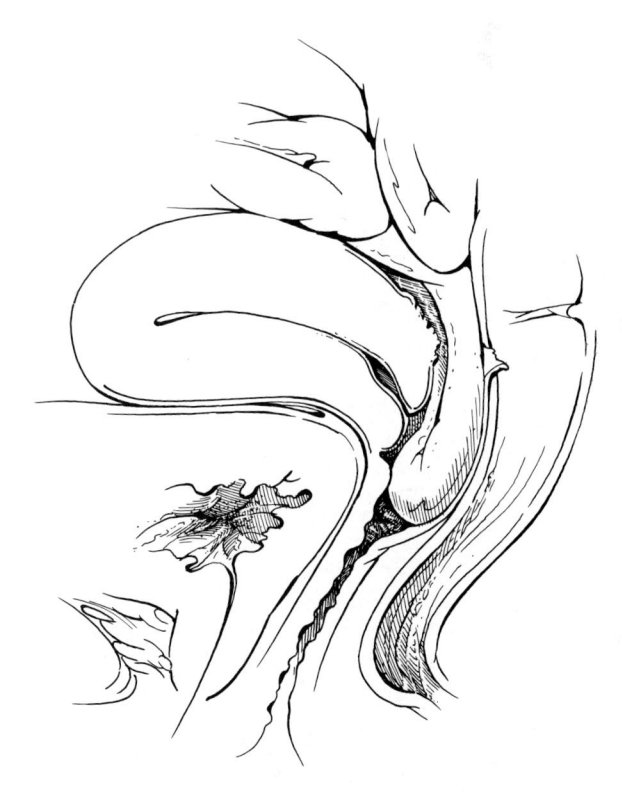

FIGURE 25–2
Evisceration after vaginal laceration.

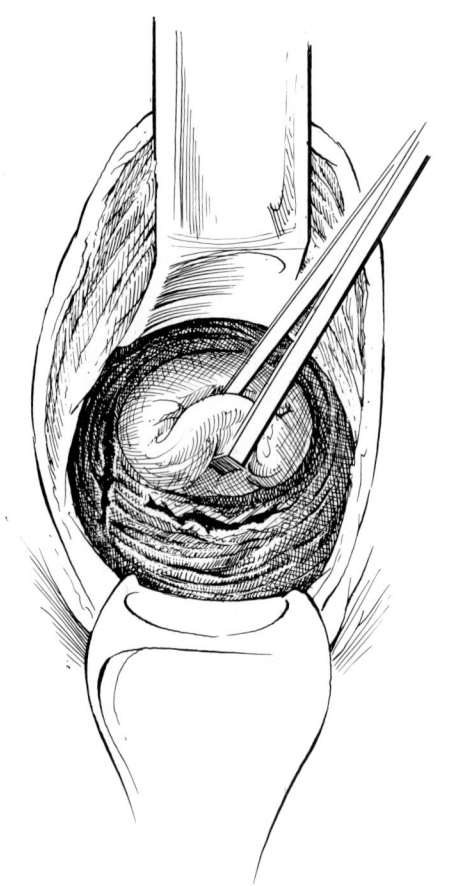

FIGURE 25–3
Laceration of lateral and posterior vaginal fornices.

the abdomen with moist sponges and with the patient in the Trendelenburg position. If the bowel has passed beyond the introitus, it should be wrapped in moist towels until the patient can be taken to the operating room. Included in the evaluation should be a digital rectal examination looking for a rectal laceration. The bladder can be evaluated by instillation of methylene blue dye and then observed for leakage. Cystourethrography may be necessary to look for intra-abdominal leakage.[12] A flat plate of the abdomen is necessary to rule out an intraperitoneal foreign body.

Once the evaluation is completed and there are no other injuries besides the vaginal rupture known to be caused by a blunt object, simple vaginal repair with observation and IV antibiotics is indicated. Rarely will significant bowel injury have occurred with this situation.[4] If further injury has been documented or evisceration outside the introitus is present, then abdominal repair will become necessary. If bleeding persists even after closure and applied pressure to a vaginal nonpenetrating laceration, then laparotomy with hypogastric artery ligation is an option.[13] A Pfannenstiel incision has been advocated when an abdominal approach becomes necessary, since it is a stronger incision than those available in the face of operating in a contaminated field. However, if bowel injury is even suspected, a vertical incision is necessary to evaluate the entire bowel fully. Upper abdominal bowel injuries have been reported after a history of blunt vaginal perforations.[12] Repair of the vaginal laceration is performed after the abdominal part of the procedure is completed. Closed suction drains should be used routinely.[12] Antibiotics are appropriate in all cases after cultures are taken. Prophylaxis with tetanus toxoid should also be considered. Complications from penetrating vaginal wounds include pelvic abscess, vaginal stricture, vesicovaginal and rectovaginal fistula.[12]

Anal intercourse is a practice of the heterosexual as well as the homosexual community. Women can present with various forms of trauma from this. Proctitis can occur and is generally the result of inflammation caused by trauma but may be due to chlamydia or herpes. Patients may present with rectal bleeding from a rectal mucosal laceration. If a history of anal intercourse is obtained, then evaluation should include an upright abdominal film to rule out pneumoperitoneum and retained foreign body. Proctoscopy is then performed to determine the extent of the lesion. Most patients require no treatment, though transanal repair is occasionally necessary. Stool softeners and sitz baths are recommended. If disruption of the anal sphincter occurs from this form of sexual activity, repair should be done in the operating room. Occasionally, a patient will present to the emergency department reporting loss of a sexual aid used in anal-rectal stimulation. Most foreign objects can be removed in the emergency department with appropriate instruments. Occasionally general anesthesia will be necessary to promote relaxation and patient comfort.[10] If a vacuum has been created, passage of a Foley catheter around the object can break the seal (Fig. 25-4). The inflated bulb of the Foley can then help provide

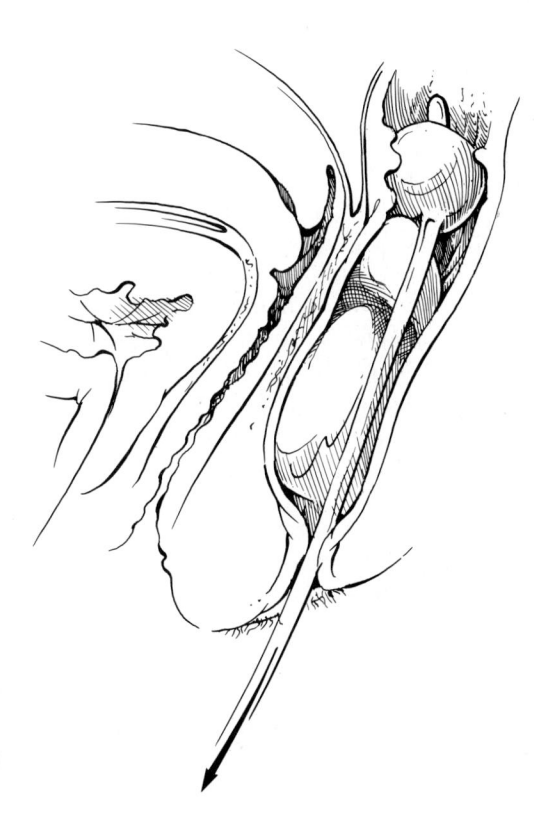

FIGURE 25–4
Foley catheter removal of intrarectal foreign body.

traction downward.[4] If the object is beyond reach, the patient may be observed for 24 hours. The object will generally descend into the rectum within that time. Sigmoidoscopy should be performed after removal to rule out significant lacerations. If none are found and there are no signs of peritonitis, the patient can be discharged with close follow-up. Rectosigmoid colon perforations are rare but can be caused by foreign body manipulation. Peritonitis is generally the result. Attempts should be made to make the diagnosis without the use of barium enemas or gastrografin enemas, since these increase irritation and can increase bowel content spillage.[4] A diversionary colostomy is necessary at the time of repair to allow the laceration to heal. Generous irrigation and broad-spectrum antimicrobial coverage are indicated. Perforations occurring below the peritoneal reflection will not cause a peritonitis, thus possibly delaying their presentation and diagnosis.[4] Treatment, however, is the same.

Nonsexually Related Trauma

Many mechanical causes of vaginal lacerations have been reported in the literature, not always related to sexual stimulation. Tampons with plastic applicators have been incriminated.[14] Patients can present acutely with bright red bleeding, or chronically, with a several-week history of bleeding.[14] Examination will generally show a linear lesion through full thickness of the vaginal mucosa. Lesions tend to heal on their own with an extended absence of tampons in the vagina.

Pressurized water entering the vagina can also cause laceration or rupture. Case reports exist of water skiing injury, as well as attempting to stop the flow of water from a fountain.[13,15-17] The typical fall while water skiing is backward, with legs abducted. Thus the speed at impact dictates the amount of pressurized water that will enter potential spaces such as the vagina and rectum.[16] The pressurized water has been documented to cause significant lacerations with significant blood loss.[15,16] The douche can also cause less visible injuries to the cervix, uterus, and fallopian tubes, such as salpingitis, tubo-ovarian abscesses, and precipitation of a miscarriage.[17] Laparoscopy or laparotomy should be considered when uncertainty as to intraperitoneal injury is present.

More serious gynecologic injuries are seen in automobile accident victims with pelvic fractures. Pelvic fractures in females can be associated with significant intra-abdominal gynecologic injury.[18] Intra-abdominal soft-tissue injuries are generally caused by tears and lacerations from sharp, bony fragments. Lacerations have been seen in the intestines and genitourinary tract, including the vagina and urethra.[18,19] There have been reported cases of laceration to the uterus, tube, and ovary after a pelvic fracture as well as avulsion of the uterus.[18,20] Retroperitoneal hematoma may result from such injuries.[18] Avulsion of the uterus may result in hysterectomy.[20] Infertility and obstetric complications are potential consequences of pelvic fractures as well as vaginal stricture, dyspareunia, osteomyelitis, and pelvic abscess.[21] A gentle pelvic examination is warranted in women with pelvic fractures.[18] The gentleness is emphasized because one could create an open fracture through the vaginal wall. Delay in identifying lacerations could result in pelvic abscesses and higher rates of mortality. Once an abscess occurs, multiple operations are often necessary before complete cure occurs.[21] Future complications after apparent resolution of abscesses includes urethrovaginal fistula, vesicovaginal fistula, and rectovaginal fistula.[21] Sudden bladder rupture has been reported secondary to osteomyelitis.[21]

Mechanisms by which pelvic fractures cause vaginal lacerations are multiple. Most obvious is penetration of a bone fragment through the vaginal wall.[21] Diastasis of the symphysis pubis tends to result from straddle injuries.[21] The lateral tearing force of this injury lacerates deep pelvic soft tissues and sometimes extends to the vaginal wall. Bilateral ischiopubic rami fractures result in the anterior pelvic ring being freed from the weight-bearing portion of the pelvis. This can cause an avulsion of the vaginal vault or urethra.[19] Finally, crushing injuries are capable of producing vaginal wall lacerations. Foreign bodies such as tampons or contraceptive devices can increase the chances of a vaginal laceration.[21]

Niemi and colleagues recommended repair of vaginal lacerations as early as possible.[21] A severely comminuted open pelvic fracture with associated rectal injuries and fecal contamination requires a diverting colostomy to allow the best chance of healing.[21] Urethral avulsions have been reported to heal after primary end-to-end reanastomosis.[19] Of course IV antibiotics are always indicated with an open fracture.

In one study of 102 major pelvic fractures, there was a 16% mortality rate. They suggested that the most significant determinant of mortality was the life-threatening injuries, along with the hemorrhage from lacerated pelvic vessels. Promptly recognizing and treating injuries to the bowel or bladder is also important.[21]

Rarely, one will find gynecologic injury after blunt abdominal trauma unassociated with pelvic fracture. Stone and colleagues, in their study of 220 patients with blunt abdominal trauma, found the most frequent gynecologic injury was a ruptured and bleeding corpus luteum.[22] The ovarian laceration can be simply oversewn, thus preserving the ovary.

Vulvar injuries and hematomas are another major area of gynecologic trauma. Injuries to the vulva and perineum of young girls are fairly common. Often they consist of slight tears that heal on their own. However, more severe cases, including urinary retention from vulvar injury following straddling the bar on a boy's bike or other toy, have been reported.[23] Even a small mucosal tear of the vulva or vestibule can cause intense pain or burning on urination and so inhibit a child from voiding. This cause should be considered in young girls with urinary retention. They often will not volunteer information about the injury, and so may not be diagnosed unless suspected. Lidocaine gel to the tear with each urge to void, as well as voiding in a tub of warm water, is helpful and may prevent the need for catheterization.

Vulvar hematomas are seen from trauma in both young girls and women (Fig. 25-5). Naumann and colleagues reported on two cases of vulvar hematoma that occurred while riding a "mechanical bull," although they can result from any blunt trauma.[24–26] Both women experienced abrupt pain and bleeding. One woman had a small hematoma merely treated with ice packs as an outpatient. The second woman had a large vulvar hematoma, producing urethral obstruction, that required a Foley for 7 days. She initially had a significant drop in her hematocrit, which stabilized after 24 hours of conservative management of ice packs and observation. The ice pack is the primary treatment, with surgical evacuation reserved for a rapidly enlarging hematoma or drainage of large hematomas following clot lysis.[24–26] It is important to make the correct diagnosis, since evacuation in the first 24 hours could decompress the bleeding vessel, resulting in further blood loss. However, as

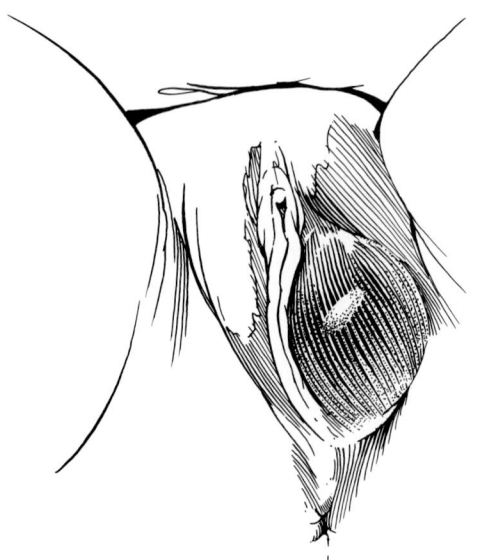

FIGURE 25-5
Vulvar hematoma.

mentioned earlier in the chapter, an infected vulvar hematoma must be incised, drained, and debrided as soon as possible. The bleeding site in this case must be localized quickly and ligated.

One final topic is iatrogenic gynecologic trauma. One reported case is of bilateral vaginal tears causing the loss of approximately 1000 mL of blood from a routine speculum examination in a patient with vaginismus.[27] No gross vaginal abnormality was apparent. The patient had to be taken to the operating room for repair and was transfused with two units of blood.

Genital trauma in women can have multiple etiologies. Accurate information obtained from a cooperative patient is imperative to guarantee proper management. Compassion and a nonjudgmental manner are therefore all-important in ensuring that the required management is rendered.

REFERENCES

1. Claytor RN, Barth KL, Shubin CI. Evaluating child sexual abuse, observations regarding ano-genital injury. Clin Pediatr 28:9, 1989
2. Muram D. Child sexual abuse: relationship between sexual acts and genital findings. Child Abuse Negl 13:211, 1989
3. Slaughter L, Brown CRV. Cervical findings in rape victims. Am J Obstet Gynecol 164:528, 1991
4. Elam AL, Ray VG. Sexually related trauma: a review. Ann Emerg Med 15:576, 1986
5. Christiansen WC, Danzl DF, McGee HJ. Pneumoperitoneum following vaginal insufflation and coitus. Ann Emerg Med 9:480, 1980
6. Smith NC, Van Coeverden De Groot HA, Gunston DK. Coital injuries of the vagina in nonvirginal patients. S Afr Med J 64:746, 1983
7. Paraskevaides EC. Severe post-coital puerperal vaginal tear. Br J Clin Pract 44:777, 1990
8. Cullins V, Anasti J, Huggins GR. Vaginal evisceration with pneumoperitoneum, a case report. J Reprod Med 34:426, 1989

9. Metsala P, Nieminen U. Traumatic lesions of the vagina. Acta Obstet Gynecol Scand 47:482, 1986
10. Cummings PH, Cummings SP. Foreign object-induced sexual trauma. J Emerg Nurs 7:24, 1981
11. Mathelier AC. Vulvar hematoma secondary to a human bite, a case report. J Reprod Med 32:618, 1987
12. Grindlinger GA, Vester SR. Transvaginal injury of the duodenum, diaphragm and lung. J Trauma 27:575, 1987
13. Druzin ML, Gottesfeld SA. Management of serious vaginal injury, a case report. J Reprod Med 31:151, 1986
14. Gray MJ, Norton P, Treadwell K. Tampon-induced injuries. Obstet Gynecol 58:667, 1981
15. Gray HH. A risk of waterskiing for women. A letter to the editor. West J Med 136:169, 1982
16. Kalaichandran S. Vaginal laceration: a little-known hazard for women water skiers. A letter to the editor. Can J Surg 34:107, 1991
17. Kizer KW, Medical hazards of the water skiing douche, a case report. Ann Emerg Med 9:268, 1980
18. Doman AN, Hoekstra DV. Pelvic fracture associated with severe intra-abdominal gynecologic injury. J Trauma 28:118, 1988
19. Netto NR, Ikari O, Zuppo VP. Traumatic rupture of the female urethra, case reports. Urology 22:601, 1983
20. Smith RJ. Avulsion of the nongravid uterus due to pelvic fracture, a case report. South Med J 82:70, 1989
21. Niemi TA, Norton LW. Vaginal injuries in patient with pelvic fractures. J Trauma 25:547, 1985
22. Stone NN, Ances IG, Brotman S. Gynecologic injury in the nongravid female during blunt abdominal trauma. J Trauma 24:626, 1984
23. Manaker JS. Gynecologic trauma, non-obstetrical vulvar, urethral, and vaginal injuries. J Kans Med Soc 81:329, 1980
24. Naumann RO, Droegmueller W. Unusual etiology of vulvar hematomas, a communications in brief. Am J Obstet Gynecol 142:357, 1982
25. Shesser R, Shulman D, Smith J. A nonpuerperal traumatic vulvar hematoma, a case report. J Reprod Med 32:618, 1987
26. Vermesh M, Deppe G, Zbella E. Non-puerperal traumatic vulvar hematoma, case reports. J Gynaecol Obstet 22:217, 1984
27. Rafla N. Vaginismus and vaginal tears, a case report. Am J Obstet Gynecol 158:1043, 1988

Obstetric and Gynecologic Emergencies, edited by
Guy I. Benrubi. J.B. Lippincott Company,
Philadelphia © 1994.

CHAPTER 26

Imaging in Gynecologic Emergencies

Marcia E. Murakami and Gregory C. Wynn

Ultrasound has proved to be the most useful imaging modality in the evaluation of gynecologic emergencies. It displays the female reproductive organs with great consistency and clarity without the risks of ionizing radiation in the potentially pregnant patient. Plain radiographs rarely provide useful information as the initial screening study. Computed tomography (CT) in selected cases can provide more global information to assess extensive disease, especially when the pathologic process extends out of the pelvis. With the advent of transvaginal ultrasound, the uterus and ovaries can be examined with exquisite detail, often rendering a specific diagnosis with great confidence.

Although some authors feel that transvaginal scanning (TV) alone is sufficient for defining pelvic pathology,[1,2] it is our view that transabdominal scanning (TA) should be performed first. In patients who are suspected of having an emergent gynecologic problem and require imaging studies, a Foley catheter should be inserted in the urinary bladder prior to arrival in the ultrasound suite. While fluid is instilled into the bladder via the catheter, the sonographer can scan the upper abdomen to exclude free intraperitoneal fluid, which is highly suspicious for hemoperitoneum in this patient population. Scanning through the distended urinary bladder affords a wide field of view and a survey of the entire pelvis. Often the diagnosis can be made using transabdominal scanning alone (Fig. 26-1). If a mass or a nonspecific fluid collection is detected either within the uterus or in the adnexal regions, transvaginal ultrasound is performed to characterize the transabdominal

366 ♦ OBSTETRIC AND GYNECOLOGIC EMERGENCIES

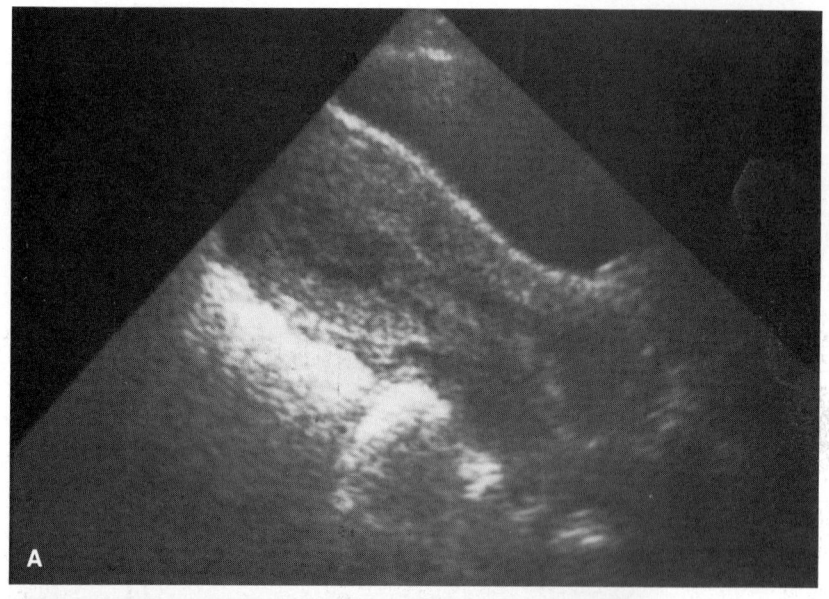

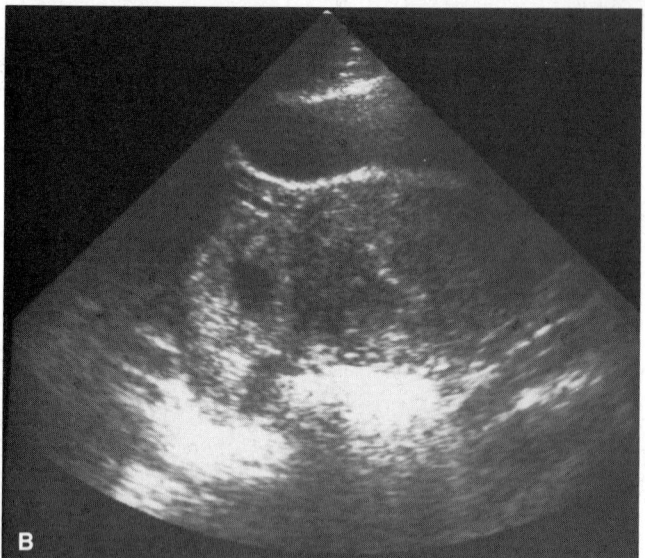

FIGURE 26-1
Value of transabdominal technique. (**A**) Midline sagittal scan shows empty uterus with hypoechoic endometrial lining and echogenic fluid in the cul-de-sac. (**B**) Transverse scan through the fundus of the uterus shows echogenic ring in the right adnexal region. (**C**) High-resolution image of the right adnexa shows embryonic pole. Cardiac activity was observed, diagnostic of a living ectopic pregnancy. Transvaginal scanning, even with knowledge of the transabdominal findings, could not visualize the ectopic pregnancy.

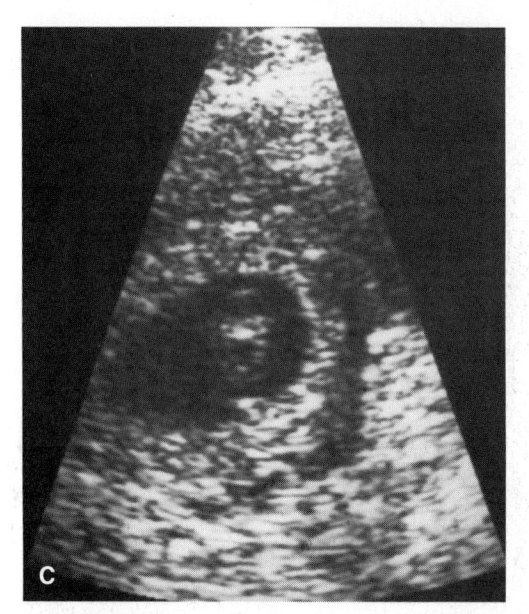

FIGURE 26-1
(Continued)

findings better (Fig. 26-2). The transvaginal examination is therefore directed and performed with the confidence that pathology is not outside the limited field of view of the transvaginal probe. Other authors suggest that transvaginal scanning may be performed first, with the addition of transabdominal scanning as needed.[3–5]

The Pregnant Patient

The development of an accurate and rapid pregnancy test has narrowed the differential diagnostic possibilities of otherwise nonspecific clinical findings. Still, the list of diagnostic possibilities in the early stages of pregnancy remains long and includes intrauterine pregnancy, ectopic pregnancy, embryonic or fetal demise with missed or incomplete abortion, completed abortion, and molar pregnancy. Ultrasound can make a specific diagnosis in a number of cases or at least aid in the clinical management of the patient. Establishing the presence of a normal intrauterine pregnancy essentially excludes an ectopic pregnancy. Evaluation of the gestational sac and its contents can often confirm embryonic demise. Often correlation of the ultrasound findings with the clinical history may strongly suggest incomplete or completed abortion.

Normal Early Intrauterine Pregnancy

At the time of implantation, between day 20 and day 23 (menstrual age), the conceptus is only about 0.1 mm in diameter,[6] much too small to detect using transabdominal or transvaginal techniques. The earliest an intradecidual sac may be seen

368 ♦ OBSTETRIC AND GYNECOLOGIC EMERGENCIES

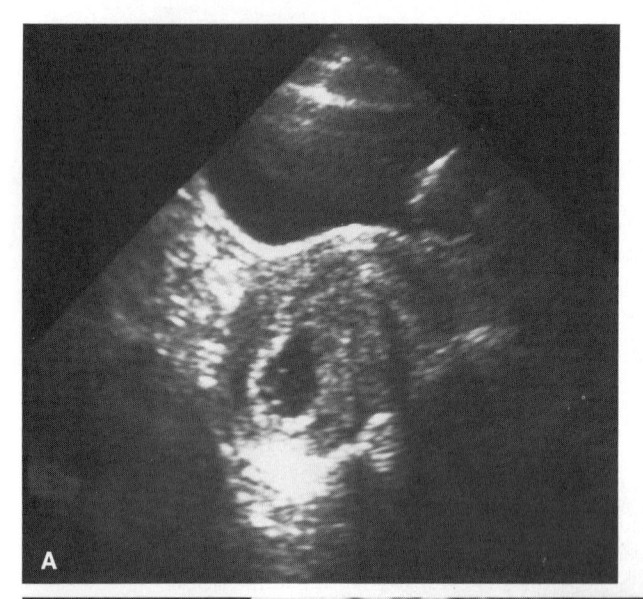

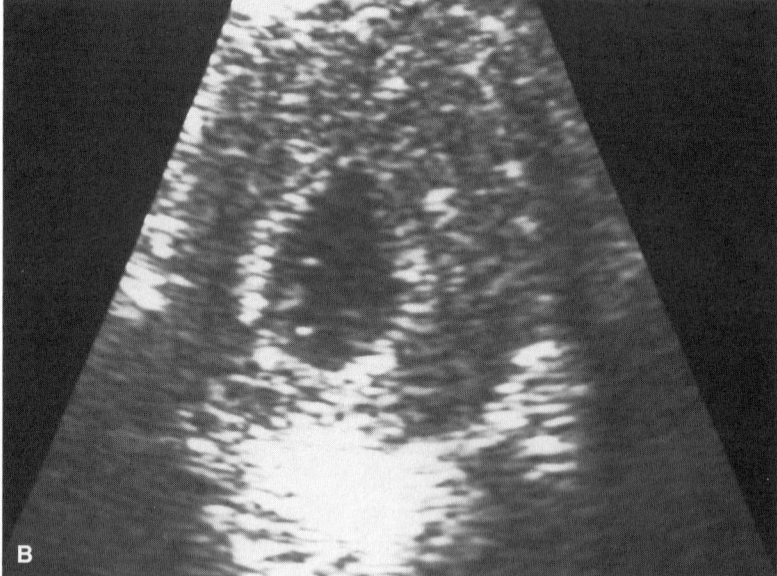

FIGURE 26-2
Value of transvaginal technique. (**A**) Transabdominal sagittal scan shows retroverted uterus with an intrauterine gestational sac corresponding to 6.8 weeks. (**B**) Magnified transabdominal image adds little diagnostic information. (**C**) Transvaginal image shows abnormally large 10 mm yolk sac. No cardiac activity was observed within the small adjacent embryo, diagnostic of embryonic demise.

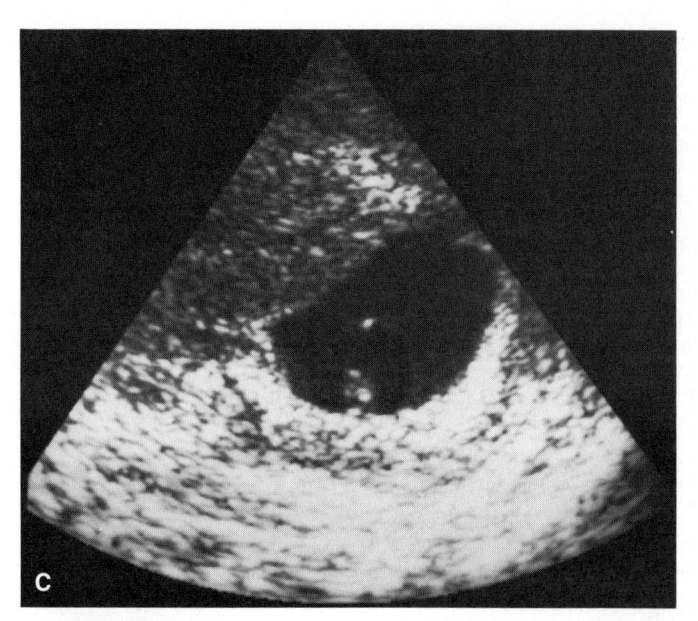

FIGURE 26–2
(Continued)

within the uterus is at 3.5 weeks.[7] More commonly, an early gestational sac is reliably detected at approximately 4.5 weeks menstrual age transvaginally and 5 weeks transabdominally (Fig. 26-3).[8] Correlation with serum human chorionic gonadotropin (HCG) levels is extremely helpful. Sac detection threshold levels of 1800 IU/L (Second International Standard [IS]) or 3240 IU/L (International Reference Preparation [IRP]) transabdominally[9,11] and 1000 IU/L (2nd IS) or 1800 IU/L (IRP) transvaginally[10,11] have been established. At these levels or greater, a definite intrauterine gestational sac should be visualized. Below these threshold levels, a normal intrauterine gestation may be too small to be detected. If the HCG level is disproportionately low relative to gestational sac size, an abnormal pregnancy should be suspected (see Table 26-1).[9] In general, the intrauterine findings of an early pregnancy will be visualized on transvaginal imaging approximately 1 week earlier than on transabdominal scanning.[12]

The double decidual sac sign[13] may be the earliest confirmatory sign of an intrauterine pregnancy transabdominally or transvaginally (Fig. 26-4).[14,15] Although a definite double decidual sac sign is not identified in all normal intrauterine pregnancies, when this sign is clearly present, it is a very useful indicator of intrauterine pregnancy.[16] It is based on the visualization of the chorionic cavity surrounded by two layers of echoes, the inner echogenic ring representing the decidua capsularis and chorion, and the outer echogenic ring, the decidua parietalis. The combination of the gestational sac plus the decidual layers forms a much larger complex than the chorionic cavity itself and may be more readily identified at an earlier stage.

Normally, the yolk sac is the first structure visualized within the gestational sac (Fig. 26-5). It should always be visualized with a mean sac diameter of 20 mm transabdominally[17] and 8 mm transvaginally.[18] Whereas the double decidual sac sign is

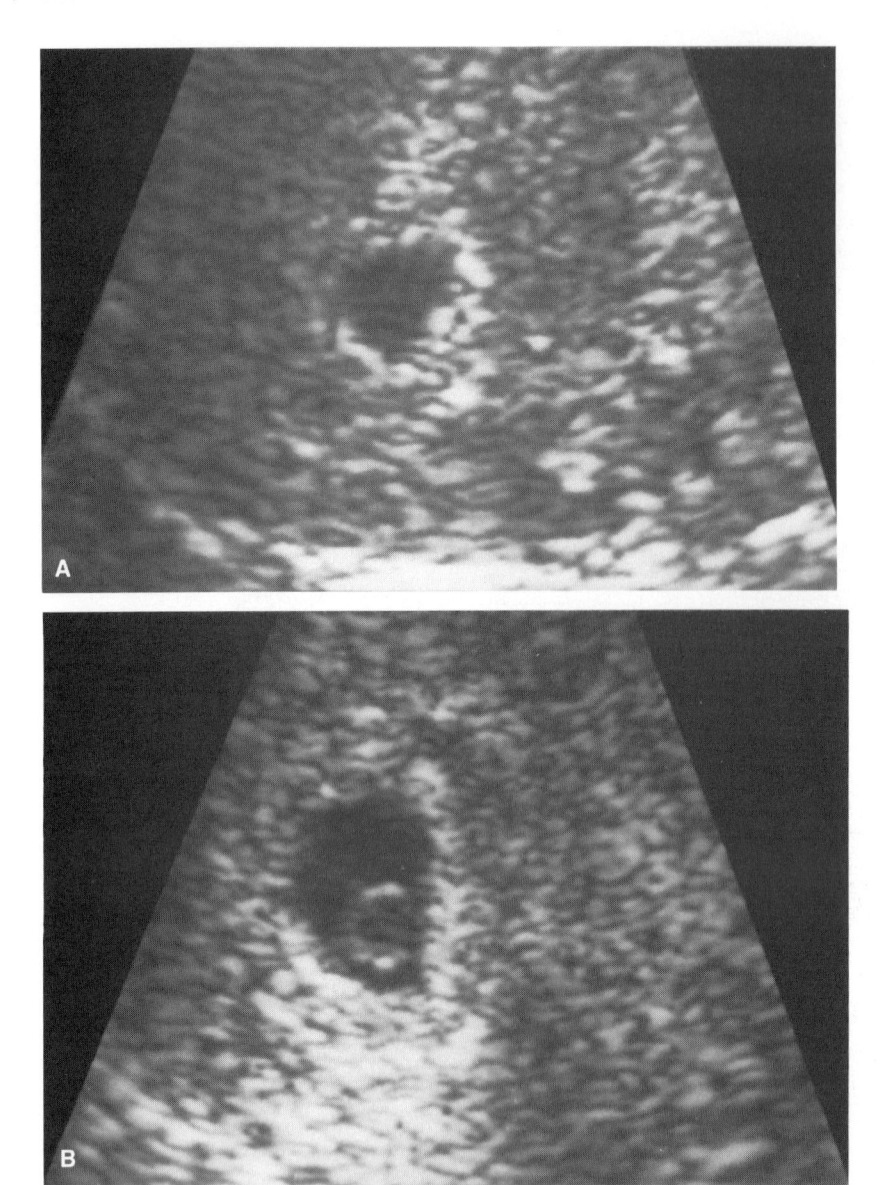

FIGURE 26-3
Very early intrauterine pregnancy. (**A**) Transvaginal image shows a 5 mm intrauterine fluid collection. (**B**) One week later, MSD of 9.3 mm corresponds to an IUP of just less than 5 weeks. A definite yolk sac and double decidual sac sign are now seen.

TABLE 26-1

	Uterus Empty	Uterus With Nonspecific Fluid
HCG [2nd IS] <1800 mIU/mL TA <1000 mIU/ml TV	1. Very early IUP 2. Nonvisualized ectopic 3. Completed abortion	1. Early IUP 2. Pseudosac of ectopic 3. Incomplete abortion
HCG [2nd IS] ≥1800 mIU/mL TA ≥1000 mIU/mL TV	1. Nonvisualized ectopic 2. Completed abortion	1. Non-visualized ectopic 2. Incomplete abortion

TA-transabdominal
TV-transvaginal

not absolutely specific for an intrauterine gestation, the presence of a yolk sac is definitive.[14] Between 5 and 10 menstrual weeks, a yolk sac should never exceed 5.6 mm in diameter.[19] As early as 5.5 weeks, a second sac may be seen adjacent to the yolk sac. This second sac represents the amnion, and this, together with the yolk sac, is known as the double bleb sign.[20] The embryonic disc lies between the two sacs. The amnion continues to grow and eventually fills the chorionic cavity by weeks 14 to 16. Normally, the amnion may be seen as a separate membrane until this time (Fig. 26-6).[20]

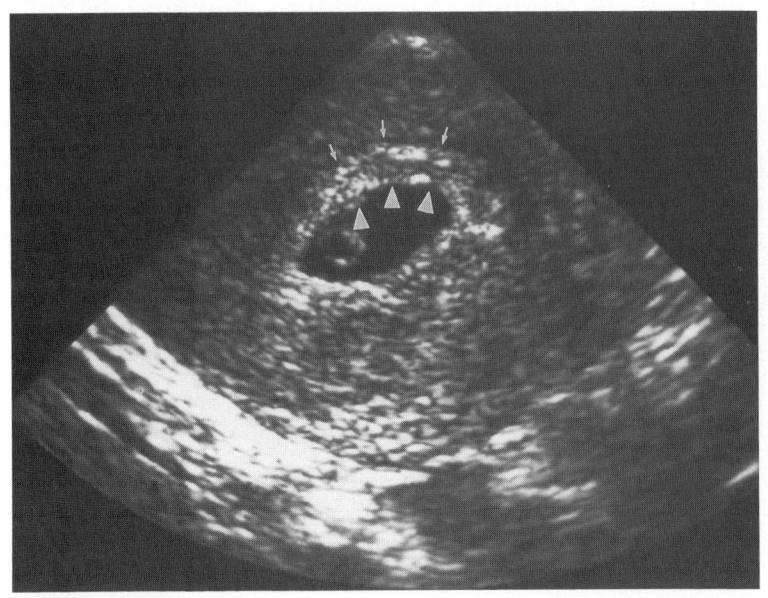

FIGURE 26-4
Double decidual sac sign. Decidua capsularis and chorion (**arrowheads**) and decidual parietalis (**arrows**) form the two arcs of the double decidual sac in a 5.2 week gestation. Yolk sac is clearly visible.

372 ♦ OBSTETRIC AND GYNECOLOGIC EMERGENCIES

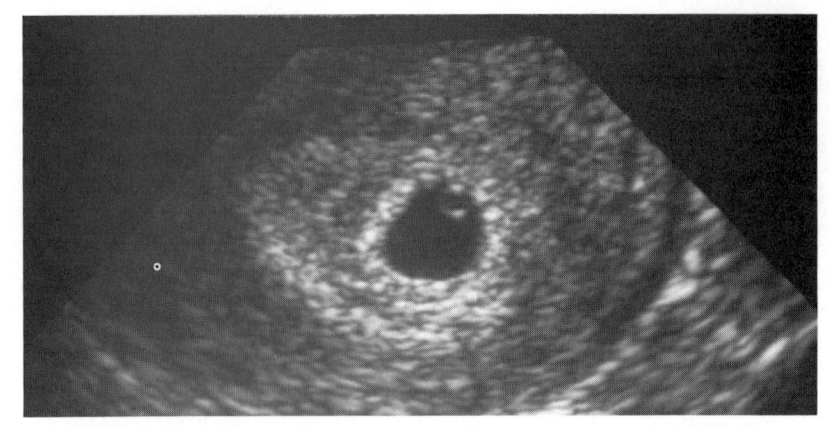

FIGURE 26–5
Yolk sac. Perfectly spherical, thin-walled yolk sac is noted in the periphery of the gestational sac. Ten-millimeter MSD corresponds to 5 week gestation. Note double decidual sac sign.

Once a yolk sac is visualized within the gestational sac, a search should be made for an embryo immediately adjacent to the yolk sac (Fig. 26-7). Transabdominally, pulsation of the embryonic heart may be identified at real-time, establishing a live pregnancy, even though a distinct embryo is not visible.[21] An embryo should definitely be visualized with a mean sac diameter of 25 mm transabdominally[9] and 16 mm transvaginally.[10] An embryo is consistently detected transabdominally once it has reached a crown-rump length of 5 mm or more. Cardiac activity is often visible transvaginally in embryos with a crown-rump length of 2 to 4 mm (about 6 weeks).

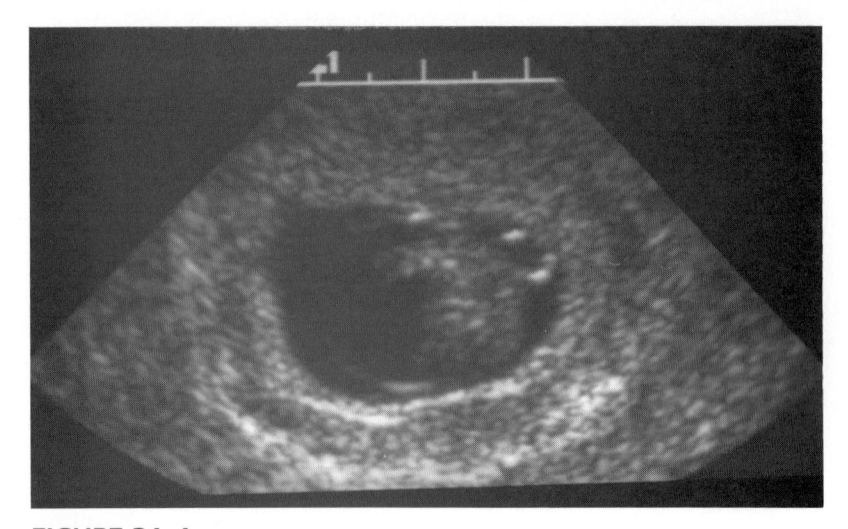

FIGURE 26–6
Yolk sac and amnion. Delicate amniotic sac envelops an 8 week embryo. The amnion has not yet fused with the chorion. Note yolk sac adjacent to the embryo.

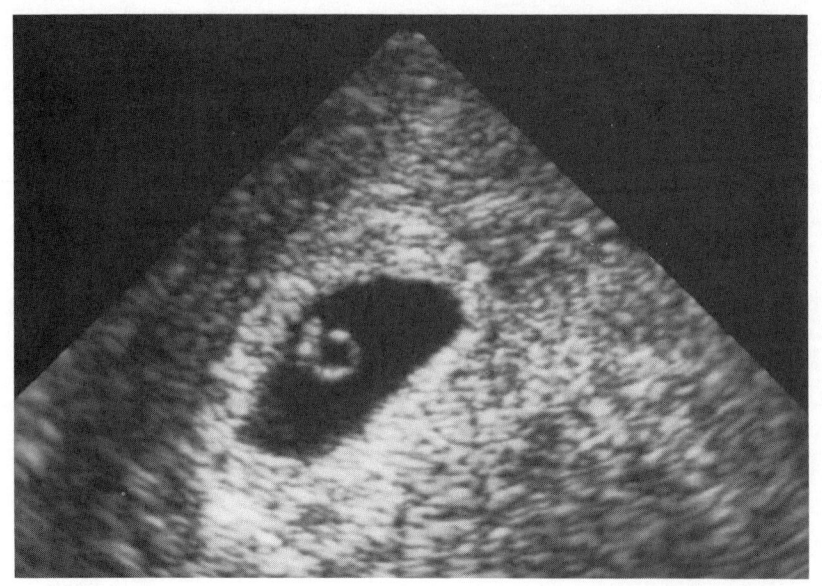

FIGURE 26-7
Embryo. Gestation of 5.5 weeks (13 mm MSD) with yolk sac and adjacent embryo. Cardiac activity was present.

However, it should be noted that transvaginal ultrasound can identify normal embryos without cardiac activity, when they are less than 5 mm.[22] The absence of cardiac activity in these small embryos should not be construed as embryonic demise.

Subchorionic hemorrhage is a common finding late in the first trimester and may be associated with vaginal bleeding. The hemorrhage causes elevation of the chorionic membrane appearing as a fluid collection more echogenic than amniotic fluid acutely (Fig. 26-8), becoming more hypoechoic in 1 to 2 weeks. The significance of these hematomas is somewhat controversial. Some believe that prognosis depends upon the volume of the hemorrhage, with a better prognosis associated with the smaller hematomas. Others suggest that in pregnancies with subchorionic hemorrhage detected before 20 menstrual weeks, the vast majority end in a normal term delivery.[23]

Corpus luteum cysts are commonly detected in the first trimester. The cysts may be simple or hemorrhagic (Fig. 26-9). They are usually 3 to 6 cm but may be as large as 10 cm. These cysts usually resolve spontaneously by 16 weeks.[24]

Abnormal Early Intrauterine Pregnancy

Ultrasound has proved to be extremely helpful in the evaluation of the failed pregnancy. With the development of transvaginal scanning, a single examination is often conclusive in establishing embryonic demise. A large gestational sac (MSD > 25 mm TA[9] or 16 mm TV[10] without an embryo; MSD > 20 mm TA[9] or 8 mm TV[10] without a

374 ♦ OBSTETRIC AND GYNECOLOGIC EMERGENCIES

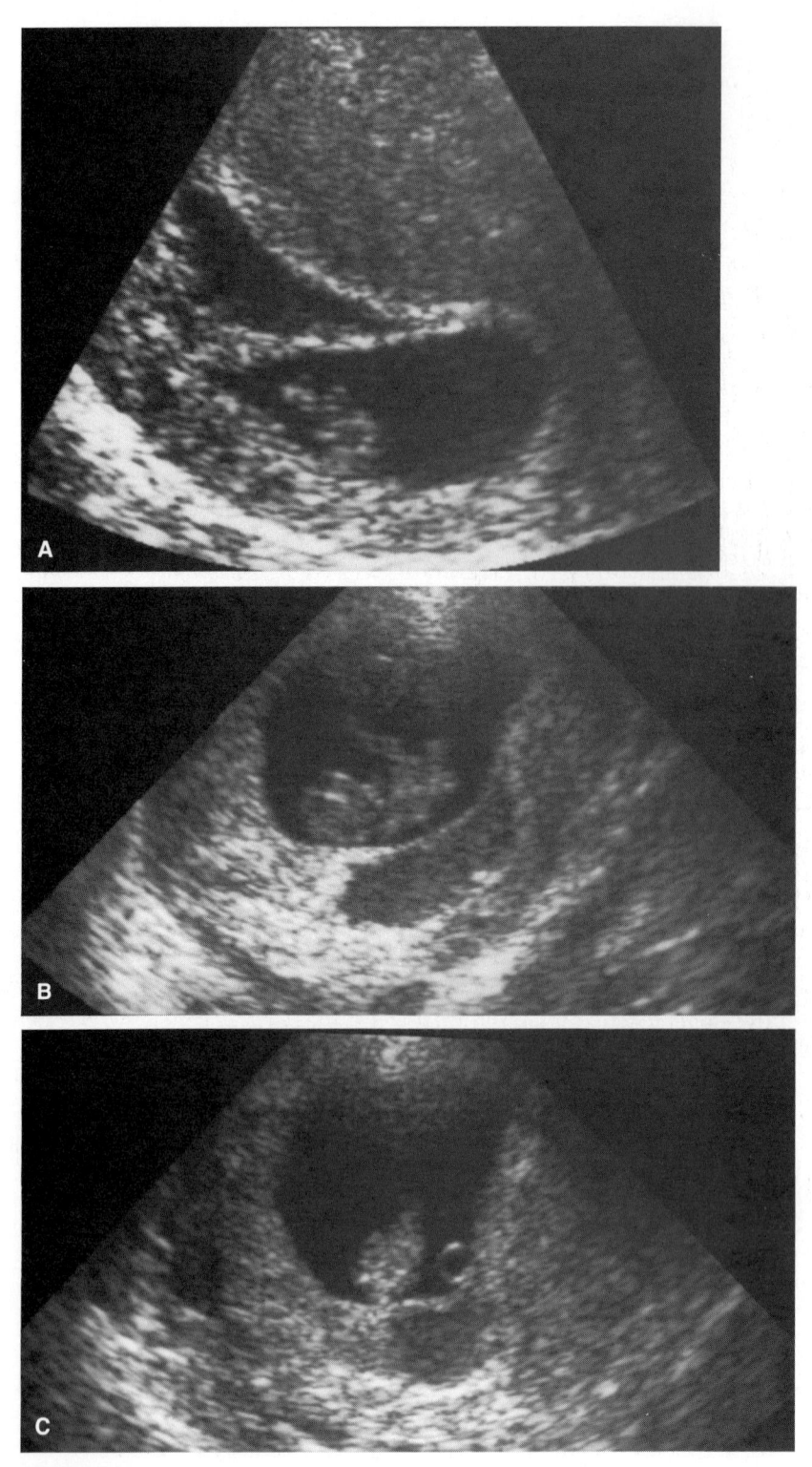

FIGURE 26–8

◀ **FIGURE 26–8**
Subchorionic hemorrhage. (**A**) Seven-and-one-half-week living IUP, (**B,C**) Nine-and-one-half week living IUP in two patients who presented with acute vaginal bleeding. Both hemorrhages are more echogenic than the fluid within the gestational sac.

yolk sac) is diagnostic of an anembryonic gestation or blighted ovum (Fig. 26-10). Distorted gestational sac shape is also highly specific for abnormal pregnancy, although a somewhat subjective feature and relatively insensitive. Suggestive, but less specific, findings include a thin (<2 mm), weakly echogenic or irregular choriodecidual reaction, absent double decidual sac sign, and low position of the sac within the endometrial cavity.[9]

The yolk sac itself should not measure more than 5.6 mm in diameter between 5 and 10 weeks and not less than or equal to 2 mm between 8 and 12 weeks.[19] If a normal embryo cannot be identified adjacent to an abnormally large yolk sac, the diagnosis of blighted ovum or anembryonic pregnancy is made (Fig. 26-11). Conversely, it is also abnormal if a yolk sac is not visualized in the presence of an embryo demonstrated by transvaginal scanning.[8] This is associated with embryonic demise

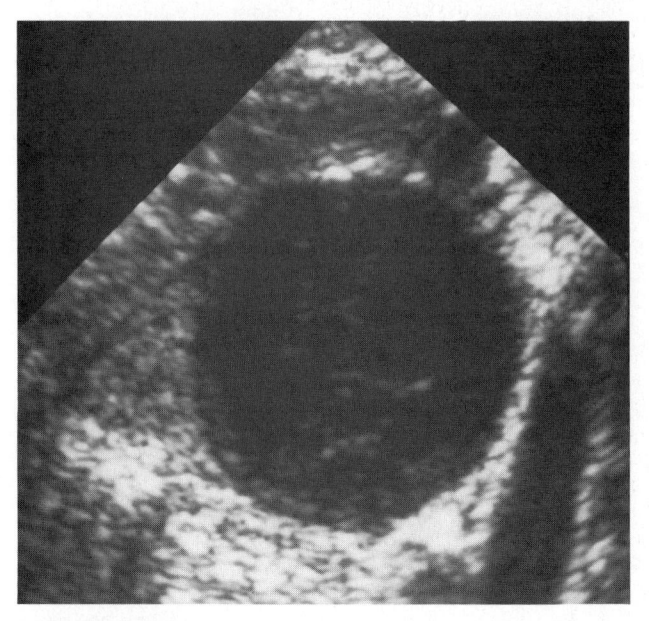

FIGURE 26–9
Hemorrhagic corpus luteum cyst. Transvaginal image shows 3 cm complex mass arising from the ovary compatible with a hemorrhagic cyst. Tubular structure adjacent to the cyst is an internal iliac vessel, a landmark for localization of the ovaries.

376 ♦ OBSTETRIC AND GYNECOLOGIC EMERGENCIES

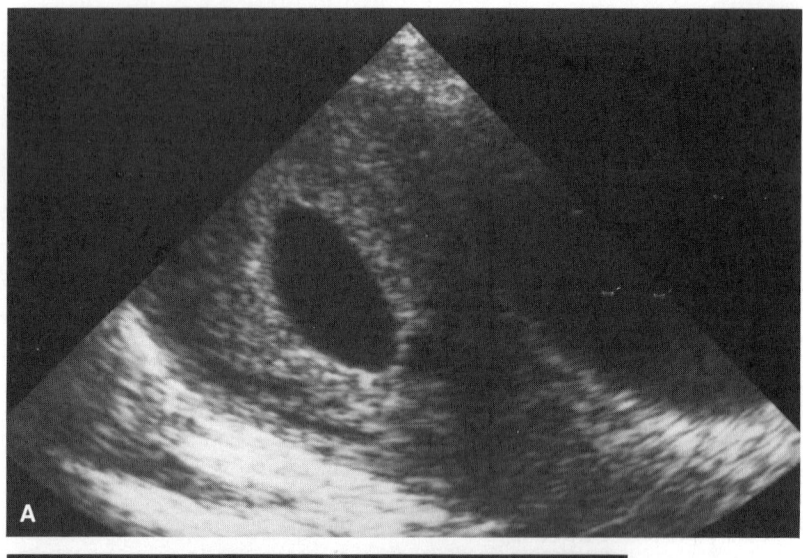

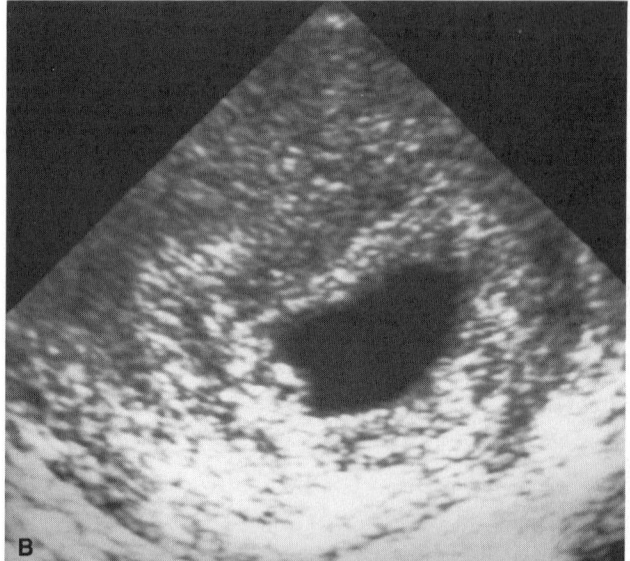

FIGURE 26–10
Blighted ovum: empty gestational sac. (**A**) Transabdominal, and (**B**), transvaginal images of two different patients. In **A** no embryo was visualized, and the decidual reaction is weak. **B** shows definite double decidual sac sign. With an MSD of 20 mm, a yolk sac should be visualized.

IMAGING IN GYNECOLOGIC EMERGENCIES ◆ 377

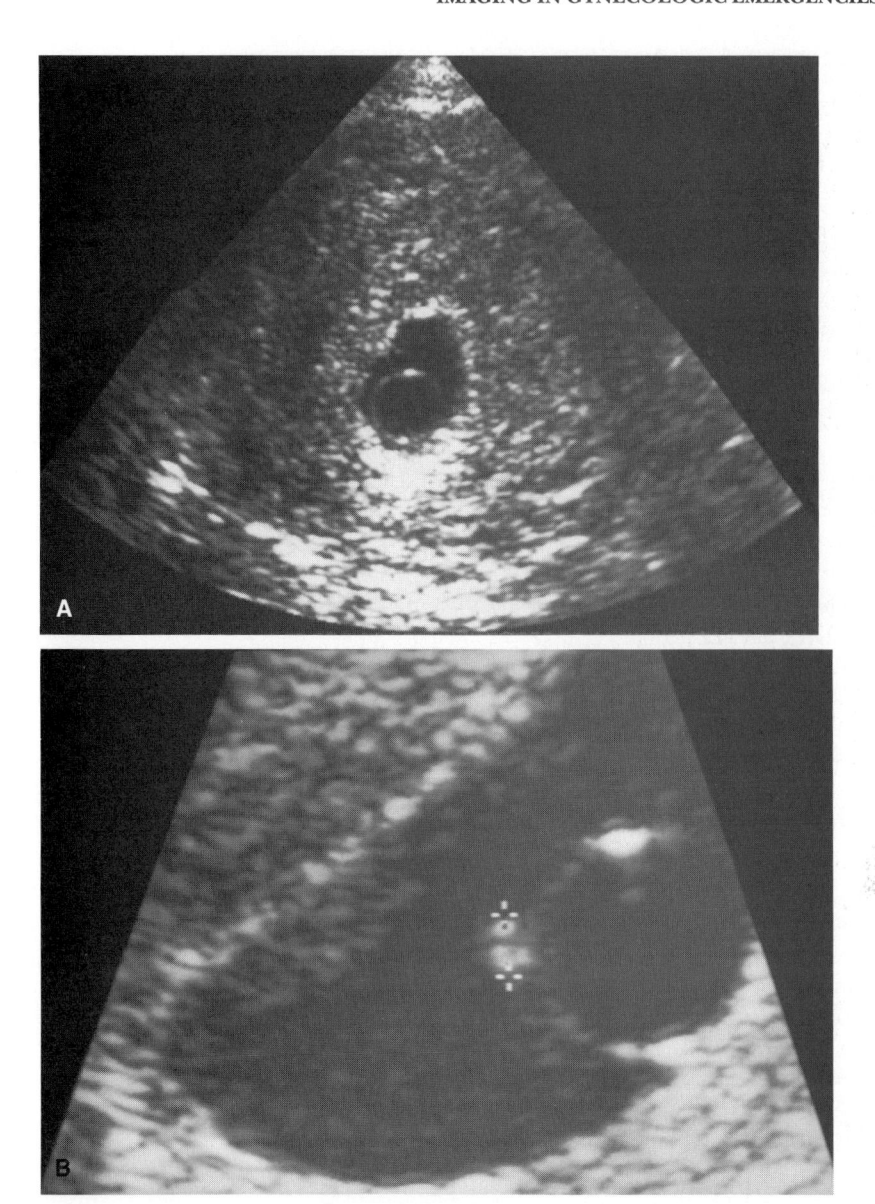

FIGURE 26-11
Blighted ovum: abnormally large yolk sac. (**A**) Yolk sac of 9 mm occupies about one half the volume of the gestational sac, and no embryonic pole could be detected. (**B**) Yolk sac of 11 mm is too large. Tiny adjacent embryo showed no cardiac activity.

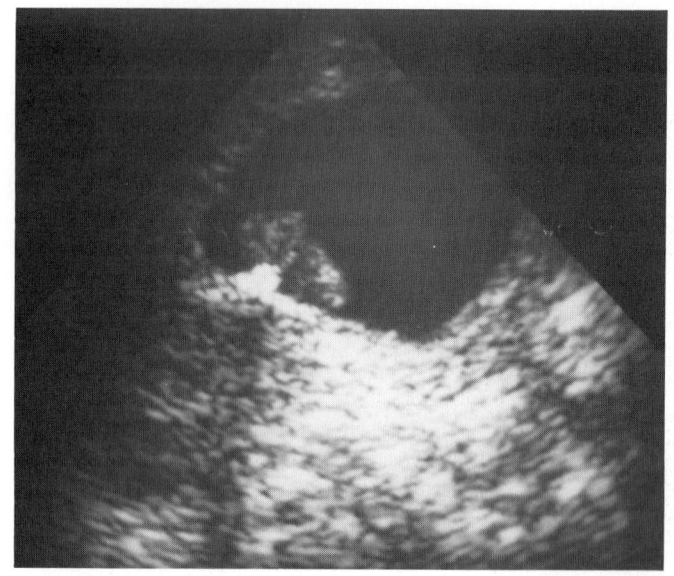

FIGURE 26–12
Embryonic demise: calcification of the yolk sac. Densely echogenic structure with shadowing is presumed to be shadowing within a calcified yolk sac immediately adjacent to the embryo. No cardiac activity was visualized.

either at the time of the scan or on follow-up examination. Calcification of the yolk sac is also seen with embryonic demise (Fig. 26-12).[24] Just as a gestational sac too large for its contents is abnormal, a too small gestational sac also carries a poor prognosis (Fig. 26-13). Despite the presence of cardiac activity within embryos between 6 and 9 weeks, those with a gestational sac size too small for the crown-rump length almost always end in miscarriage.[25] Therefore the management of these pregnancies should be cautious.

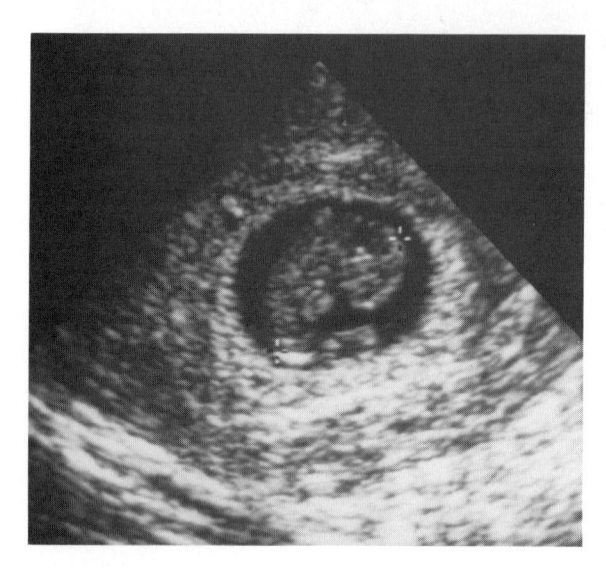

FIGURE 26–13
Embryonic demise: missed abortion. Embryo of 8.2 weeks' gestation is too large for the gestational sac size that corresponds to a 6.7 week gestation. Cardiac activity was not present.

IMAGING IN GYNECOLOGIC EMERGENCIES ♦ 379

Cardiac activity establishes embryonic life. In a high-quality transabdominal scan, once an embryo is visualized, cardiac activity should always be present (Fig. 26-14). Transvaginally, however, a normal embryo of less than 5 mm in crown-rump length may or may not exhibit cardiac activity, and follow-up sonography may be of benefit to establish normal development.[22]

Embryonic bradycardia is also a sign of impending fetal demise. The normal embryonic heart rate at 5 to 6 menstrual weeks is approximately 100 beats per minute. At 8 to 9 menstrual weeks, the rate is approximately 140 beats per minute. It has

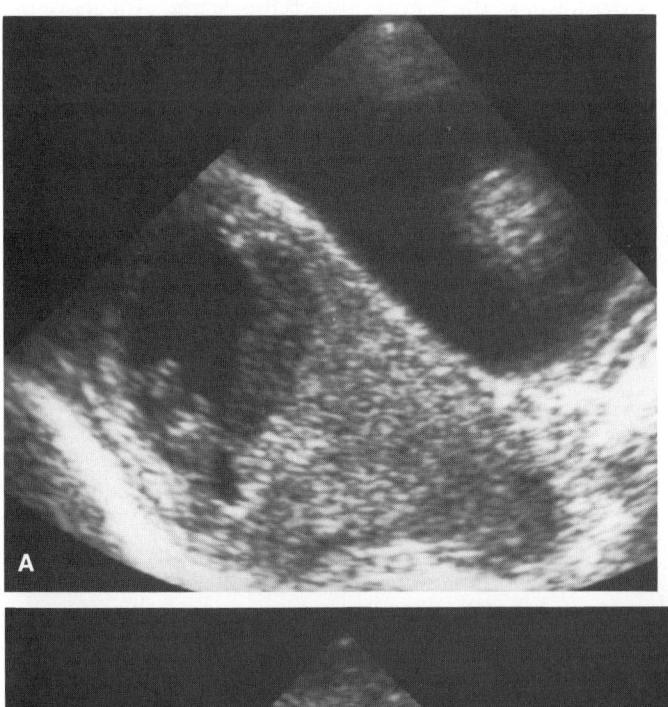

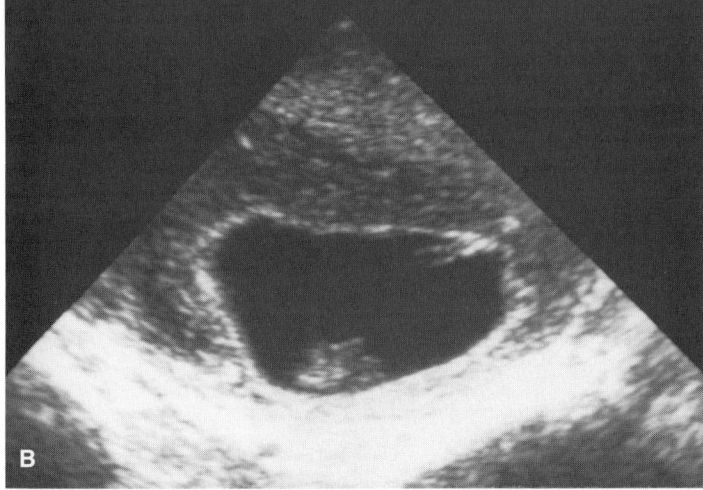

FIGURE 26-14
Embryonic demise: missed abortion. (**A**) Sagittal transabdominal and (**B**) transvaginal scans did not detect cardiac activity within the embryo. Note the large associated subchorionic hemorrhage.

been demonstrated that embryos between 5 and 8 weeks of menstrual age with heart rates of less than 85 beats per minute ended in fetal loss.[26]

Retained products of conception from an incomplete abortion are quite variable in appearance and are often difficult to differentiate from a pseudogestational sac or decidual cast of an ectopic pregnancy. The endometrium may appear abnormally thick (>5 mm), with fluid and debris within the uterine cavity (Figs. 26-15, 26-16). If the endometrial stripe is thin (<2 mm), there is little likelihood of retained products.[27]

At times, an abortion in progress can be observed at real-time ultrasound. The uterine contents move lower in the uterus, toward the cervix, with active contraction of the uterus, and the cervical canal may be fluid-filled and dilated (Fig. 26-17). A completed abortion is often identical in ultrasound appearance to a normal empty uterus. In the presence of a positive pregnancy test, the differential diagnosis must include very early intrauterine pregnancy or nonvisualized ectopic.

Early trophoblastic disease is usually indistinguishable from an incomplete abortion, demonstrating abnormal echogenicity within the uterine cavity. Hydropic villae may not develop vesicles until 12 weeks or more, making detection by even transvaginal sonography difficult until that time.[28]

Ectopic Pregnancy

The sine qua non for diagnosis of an ectopic pregnancy is demonstration of an extrauterine embryo with cardiac activity (Figs. 26-18, 26-19). Transvaginal scanning has increased the detection of live extrauterine embryos compared to transabdominal scanning.[29,30] Practically speaking, the presence of a normal intrauterine gestation excludes ectopic pregnancy. The likelihood of coexistent intrauterine and ectopic pregnancy is variably estimated at one in 30,000 to one in 7000.[16]

A pseudogestational sac or decidual cast must be differentiated from a very early

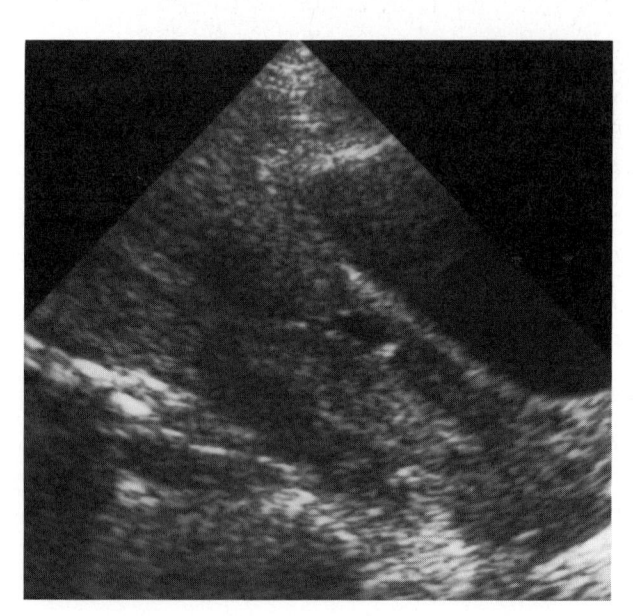

FIGURE 26–15
Incomplete abortion. Longitudinal transabdominal image shows echogenic debris and a small amount of fluid widening the lower uterine cavity and cervix.

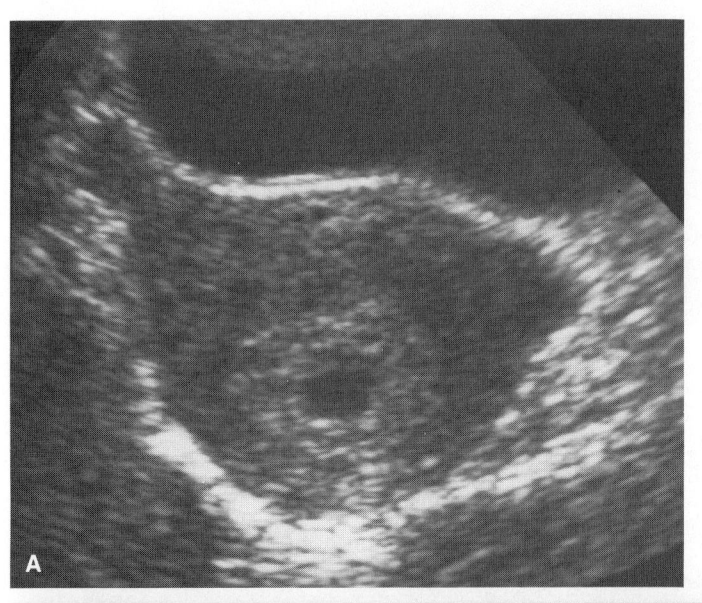

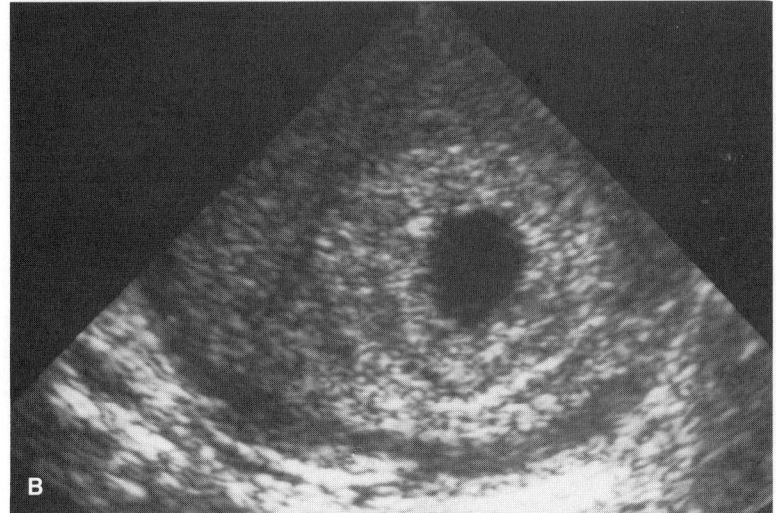

FIGURE 26-16
Incomplete abortion. (**A**) Transverse transabdominal and (**B**) transvaginal images show intrauterine fluid and markedly thickened endometrium. No embryo or yolk sac detected.

intrauterine pregnancy.[13] The pseudogestational sac represents an intrauterine fluid collection surrounded by a single decidual layer rather than the concentric arcs of the double decidual sac sign (Fig. 26-20). It may be impossible to distinguish a decidual cast from a spontaneous incomplete abortion (Fig. 26-21).

If an intrauterine pregnancy is not identified in the patient who is suspected of

(text continues on page 384)

382 ♦ OBSTETRIC AND GYNECOLOGIC EMERGENCIES

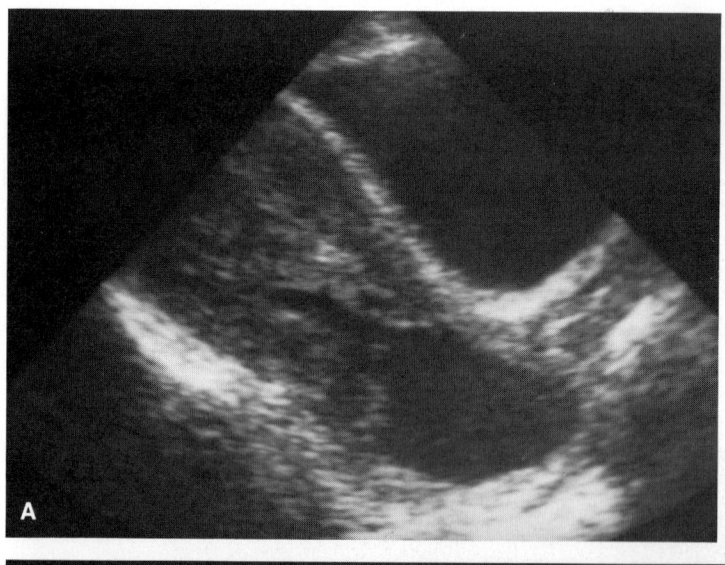

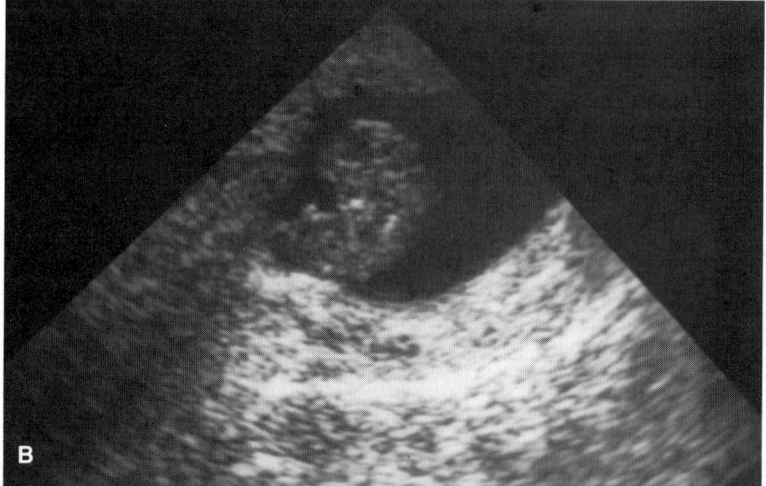

FIGURE 26-17
Abortion in progress. (**A**) A large, irregular fluid collection expands the cervix and lower endometrial cavity. (**B**) Transvaginal scan demonstrated an embryo without cardiac activity within this collection of fluid.

IMAGING IN GYNECOLOGIC EMERGENCIES ♦ 383

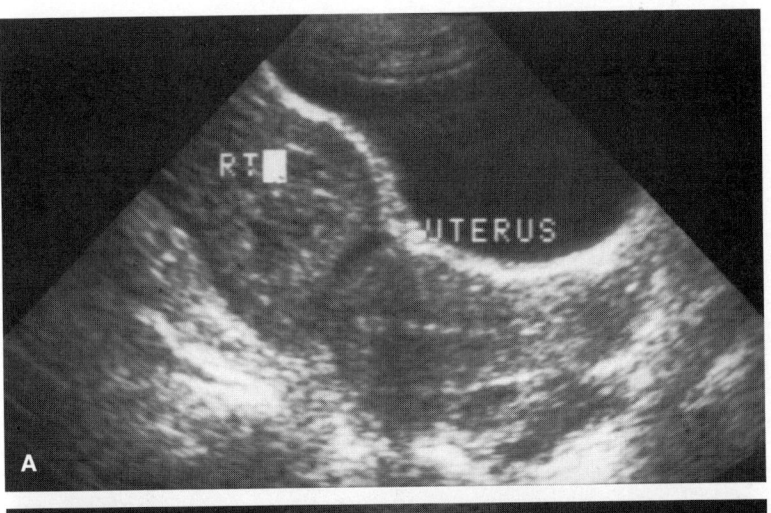

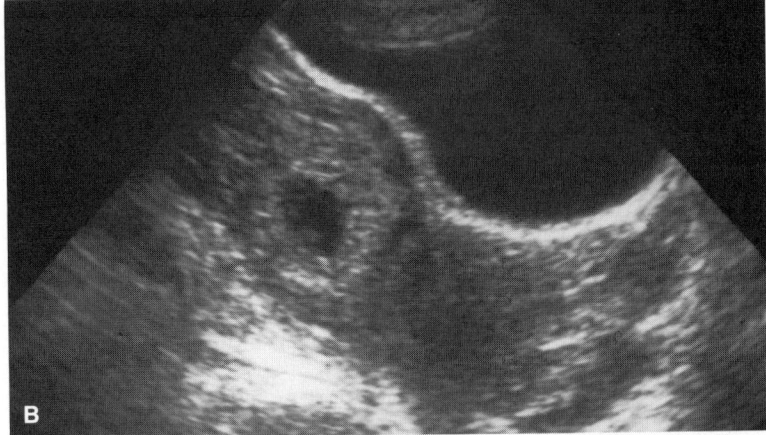

FIGURE 26-18
Ectopic pregnancy. (**A**) Sagittal scan shows empty uterus and abnormal mass just superior to the fundus of the uterus. (**B**) Right parasagittal scan revealed gestational sac containing a living embryo. Note the echogenic fluid in the cul-de-sac in **A** and **B,** characteristic of acute blood.

384 ♦ OBSTETRIC AND GYNECOLOGIC EMERGENCIES

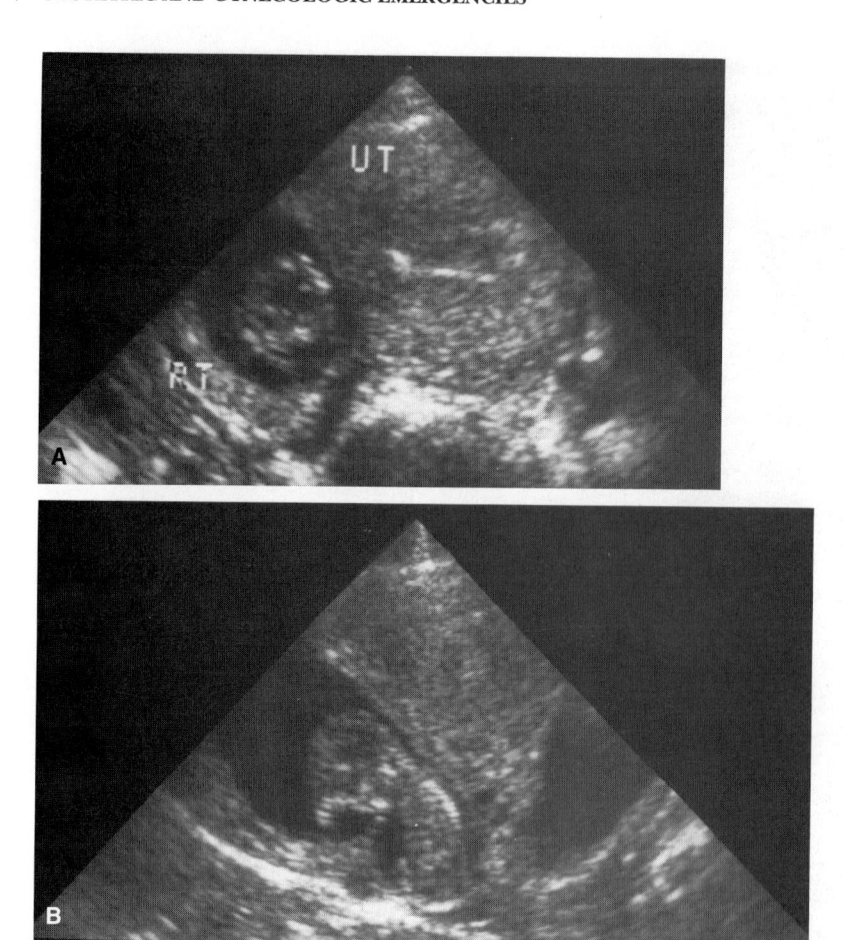

FIGURE 26-19
Ectopic pregnancy. (**A**) Transverse transabdominal image shows empty uterine cavity with extrauterine pregnancy in the right adnexal region. (**B**) A better view of the 11.2 week fetus. Cardiac activity was present.

having an ectopic pregnancy, the adnexal regions should be carefully examined. An adnexal mass is highly suspicious for ectopic pregnancy in this setting. The appearance of the mass is quite variable but is usually complex (Fig. 26-22). An ectopic tubal ring may be seen separate from the ovaries, a finding strongly associated with an unruptured tubal pregnancy (Figs. 26-23, 26-24).[31,32] The ring is an echogenic structure created by the trophoblast of the ectopic pregnancy. If this ring is carefully examined, a yolk sac or embryo may be identified within it.

A search for free fluid should be made in the cul-de-sac, over the fundus of the uterus,[33] in both paracolic gutters, in the hepatorenal space, and about the spleen (Figs. 26-25, 26-26). The fluid of hemoperitoneum is often echogenic. The presence of even relatively small amounts of echogenic fluid should alert the examiner to the strong possibility of an ectopic pregnancy, despite the absence of other abnormal

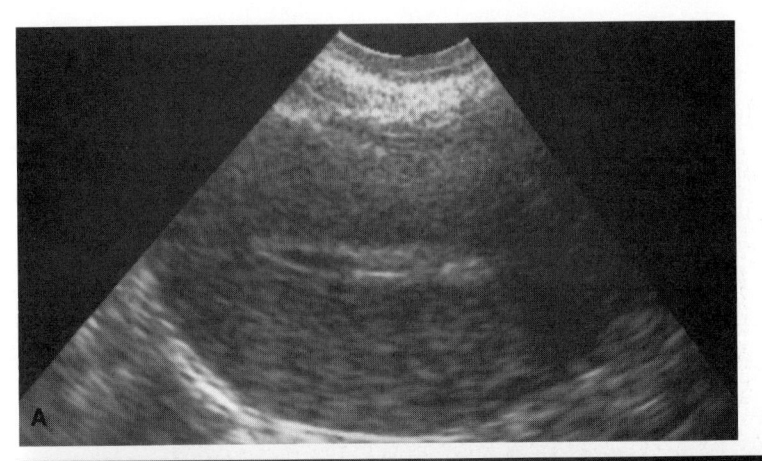

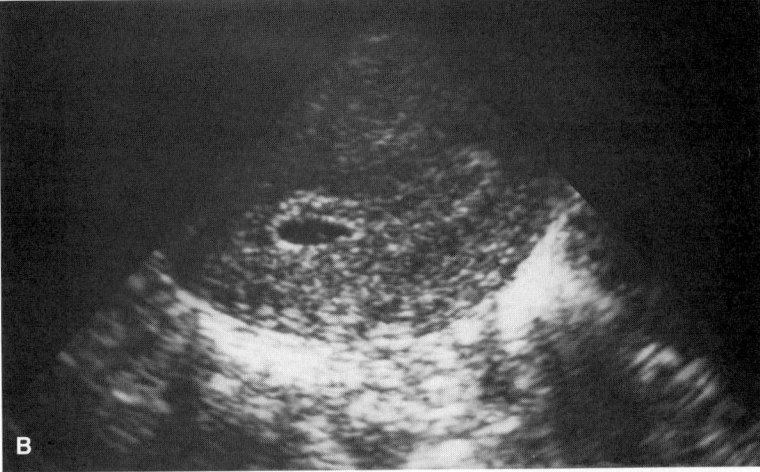

FIGURE 26-20
Pseudogestational sac vs early intrauterine pregnancy. (**A**) Small fluid collection within the uterus surrounded by a single echogenic layer in a patient with a proven ectopic pregnancy. Compare to (**B**), a less than 5 week intrauterine pregnancy with double decidual sac sign.

findings (Fig. 26-27).[34] Small amounts of free, simple, nonechogenic fluid can be normal and do not necessarily indicate hemoperitoneum.

Interstitial or cornual pregnancies are suggested by an eccentric location of the gestational sac within the fundal region of the uterine cavity (Fig. 26-28). The myometrium surrounding the sac may be thin or incomplete, with the gestational sac within 5 mm of the uterine serosa.[31,35] A high degree of clinical suspicion should be maintained, since these pregnancies tend to rupture later than other tubal gestations, often with massive intraperitoneal hemorrhage.

Cervical pregnancies are extremely rare but must be distinguished from an abortion in progress.

(text continues on page 395)

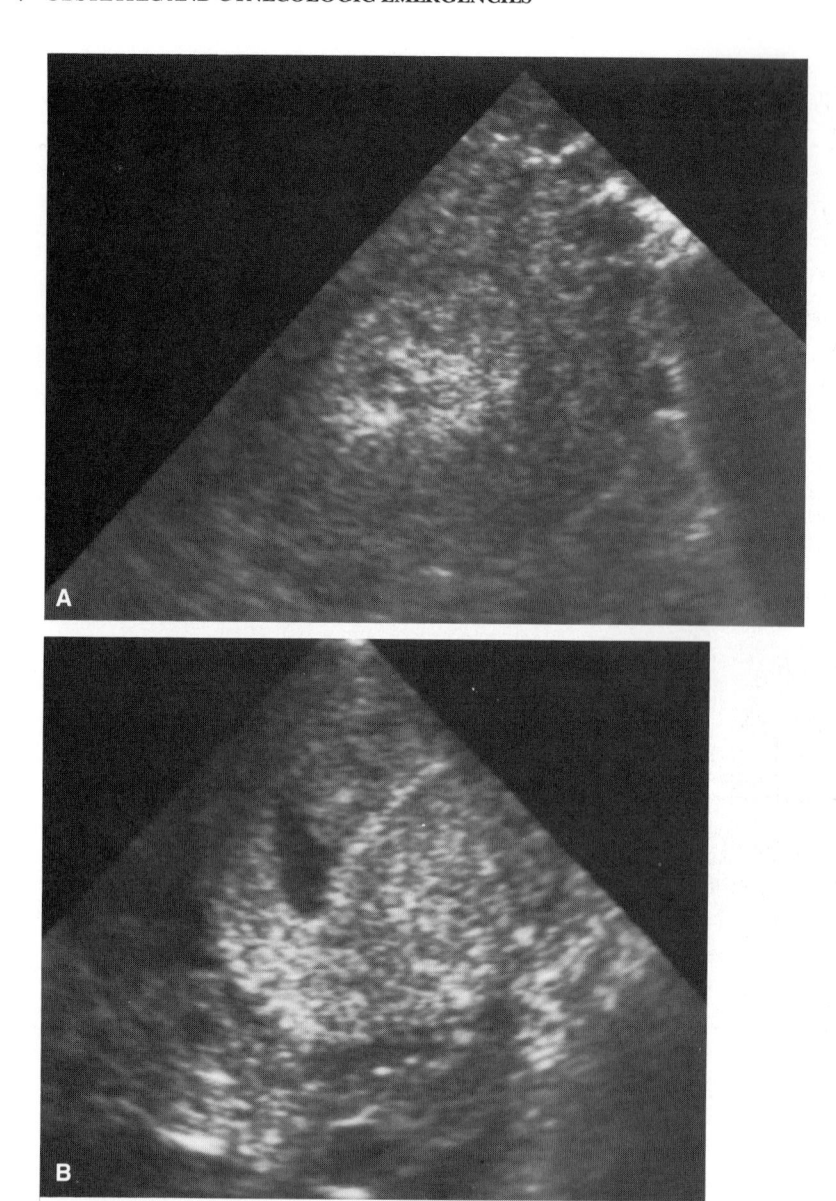

FIGURE 26-21
Decidual cast of ectopic pregnancy vs spontaneous incomplete abortion. Four different patients. (**A,B**) Decidual cast of ectopic pregnancy. (**C,D**) Incomplete abortion. The nonspecificity of the intrauterine findings is quite evident.

IMAGING IN GYNECOLOGIC EMERGENCIES ♦ 387

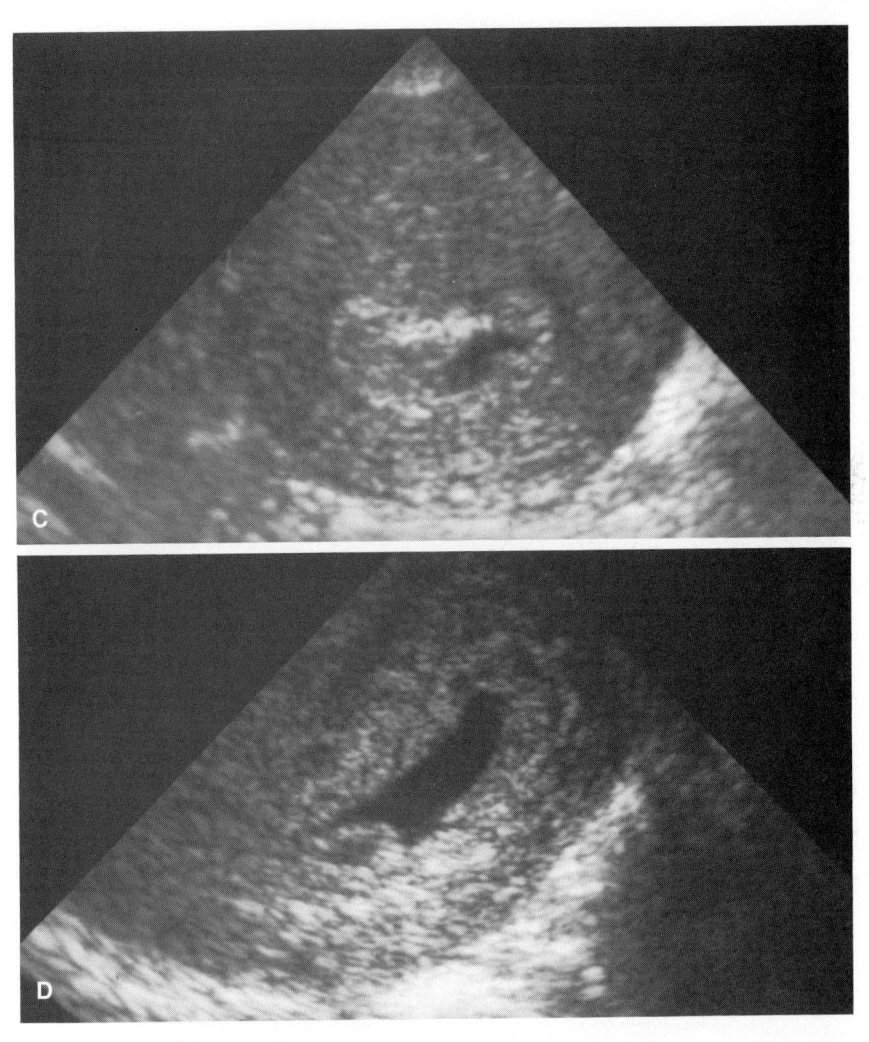

FIGURE 26–21
(Continued)

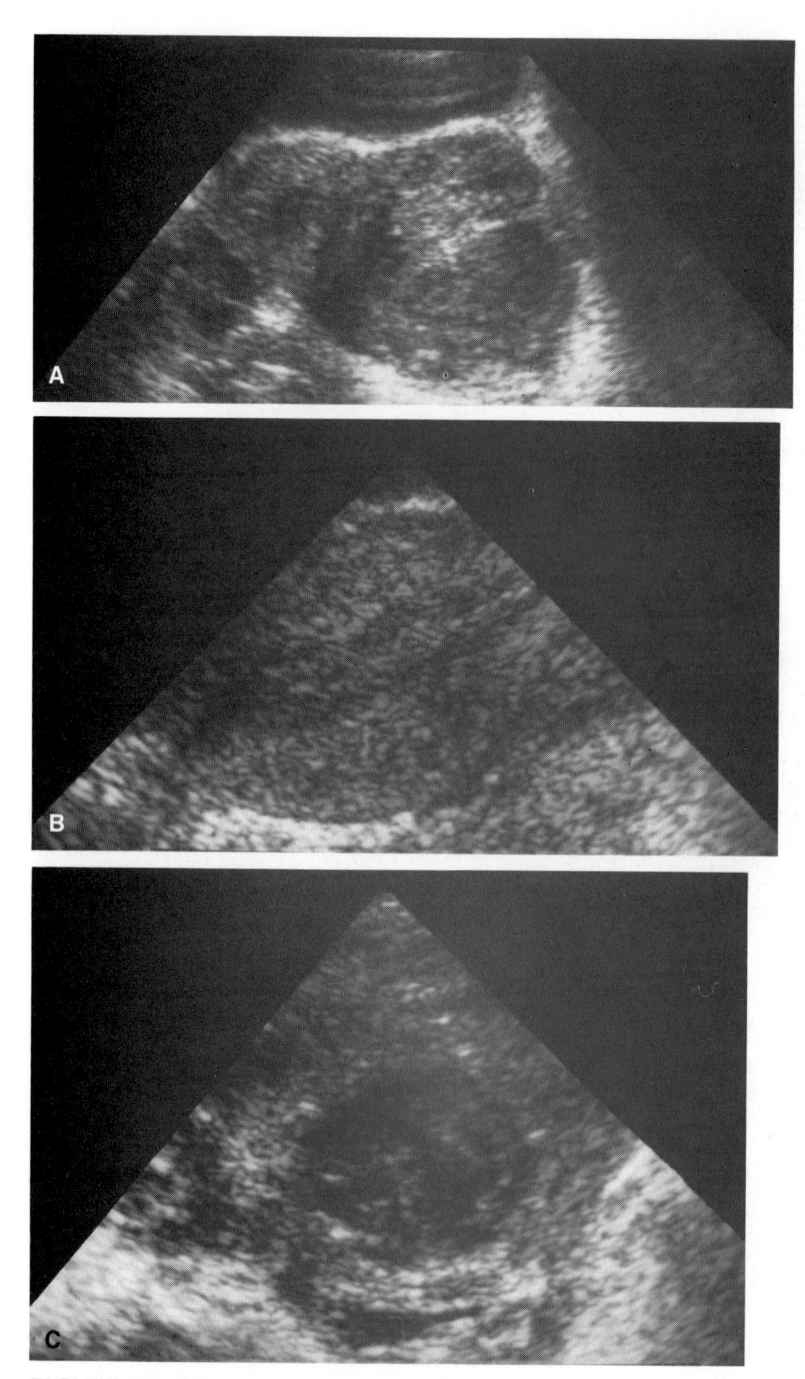

FIGURE 26–22
Ectopic pregnancy: nonspecific adnexal mass. (**A**) Transverse, transabdominal image to the left of midline shows large complex, predominantly solid mass in the left adnexa. (**B**) Tranvaginal image shows empty uterus. (**C**) Transvaginal scan through the left adnexal region better characterizes the mass and shows a small amount of fluid about the mass. Left ectopic pregnancy was found at surgery.

IMAGING IN GYNECOLOGIC EMERGENCIES ♦ 389

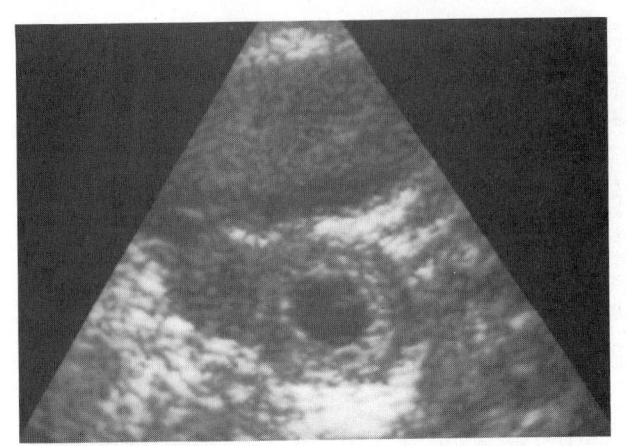

FIGURE 26–23
Tubal ring of ectopic pregnancy. Transvaginal image shows echogenic ring less than 2 cm in diameter found to be tubal pregnancy at surgery.

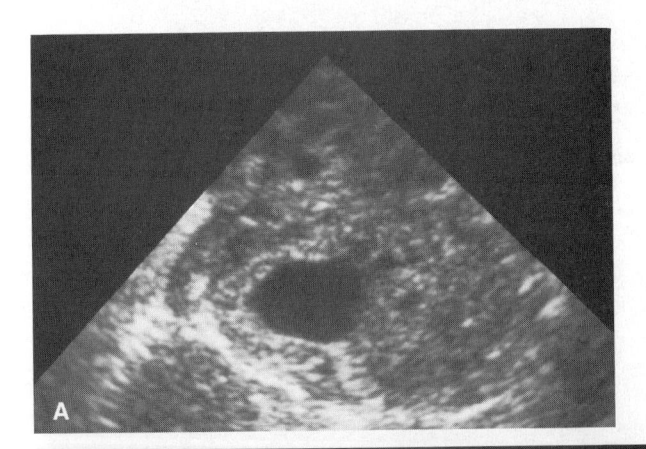

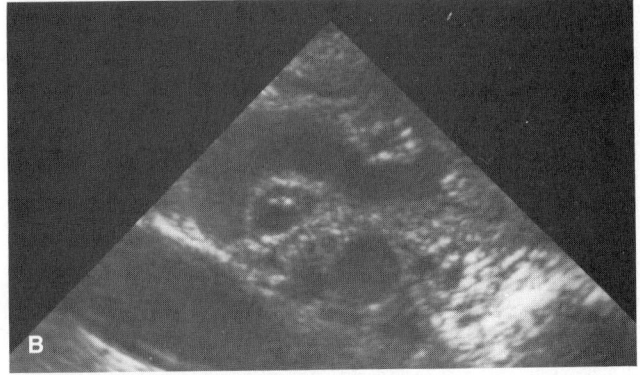

FIGURE 26–24
Tubal ring of ectopic pregnancy. (**A**) Echogenic ring adjacent to but separate from the ovary. (**B**) Undulating tubular structure containing low-level echoes compatible with hematosalpinx in the same patient with proven ectopic pregnancy.

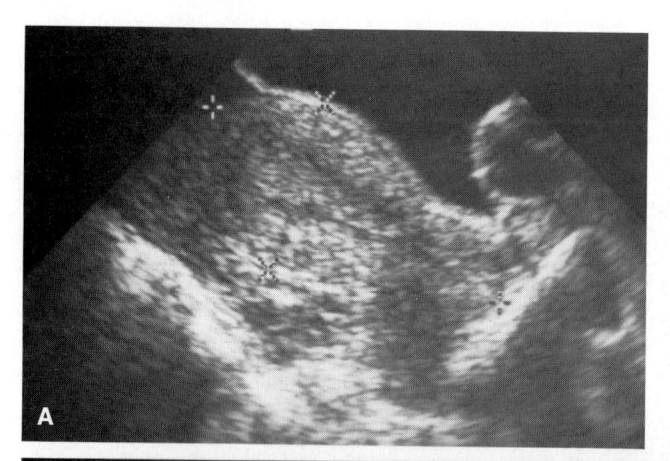

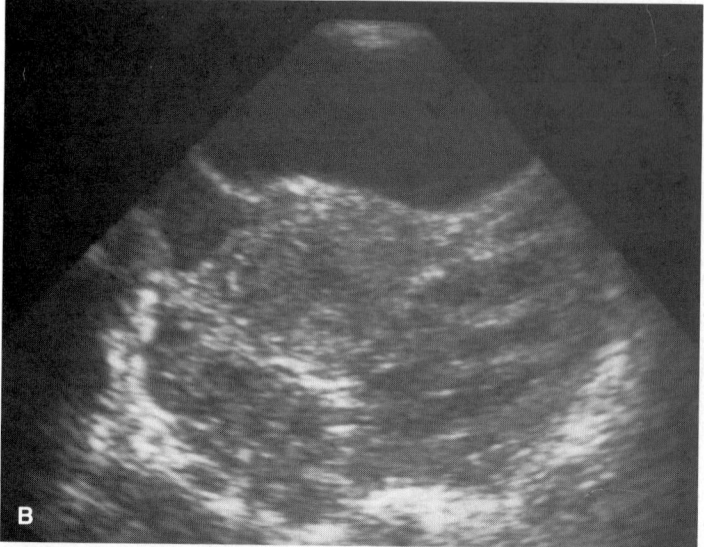

FIGURE 26–25
Ectopic pregnancy and hemoperitoneum. (**A**) Sagittal image of the uterus shows prominent decidual reaction and echogenic fluid just superior to the uterus and within the cul-de-sac. (**B**) Transverse image shows bilateral complex adnexal masses, larger on the left than on the right. More echogenic fluid is noted just to the right of the uterus. (**C**) Free fluid extends between the liver and right kidney in Morison's pouch. (**D**) Image of the right iliac fossa shows bowel loops floating in echogenic fluid compatible with the large hemoperitoneum in this patient with ruptured left ectopic pregnancy.

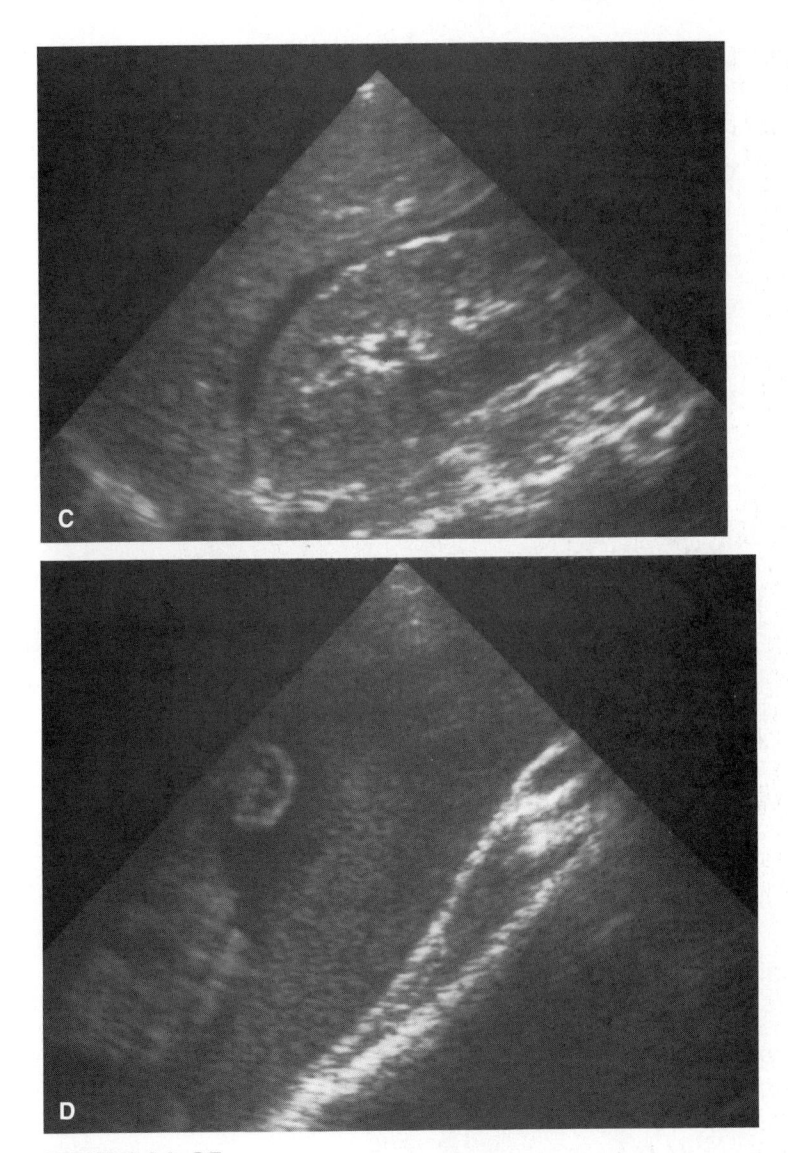

FIGURE 26–25
(Continued)

392 ♦ OBSTETRIC AND GYNECOLOGIC EMERGENCIES

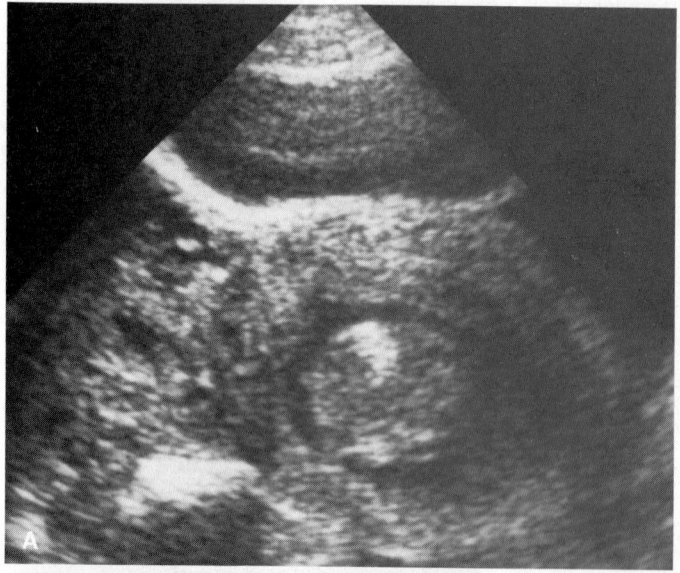

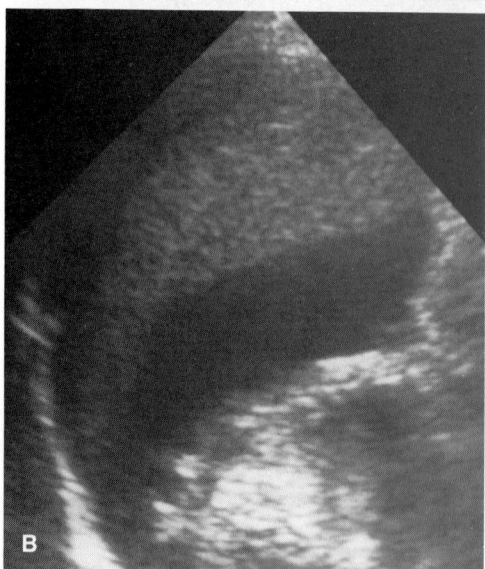

FIGURE 26-26
Ectopic pregnancy. (**A**) Transverse image shows a large fluid collection and amorphous mass within the uterine cavity. A tubal ring is noted in the right adnexal region. (**B**) Large amount of free fluid is visualized about the spleen. At surgery there was a ruptured right infundibular ectopic pregnancy and an 800 cc hemoperitoneum. Amorphous material within the uterus represented blood clot and debris.

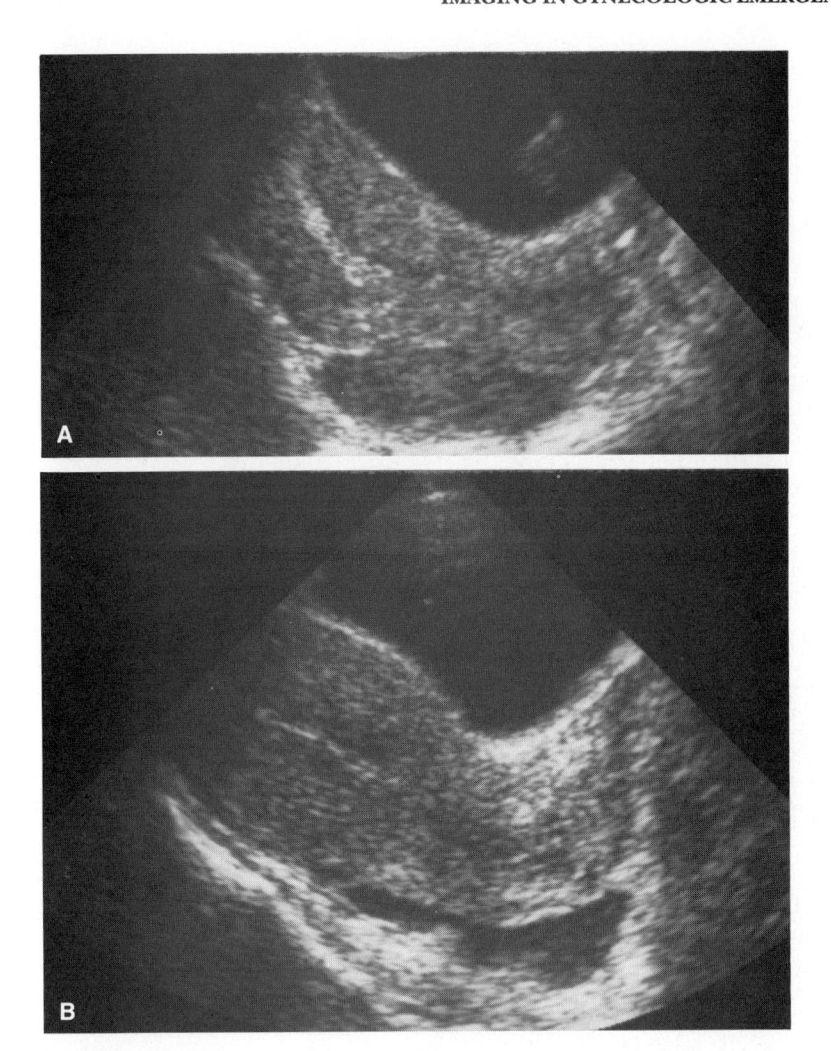

FIGURE 26-27
Hemoperitoneum. (**A**) Sagittal scan in a patient with ectopic pregnancy shows echogenic fluid in the cul-de-sac. Decidual reaction within the uterus is prominent. (**B**) Sagittal scan in another patient shows an anechoic fluid collection in the cul-de-sac. This is more nonspecific in appearance and could represent simple fluid or hemoperitoneum.

394 ♦ OBSTETRIC AND GYNECOLOGIC EMERGENCIES

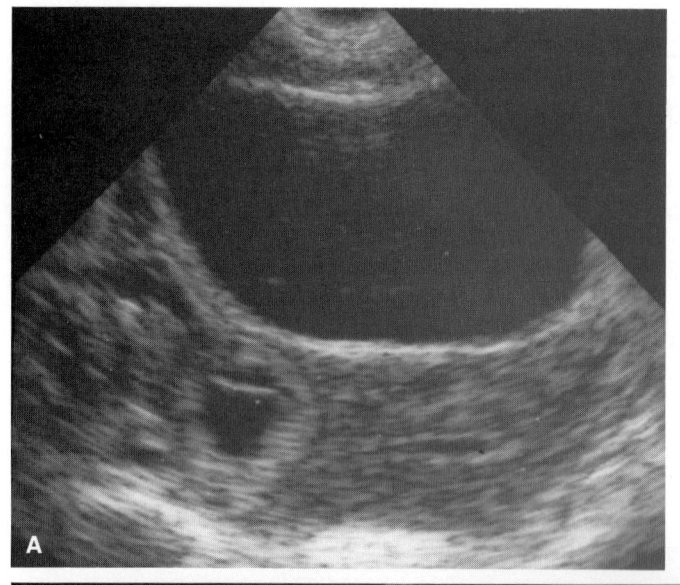

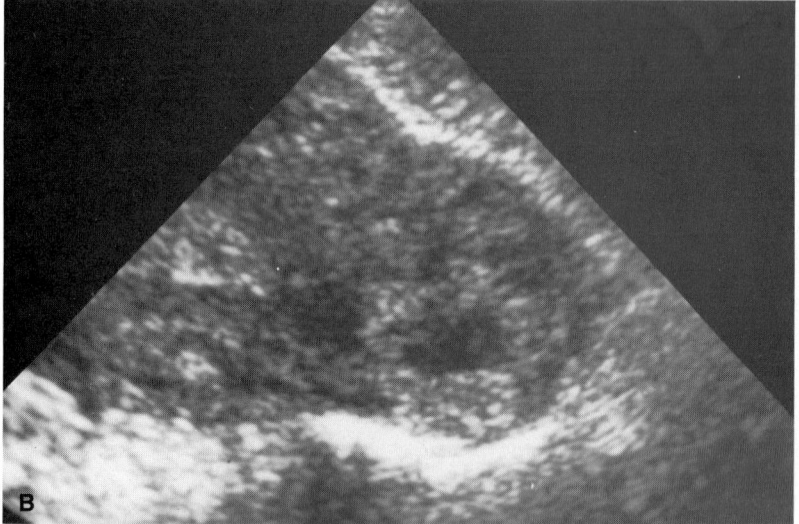

FIGURE 26-28
Interstitial ectopic. (**A**) Transverse, transabdominal image shows a highly echogenic ring eccentrically located in the periphery of the right side of the fundus of the uterus. (**B**) Tranvaginal image of a second patient shows similar findings in the left fundal portion of the uterus. Note that myometrium extends incompletely about both rings.

Gynecologic Infections

Pelvic Inflammatory Disease

Pelvic inflammatory disease is usually caused by tubal infection with *Neisseria gonorrhoeae* or chlamydia followed by infection with anaerobic bacteria. It is an ascending infection that begins in the lower genital tract and spreads to the adnexae. The adnexae may also be involved by direct spread from inflammatory processes in other organs in close proximity.

Ultrasound is the primary diagnostic imaging modality used to evaluate the gynecologic organs in cases of infectious disease and may be of particular assistance when patient tenderness limits the physical examination. In mild infections the sonogram is often normal. Inability to resolve the pelvic structures clearly and delineate organ margins may be the only findings. Mild ovarian enlargement is another possible sonographic clue.[36]

Endometritis

Interestingly, with infections that are sexually transmitted there is relative sparing of the endometrium. The incidence of endometritis is greater with the less common infections caused by streptococci and staphylococci that may complicate abortions or delivery.[37] The sensitivity of ultrasound in detecting endometritis is not high but signs that have been described include uterine enlargement and indistinct uterine contours.[38] Prominent echogenicity of the endometrium, endometrial fluid, and gas may also be seen. Computed tomography (CT) shows similar findings.

Salpingitis

In the adult, the fallopian tubes are the primary sites of sexually transmitted pelvic inflammatory disease. This is also the main location of hematogenously spread gynecologic tuberculosis. Acute salpingitis may progress to a more chronic form, particularly if left untreated. If the fimbriated end of the tube is blocked, pyosalpinx results.[37] Sonographically, one may identify a serpiginous, tubular structure in the adnexal region containing low-level echoes (Fig. 26-29). With time the purulent contents of the tube undergo proteolysis, causing hydrosalpinx.[37] At this point the dilated tube appears anechoic (Fig. 26-30). Hydrosalpinx may also occur following surgical ligation and secondary to obstruction of the fallopian tube by tumor. Hysterosalpingography can demonstrate hydrosalpinx, but it is most useful when documentation of the site of obstruction is necessary. It should not be performed during acute infection, as it may worsen the disease.[39]

Tubo-ovarian Abscess

The ovary may become adherent to the fallopian tube in advanced infection and a tubo-ovarian abscess may form. Although the superficial layers of the ovary are in-

396 ♦ OBSTETRIC AND GYNECOLOGIC EMERGENCIES

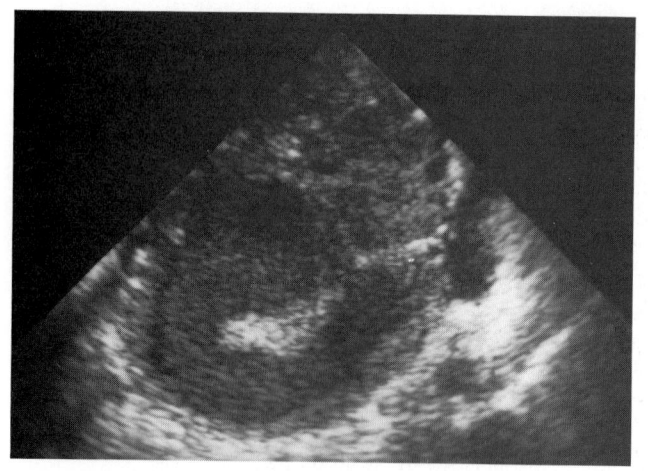

FIGURE 26–29
Pyosalpinx. Endovaginal ultrasound demonstrates a tubular adnexal structure filled with low-level echoes immediately adjacent to the ovary.

volved, the deeper tissue is notably spared.[37] A tubo-ovarian abscess typically appears sonographically as a complex cystic mass.[40] It often contains septations, irregular borders, and thick walls.[39] Debris within the collection is common and may lead to a fluid/debris level (Fig. 26-31). However, the appearance is not specific for tubo-ovarian abscess and may also be seen in cases of ectopic pregnancy, endometrioma, and cystic ovarian neoplasms. When CT is performed in cases of tubo-ovarian abscess, the most frequent finding is a thick-walled, fluid density mass commonly containing septations.[41] This appearance, as on ultrasound, is nonspecific. CT, however, is more sensitive for very small quantities of gas, which, although present only uncommonly, greatly raises the specificity for diagnosing a tubo-ovarian abscess.

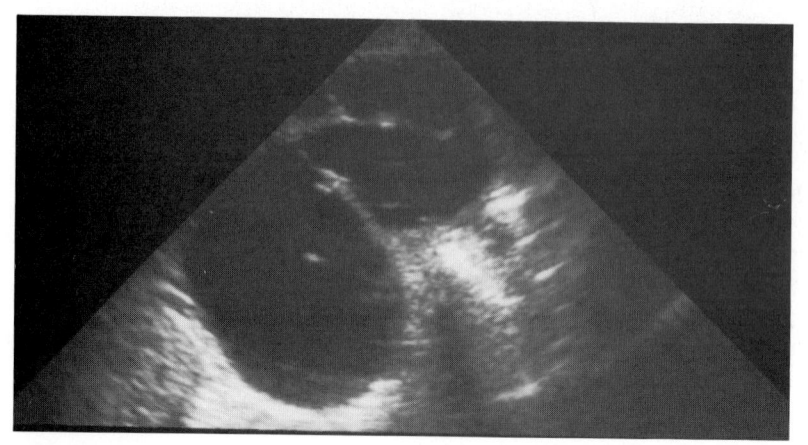

FIGURE 26–30
Hydrosalpinx. Endovaginal ultrasound illustrates an anechoic adnexal region that is tubular and tortuous in configuration. The good through transmission of sound is further evidence of its fluid content.

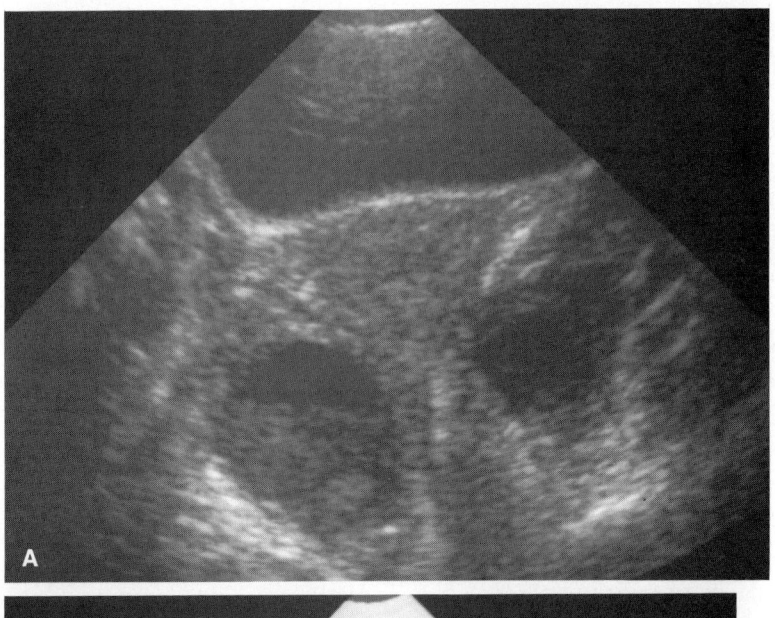

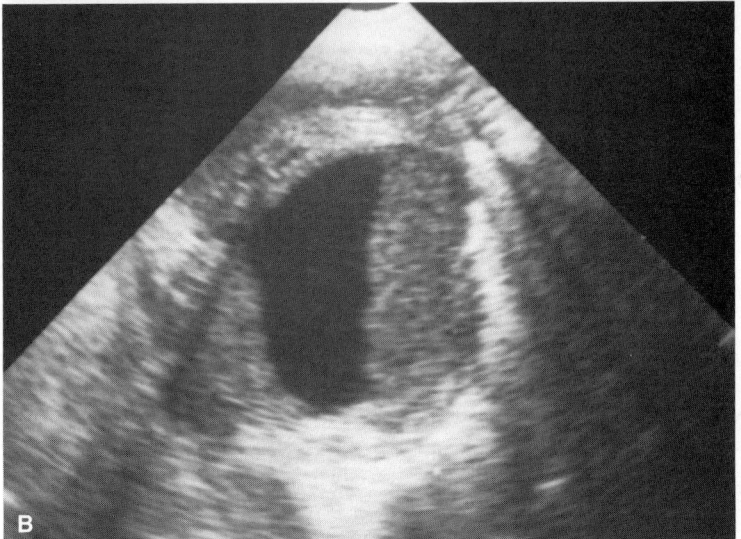

FIGURE 26-31
Bilateral tubo-ovarian abscesses. (**A**) Transabdominal sonography performed in the transverse plane reveals thick-walled, rounded hypoechoic areas adjacent to the posterolateral margins of the uterus. Both demonstrate fluid/debris levels. (**B**) Endovaginal examination on the same patient again shows the fluid/debris level of the right lesion.

Ovarian Torsion

Torsion of the ovary is seen most commonly in young women and girls with ovarian cysts, tumors, or other masses[36] but may be seen in patients with normal ovaries.[43,44] Sonographic findings are nonspecific, but usually an adnexal mass, either complex or predominantly cystic, can be demonstrated (Fig. 26-32). If the ovary is identified, it is enlarged and may have multiple prominent peripheral follicles, presumably from transudation of fluid from vascular congestion.[45]

Ruptured Ovarian Cyst

The patient with a ruptured cyst may present with extreme pain, clinically similar to torsion. The collapsed cyst may or may not be visualized on ultrasound examination. Hemoperitoneum, identical in appearance to that from a ruptured ectopic pregnancy, can be present (Fig. 26-33).[46]

Appendicitis

Appendicitis may be confused clinically with acute pelvic inflammatory disease and rupture or torsion of ovarian cysts. Transabdominal scanning may reveal an abnormal right lower quadrant mass in a patient with appendicitis. High-resolution transabdominal imaging using higher-frequency transducers does not routinely visualize the normal appendix. An inflamed appendix is thickened and noncompressible. In cross section it has a target appearance and a transverse diameter greater than 6 mm (Fig. 26-34). An appendicolith may be seen as an echogenic focus within the appendix, casting an acoustic shadow, and its presence is considered diagnostic of acute appendicitis.[47] Localized periappendiceal fluid may also be seen.

Renal Pathology

Examination of the kidneys should be part of the routine pelvic examination. Renal pathology can masquerade as a pelvic process, and pelvic abnormalities may produce hydronephrosis.

In uncomplicated hydronephrosis the calyces and renal pelvis are dilated with anechoic separation of the central echogenic renal sinus fat (Fig. 26-35). However, if the urinary bladder is markedly distended in the presence of hydronephrosis, postvoid examination of the kidneys should be performed, as overdistention of the bladder may give a false impression of obstruction. The retroperitoneal portion of the ureters is not routinely visualized, even if dilated.[48]

(text continues on page 403)

IMAGING IN GYNECOLOGIC EMERGENCIES ♦ 399

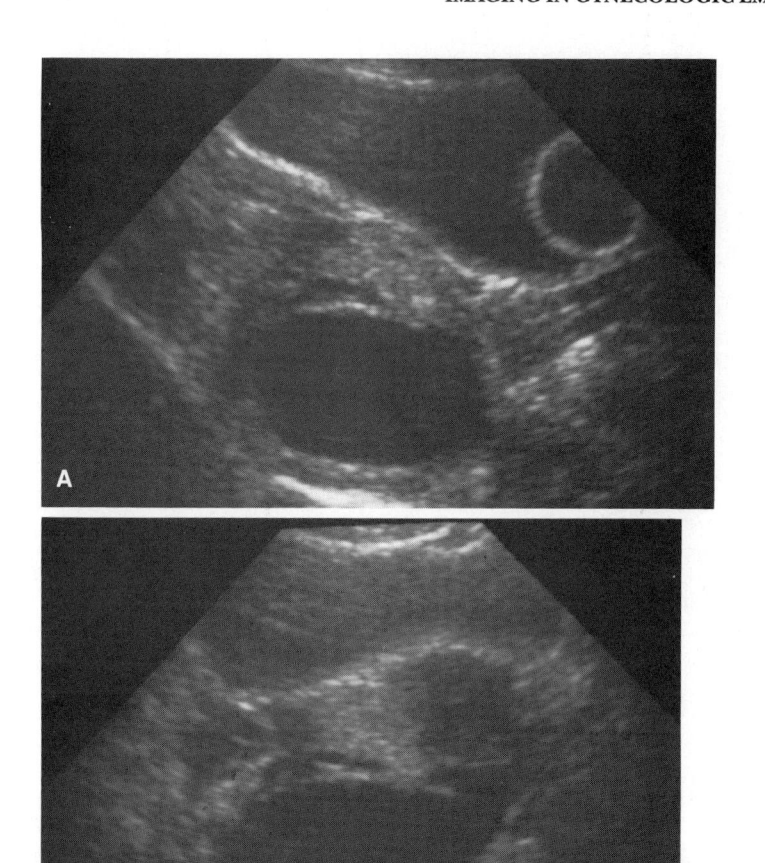

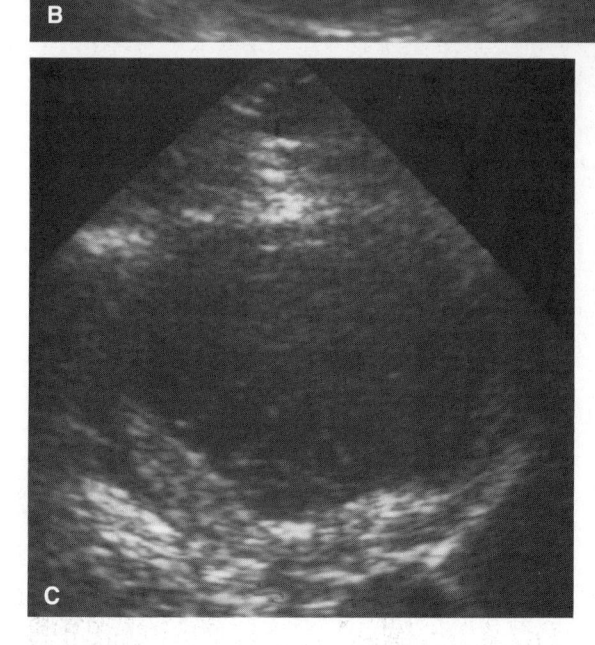

FIGURE 26–32
Ovarian torsion. (**A**) Longitudinal and (**B**) transverse transabdominal scans of a 15-year-old female, and (**C**) longitudinal transabdominal scan through the right adnexal region in a 42-year-old female. **A** and **B** show a complex, predominantly cystic mass within the cul-de-sac and slightly to the right. Note balloon of Foley catheter within the urinary bladder. At surgery, a 6 cm blue necrotic mass was found in the cul-de-sac originating from the left adnexa compatible with torsion. In **C** a residual portion of ovary is noted adjacent to a multiseptated cystic mass. Torsed necrotic right ovary and multiple pelvic adhesions were found at laparotomy.

400 ♦ OBSTETRIC AND GYNECOLOGIC EMERGENCIES

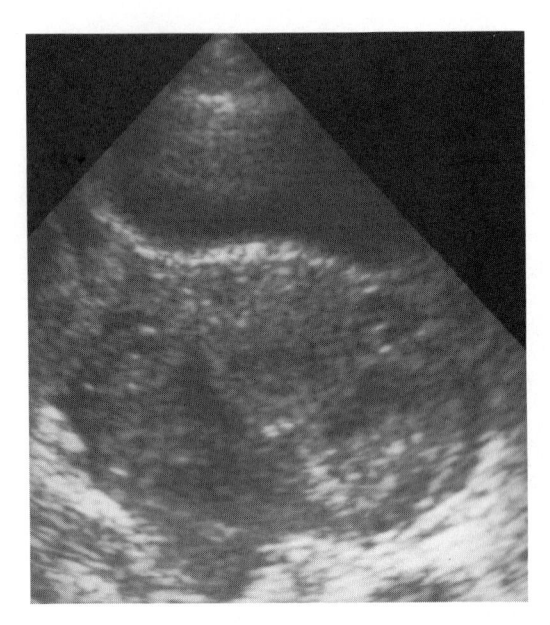

FIGURE 26–33
Ruptured hemorrhagic corpus luteum cyst. Transverse scan of the pelvis shows a large amount of echogenic fluid in the cul-de-sac outlining the posterior aspect of the uterus and both ovaries. Echogenic mass is noted in the cul-de-sac to the left, compatible with clot. At surgery, hemoperitoneum and a ruptured left ovarian cyst were found. The ultrasound appearance is indistinguishable from that of a ruptured ectopic pregnancy.

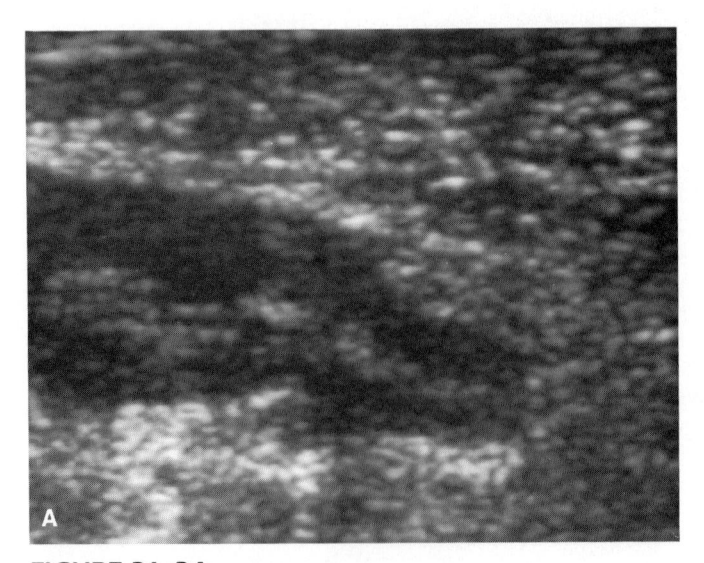

FIGURE 26–34
Acute appendicitis. (**A**) Longitudinal and (**B**) transverse scans through an inflamed appendix. The appendix was noncompressible and measured 12 mm in transverse diameter. The patient experienced maximum tenderness directly over this region during the examination.

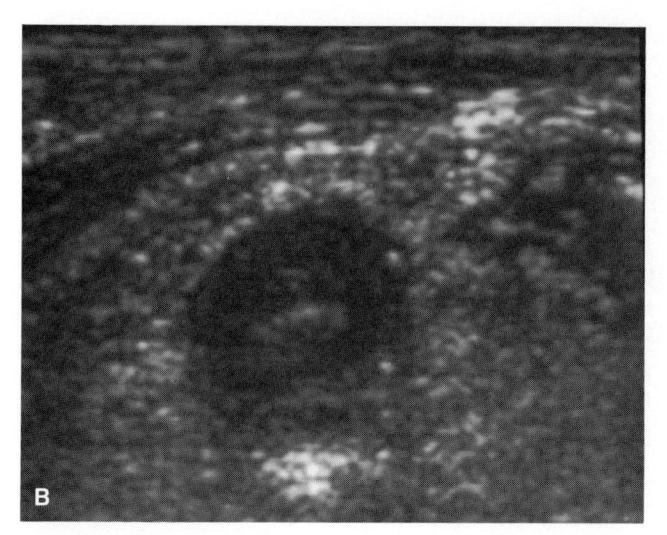

FIGURE 26–34
(continued)

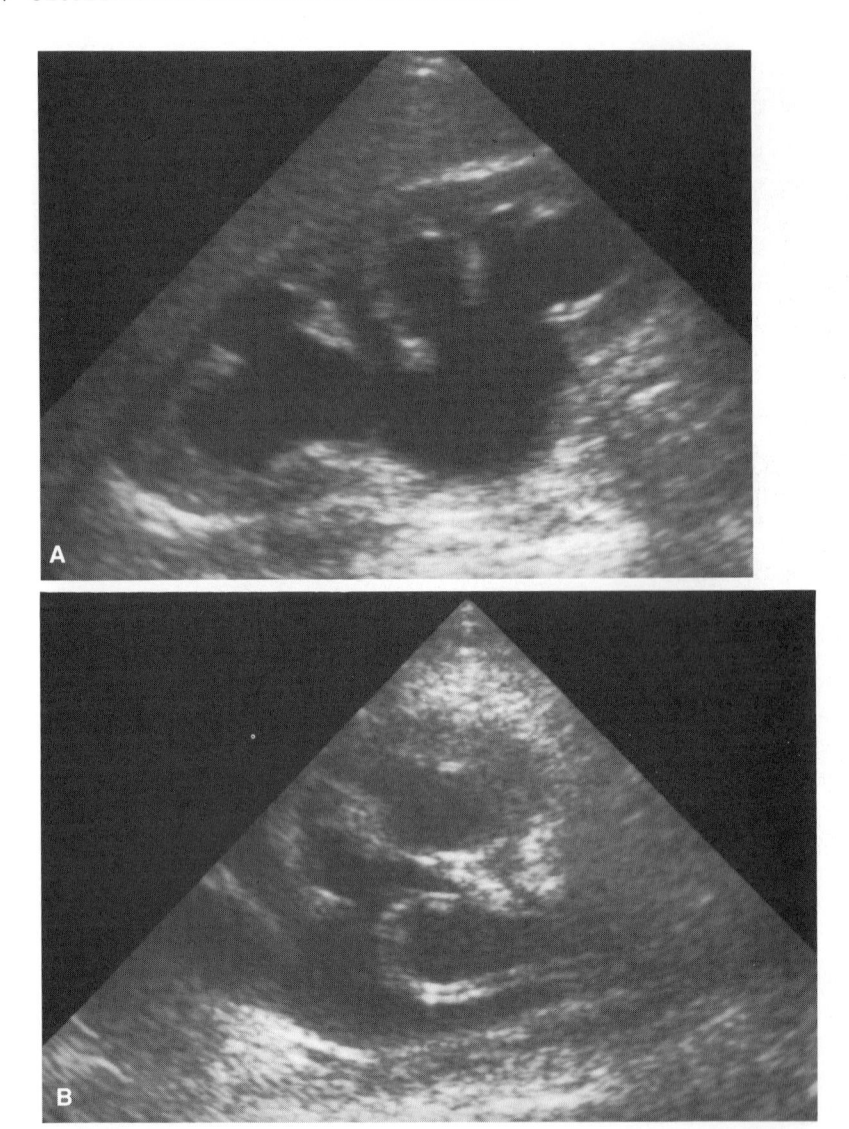

FIGURE 26-35
Hydronephrosis. (**A**) Markedly dilated calyces and renal pelvis, despite (**B**) the presence of a ureteral stent.

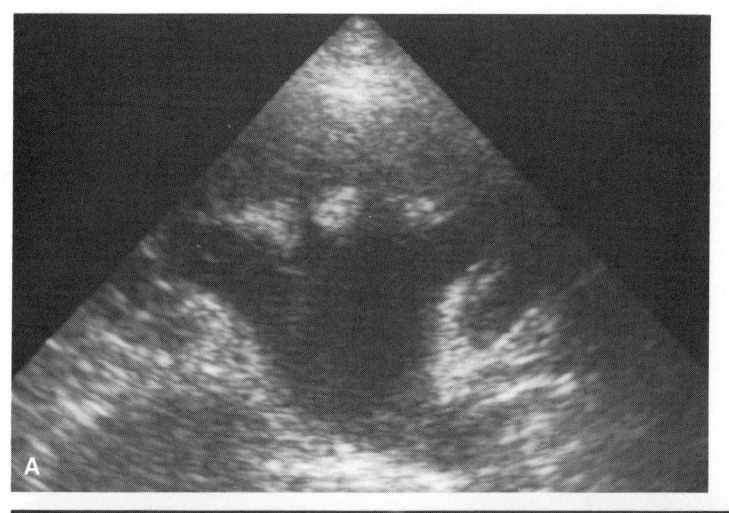

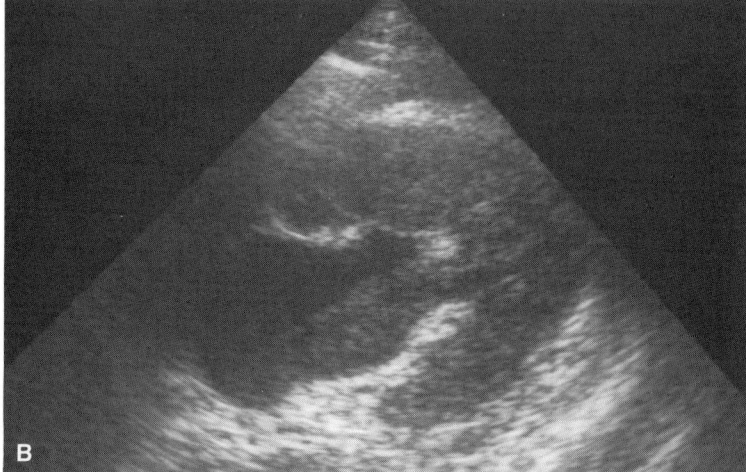

FIGURE 26-36
Pyonephrosis. (**A**) Longitudinal and (**B**) transverse scans show severe hydronephrosis with dilatation of the renal pelvis and calyces. Note fluid/debris level within dilated renal pelvis in **B**.

If low-level echoes are present within the dilated collecting system or if a fluid/debris level is noted, pyonephrosis is strongly suspected (Fig. 26-36). The presence of gas within a noninstrumented collecting system should also suggest infection.[49] It should be noted that an obstructed collecting system may still be infected without these signs.

The ultrasound examination in acute pyelonephritis is usually normal. However, suggestive signs are diffuse or focal enlargement of the affected kidney with effacement of the normally echogenic renal sinus fat (Fig. 26-37). The kidney parenchyma may be hypoechoic or rarely echogenic. Tenderness may be elicited directly over the kidney during the examination.[49]

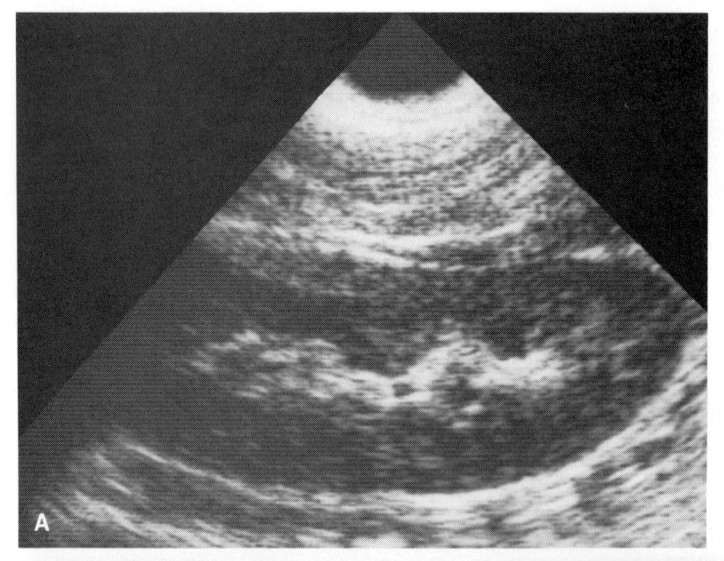

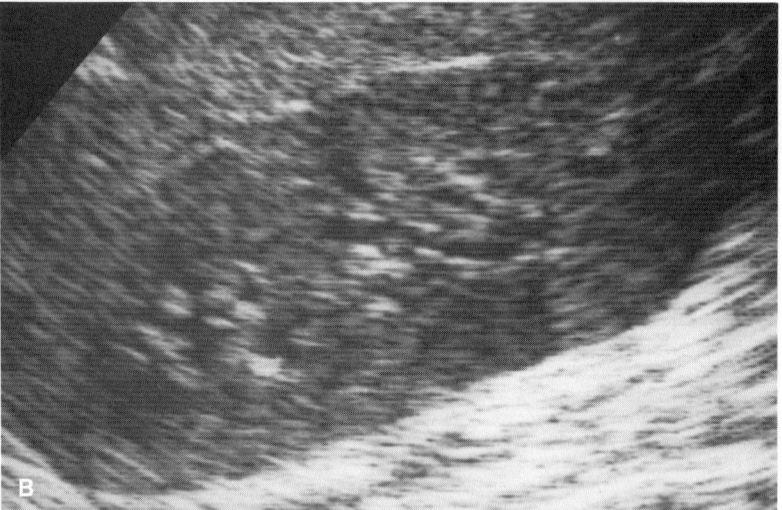

FIGURE 26-37
Acute pyelonephritis. (**A**) Normal left kidney and (**B**) enlarged swollen right kidney. Note effacement of the normally echogenic renal sinus fat echoes within the right kidney. The right kidney measures 13 × 5 cm, and the left, 10 × 4 cm.

REFERENCES

1. Dashefsky SM, Lyons EA, Levi CS, Lindsay DJ. Suspected ectopic pregnancy: endovaginal and transvesical. Radiology 169:181, 1988
2. Tessler FN, Schiller VL, Perrella RR, Sutherland ML, Grant EG. Transabdominal versus endovaginal pelvic sonography: prospective study. Radiology 170:553, 1989
3. Mendelson EB, Bohm-Velez M, Joseph N, Neiman HL. Gynecologic imaging: comparison of transabdominal and transvaginal sonography. Radiology 166:321, 1988

4. Lande IM, Hill MC, Cosco FE, Kator NN. Adnexal and cul-de-sac abnormalities: transvaginal sonography. Radiology 166:325, 1988
5. Coleman BG, Arger PH, Grumbach K et al. Transvaginal and transabdominal sonography: prospective comparison. Radiology 168:639, 1988
6. Moore KL. The beginning of development: the first week. In: Moore KL (ed): The Developing Human: Clinically Oriented Embryology, 4th ed, p 13. Philadelphia: WB Saunders, 1988
7. Yeh H-C, Goodman JD, Carr L et al. Intradecidual sign: a ultrasound criterion of early intrauterine pregnancy. Radiology 161:463, 1986
8. Levi CS, Lyons EA, Dashefsky SM. The first trimester. In: Rumack CM, Wilson SR, Charboneau JW (eds): Diagnostic Ultrasound, p 692. St Louis: Mosby Yearbook, 1991
9. Nyberg DA, Filly RA, Filho DLD, Laing FC, Mahony BS. Abnormal pregnancy: early diagnosis by US and serum chorionic gonadotropin levels. Radiology 158:393, 1986
10. Nyberg DA, Mack LA, Laing FC, Jeffrey RB. Early pregnancy complications: endovaginal sonographic findings correlated with human chorionic gonadotropin levels. Radiology 167:619, 1988
11. Laing FC. Sonographic determination of tubal rupture in patients with ectopic pregnancy: is it feasible? Radiology 177:330, 1990
12. Bree RL, Edwards M, Bohm-Velez M, Beyler S, Roberts J, Mendelson EB. Transvaginal sonography in the evaluation of normal early pregnancy: correlation with HCG level. AJR 153(July):75, 1989
13. Nyberg DA, Laing FC, Filly RA et al. Ultrasonographic differentiation of the gestational sac of early intrauterine pregnancy from the pseudogestational sac of ectopic pregnancy. Radiology 146:755, 1983
14. Nyberg DA, Mack LA, Harvey D, Wang K. Value of the yolk sac in evaluating early pregnancies. J Ultrasound Med 7:129, 1988
15. Jain KA, Hamper UM, Sanders RC. Comparison of transvaginal and transabdominal sonography in the detection of early pregnancy and its complications. Am J Roentgenol 151:1139, 1988
16. Filly RA. Ectopic pregnancy: the role of sonography. Radiology 162:661, 1987
17. Nyberg DA, Laing FC, Filly RA. Threatened abortion: sonographic distinction of normal and abnormal gestation sacs. Radiology 158:397, 1986
18. Levi CS, Lyons EA, Lindsay DJ. Early diagnosis of nonviable pregnancy with endovaginal US. Radiology 167:383, 1988
19. Levi CS, Lyons EA, Lindsay DJ. Ultrasound in the first trimester of pregnancy. Radiol Clin North Am 28:19, 1990
20. Yeh H-C, Rabinowitz JG. Amniotic sac development: ultrasound features of early pregnancy—the double bleb sign. Radiology 166:97, 1988
21. Cadkin AV, McAlpin J. Detection of fetal cardiac activity between 41 and 43 days of gestation. J Ultrasound Med 3(11):499, 1984
22. Levi CS, Lyons EA, Zheng XH, Lindsay DJ, Holt SC. Endovaginal US: demonstration of cardiac activity in embryos of less than 5.0 mm in crown–rump length. Radiology 176:71, 1990
23. Nyberg DA, Callen PW. Ultrasound evaluation of the placenta. In: Callen PW (ed): Ultrasonography in Obstetrics and Gynecology, 2nd ed, p 308. Philadelphia: WB Saunders, 1988
24. Neiman HL, Mendelson EB. Ultrasound evaluation of the ovary. In: Callen PW (ed): Ultrasonography in Obstetrics and Gynecology, 2nd ed, p 433. Philadelphia: WB Saunders, 1988
25. Bromley B, Harlow BL, Laboda LA, Benacerraf BR. Small sac size in the first trimester: a predictor of poor fetal outcome. Radiology 178:375, 1991

26. Laboda LA, Estroff JA, Benaceraff BR. First trimester bradycardia: a sign of impending fetal loss. J Ultrasound Med 8:561, 1989
27. Kurtz AB, Shlansky-Goldbert RD, Choi HY, Needleman L, Wapner RJ, Goldberg BB. Detection of retained products of conception following spontaneous abortion in the first trimester. J Ultrasound Med 10:387, 1991
28. Woodward RM, Filly RA, Callen PW. First trimester molar pregnancy: non-specific ultrasonographic appearance. Obstet Gynecol 55:315, 1988
29. Pennell RG, Baltarowich OH, Kurtz AB et al. Complicated first-trimester pregnancies: evaluation with endovaginal US versus transabdominal technique. Radiology 165:79, 1987
30. Thorsen MK, Lawson TL, Aiman EJ et al. Diagnosis of ectopic pregnancy: endovaginal vs transabdominal sonography. Am J Roentgenol 155:307, 1990
31. Fleischer AC, Pennell RG, McKee MS et al. Ectopic pregnancy: features at transvaginal sonography. Radiology 174:375, 1990
32. Cacciatore B. Can the status of tubal pregnancy be predicted with transvaginal sonography? A prospective comparison of sonographic, surgical, and serum HCG findings. Radiology 177:481, 1990
33. Nyberg DA, Laing FC, Jeffrey RN. Sonographic detection of subtle pelvic fluid collections. Am J Roentgenol 143:261, 1984
34. Nyberg DA, Hughes MP, Mack LA, Wang KY. Extrauterine findings of ectopic pregnancy at transvaginal US: importance of echogenic fluid. Radiology 178:823, 1991
35. Jafri SZH, Loginsky SJ, Bouffard JA, Selis JE. Sonographic detection of interstitial pregnancy. J Clin Ultrasound 15:253, 1987
36. Jeffrey RB. CT and Sonography of the Acute Abdomen, p 262. New York: Raven Press, 1989
37. Robbins SL. Pathologic Basis of Disease, 4th ed, p 1132. Philadelphia: WB Saunders, 1989
38. Patten RM, Vincent LM, Wolner-Hanssen P et al. Pelvic inflammatory disease endovaginal sonography with laparoscopic correlation. J Ultrasound Med 9:681, 1990
39. Hall DA, Hann LE. Gynecologic Radiology: Benign Disorders. In: Taveras JM, Ferrucci JT (eds): Radiology Diagnosis—Imaging—Intervention, p 4. Philadelphia: JB Lippincott, 1988
40. Neiman HL, Mendelson EB. Ultrasound evaluation of the oveary. In: Callen PW (ed): Ultrasonography in Obstetrics and Gynecology, 2nd ed, p 431. Philadelphia: WB Saunders, 1988
41. Wilbur AC, Aizenstein RI, Napp TE et al. CT findings in tuboovarian abscess. Am J Roentgenol 158:575, 1992
42. Helvie MA, Silver TM. Ovarian torsion: sonographic evaluation. J Clin Ultrasound 17:327, 1989
43. Han BK, Babcock DS. Ultrasonography of torsion of normal uterine adnexa. J Ultrasound Med 2:321, 1983
44. Graif M, Itzchak Y. Sonographic evaluation of ovarian torsion in childhood and adolescence. Am J Roentgenol 150:647, 1988
45. Graif M, Shalve J, Strauss S, Engelberg S, Mashiach S, Itzchak Y. Torsion of the ovary: sonographic features. Am J Roentgenol 143:1331, 1984
46. Salem S. The uterus and adenexa. In: Rumack CM, Wilson SR, Charboneau JW (eds): Diagnostic ultrasound, p 396. St. Louis: Mosby Yearbook, 1991

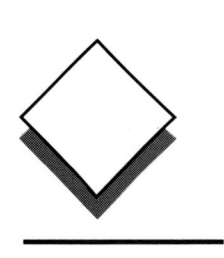

Index

Page numbers followed by f indicate figures; page numbers followed by t indicate tabular material.

Abdomen, burst, 284. *See also* Dehiscence
Abdominal hysterectomy
   complications following, 286, 288–289
   ureterovaginal fistulas as result of, 298
Abdominal pain
   acute, 25–26
   in adolescent, 335–336
   common etiologies of, 26
      appendicitis, 27–28
      biliary disease, 28–29
      intestinal obstruction, 31–32
      ovarian tumors, 33–34
      pancreatitis, 30–31
      peptic ulcer disease, 31
      urinary tract disorders, 32–33
   diagnostic testing for, 36–38
   history and physical examination in, 35–36
   pathophysiology of, 26
   role of imaging modalities in diagnosing, 179
Abdominal stab wounds, conservative management of, 72
Abdominal trauma
   blunt, 70–71
      fetal and placental injury following, 62–64f, 65f
   diagnostic peritoneal lavage for, 178
   penetrating, 71–72
Ablative therapy, for thyroid storm, 13–14
Abortion
   clinical sequelae of illegal
      evaluation and treatment of women with infection following, 199–200
      implications of restricting access, 199
   complete, 131
   deaths from, 197
   definition of, 128
   etiology of spontaneous, 128t
   incomplete, 130f, 130–131, 133
      diagnosis of, 203–204
      retained products of conception from, 380, 380f, 381f
   induced
      epidemiology in United States, 197–198
      continuing pregnancy, 198
         postabortion infection, 199
         postabortion intrauterine bleeding, 198
         retained products of conception, 198
   inevitable, 129–130
      diagnosis of, 203–204

409

Abortion (*continued*)
  missed, 131
  in progress, 380, 382*f*
  self-induced, 199
  threatened, 128–129, 133
    differential diagnosis of, 129*t*
    ultrasound in diagnosis of, 131–132
Abruptio placenta
  association with fetal distress, 136–137
  association with traumatic injuries, 178
  diagnosis of, 177
  vaginal bleeding in, 136*f*, 137*f*, 175–176
Abscess
  Bartholin's, 206
  cuff, 310
  imaging in diagnosing of tubo-ovarian, 395, 396*f*, 397*f*
    rupture of, 214
  pelvic, 292–293
Acetaminophen, during pregnancy, 193
Acquired Immune Deficiency Syndrome (AIDS), 218–222*f*, 220*f*
  psoriasis in, 235
Acrocyanosis, presence of, in asthma patient, 8
Actinomycosis, in pelvic inflammatory disease, 212
Activated partial thromboplastin time (APTT), 301
  need for frequent monitoring in heparin therapy, 5–6
Acyclovir
  for herpes, 120–121, 229
Adenopathy
  inguinal, 306
  supraclavicular, 306
Adnexa, torsion of, 275
Adnexectomy, unilateral, 279
Adolescent
  abdominal pain in, 335–336
  diagnosis of pregnancy in, 335
  examination of, 318, 321*f*, 321–324*f*, 322*f*, 323*f*
  pelvic pain in, 335–336
Adolescent years
  gynecologic emergencies
    in abdominal pain, 335–336
    pelvic pain, 335–336
    pubertal bleeding, 333–335

Adult respiratory distress syndrome, 216
  as cause of death in septic shock, 113
Advanced Cardiac Life Support (ACLS) guidelines, 81
AIDS. *See* Acquired immune deficiency syndrome (AIDS)
Air embolism, 356
Albuterol, during pregnancy, 191
Alpha-fetoprotein, as tumor marker, 266, 269
Amenorrhea, in patients with ectopic pregnancy, 44
Aminoglycoside, during pregnancy, 190
Aminophylline, for asthma, 10
Amnionitis. *See* Chorioamnionitis
Amniotic fluid infection. *See* Chorioamnionitis
Amoxicillin
  for anaerobic bacteria, 310
  for pediatric vaginitis, 327
  for pelvic mass, 271
  for postpartum infection, 158–159
Analgesics, during pregnancy, 193
Anal intercourse, trauma from, 359–360
Angiography, in diagnosing pulmonary embolism, 180–181
Anorexia, in appendicitis, 28
Anovulation, 252–253, 255, 334–335
  treatment of, 259
Antiasthmatics, during pregnancy, 191
Antibiotics
  for chorioamnionitis, 106
  for diabetic ketoacidosis, 16
  for pelvic mass, 271
  during pregnancy, 188–190
  for pyelonephritis, 110–111
  for septic pelvic thrombophlebitis, 293–294
  for septic shock, 115
  for thyroid storm, 13
Anticoagulants
  during pregnancy, 190–191
  for pulmonary emboli, 6
Anticonvulsant medications
  effect of, on fetus, 17–18
  during pregnancy, 192–193
Antiemetics, during pregnancy, 194
Antithyroid medications, for thyroid storm, 13–14
Appendiceal distention, 27–28

Appendicitis, 27–28
  acute focal stage of, 27
  imaging in diagnosis of, 398, 401f
  risk of perforation in, 27
  symptoms in, 27–28
  treatment of, 28
Appendicolith, 398
Arteriography, in diagnosing pulmonary embolus, 301
Ascites, with pelvic mass, 267
Asherman's syndrome, 131
Aspiration, of pelvic cysts, 271
Aspiration pneumonitis, as cause of dyspnea, 7
Asthma, 6–7
  different diagnosis of, 7
  emergency therapy for, 8
  pathophysiology of, 7–8
  pharmacologic agents for, 9–10
  status asthmaticus in, 10
Atrophy, association of lichen simplex chronicus with, 236
Atropine, during cardiopulmonary resuscitation, 82t
Auscultation, for asthma, 8
Automobile restraints, during pregnancy, 64f, 65f
Avulsion
  urethral, 361
  uterine, 360
Azythromycin (Zithromax), in preventing venereal disease, 349

β-HCG, as tumor markers, 266
β-HCG tests, in diagnosing pelvic masses, 269
β-lactamase penicillin, for postpartum infection, 159
β-mimetic therapy, in diabetic ketoacidosis, 14
Bacterial contamination, of abdomen, 26
Bacterial vaginosis, 242–243, 247
Bacteriuria, 161
Bacteroides, with symptoms of chorioamnionitis, 104
Bacteroides bivius
  in pelvic inflammatory disease, 212
  in postpartum infection, 156
Bacteroides fragilis
  in pelvic inflammatory disease, 212
  in postpartum infection, 159

Bacteroides species, as cause of postpartum infection, 156
Bactrim, for pediatric vaginitis, 327
Barium enemas, 360
Bartholin's cysts and abscesses, 206
Behçet's disease, 239
Benign uterine mass, 263–264
Benzodiazepines, for eclampsia, 19
Bicarbonate replacement, for diabetic ketoacidosis, 15–16
Bilateral ischiopubic rami fractures, 361
Biliary disease, 28–29
Biliary pancreatitis, 28–29
Bimanual examination
  in adolescent, 324
  in diagnosing vaginal bleeding, 306
Biophysical Profile, 172, 174t
Birth canal, laceration of, 152–154
Birth control pills, for menorrhagia, 256
Bleeding disorders, 255
  abnormal vaginal bleeding, 258
  endometrial cancer, 257–258
  essential menorrhagia, 256–257
  evaluation of, 258–259
  fibroids, 255–256
  pubertal, 333–335
  treatment of, 259–262
Bleomycin, 311
Blindness due to hypotension, pulmonary embolus as cause of, 4
Blood clots. *See* Pulmonary embolism
Blood volume, increase in maternal, 58
Bowel
  complications of radiated, 308
  laparoscopic injury to, 298
Bowel emergencies
  colostomy, 308
  complications of radiated, 308
  fistula formation, 308
  obstruction, 307–308
Bradycardia, embryonic, 379–380
Brain death, diagnosis of maternal, 90
Breast development, Tanner staging for, 319f
Breast feeding, and development of mastitis, 159–160f
Breech delivery, 152, 153f
Brenner tumor, 269
Bretylium, during cardiopulmonary resuscitation, 82t

Burns
  electrical, 73–74
  thermal, 73
Burst abdomen, 284. *See also* Dehiscence

CA-125, as tumor markers, 266, 269, 271
Carbamazepine, for eclampsia, 19
Cancer
  cervical, 306
  childhood, following radiation exposure, 4–5
  embryonal cell, 266
  endometrial, 257–258
  ovarian, 33–34, 307
  uterine, 264–265
Candida albicans, 243–244
Candida glabrata, 244
Candidiasis, 243–244
"Cannonball" position, genital examination of child in, 322
Cantor tube, 296
Carbamazepine
  during pregnancy, 192
  for seizures, 18
Carboplatinum, 311
Cardiac activity, visualization of, in embryo, 372–373
Cardiac arrest, maternal
  anatomic and physiologic considerations in mother and fetus in, 77–79
  common etiologies of, 78t
  effect of, on fetus, 79–80
  incidence of, during pregnancy, 77
Cardiac resuscitation, during perimortem cesarean section, 91
Cardiopulmonary resuscitation, 80
  complications of, 82–83
  drugs used in, 81–82t
  technique in, 80–81
Cardiovascular abnormalities, in thyroid storm, 11
Cardiovascular collapse, as complication in pulmonary emboli, 4
Cardiovascular system
  anatomic and physiologic changes associated with pregnancy in, 58–61

  anatomic and physiologic considerations of mother and fetus in, 77–79
Cefazolin, for urinary tract infection, 161
Cefotetan, for postpartum infection, 159
Cefoxitin, for postpartum infection, 159
Ceftriaxone
  for pelvic mass, 271
  in preventing venereal disease, 349
Cellulitis
  pelvic, 292–293
  vaginal cuff, 310
Central nervous system dysfunction, in thyroid storm, 11
Cephalexin
  for mastitis, 160
  for urinary tract infection, 161
Cephalosporin
  for mastitis, 160
  for postpartum infection, 159
  during pregnancy, 189
  for urinary tract infection, 161
Cephradine, for mastitis, 160
Cervical cancer, vaginal bleeding in, 306
Cervical incompetence, 132–133
Cervical infections, 133
Cervical pregnancy, 254f
  diagnosing, 391
Cesarean delivery
  and penetrating abdominal trauma, 71
  performance for ominous fetal heart rate patterns in, 105
  perimortem, 74
    and cardiopulmonary resuscitation, 83–84f
    changing concepts regarding, 88–90
    site of incision for, 84f
    special considerations during resuscitation, 91
Chadwick's sign, in diagnosing ectopic pregnancy, 48
Chain of custody, in sexual assault cases, 341
Chancroid, 230, 239–240
Chemotherapy, complications of, 311
Chest radiograph, in diagnosing pulmonary emboli, 4–5
Chickenpox. *See* Varicella, primary

INDEX ◆ 413

Children
    anatomy and physiology of developing, 315–318f, 317f, 319f
    dermatologic lesions presenting as vaginal bleeding in, 331
    examination of, 318, 321f, 321–324f, 322f, 323f
        for alleged sexual abuse in, 346–349, 347f
    genital trauma in, 327–329f, 328f
    normal vaginal flora of prepubertal, 316t
    psychosocial and developmental issues in emergency care of, 336–337
    risk of cancer in, following radiation exposures, 4–5
    sedation in, 324–325t
    vaginal bleeding in, 325–331, 326t, 328f, 329f, 330f, 332f, 333f
        urologic causes of, 330f, 330–331
Chlamydia trachomatis
    acute salpingitis in, 43
    as cause of postpartum infection, 156–157
    in children, 3, 16, 318
        treatment of, 350t
    cultures for, 345–346, 349
    in pelvic inflammatory disease, 212
    in postpartum infections, 158
    and presence of foreign object, 247
    prevention of, 349–350f
    screening for, in adolescents, 335–336
    in sexual assault, 341
Cholecystitis, 226
    incidence of, 28–29
Choledocholithiasis, 28–29
Cholelithiasis, 28–29
Chorioamnionitis, 103–104
    for diabetic ketoacidosis, 16
    diagnosis of, 104
    management of, 105–107, 106t
    outcome and sequelae in, 105
    pathophysiology in, 104–104
Chromosomal abnormality, as cause of spontaneous abortion, 128
Ciprofloxacin, during pregnancy, 190
Cisplatin, 311
Clindamycin
    for bacterial vaginosis, 243
    for pelvic mass, 271
    during pregnancy, 190
Clostridial infections, 291–292f
Clostridial myonecrosis, 291–292
Clostridium perfringens, 291–292
Clostridium septicum, 291–292
CMV retinitis, 222
Coagulopathy, 335
Coitus, trauma with, 356
Cold shock, 112, 214–215
Collaborative Perinatal Project, 191, 193
Colostomy, 308, 360
Colovaginal fistulas, 298
Colpitis macularis, 244, 245f
Colposcopy, in examination for sexual assault, 344–345
Coma, fetal outcome in cases of irreversible maternal, 90
Computed tomography (CT) scan, 365
    in evaluating
        abdominal pain, 37
        endometritis, 395
        foreign bodies, 302
        pelvic masses, 270
        trauma, 67
        tubo-ovarian abscess, 395
        urinary tract injury, 178
Condylomata, 331, 333f
Confidentiality, in adolescent patient, 323
Congestive heart failure, in thyroid storm, 11
Cornual pregnancies, imaging in diagnosing, 385, 394f, 395
Corpus luteum cyst, 265, 373, 375f
    ruptured hemorrhagic, 400f
Corticosteroids, for septic shock, 115
Cotton ball tests, 298
Coumadin
    for pulmonary embolus, 301–302
    for septic pelvic thrombophlebitis, 293–294
    for venous thrombosis, 300
Crepitus, 291
Crowning, 140f
Cuff abscess, 310
Culdocentesis
    in diagnosing pelvic mass, 268–269
    for ectopic pregnancy, 50–52, 53
    equipment needed for, 203–204
Cunnilingus syndrome, 356
Cyclophosphamide, complications from, 311
Cyst
    aspiration of pelvic, 371
    Bartholin's, 206

Cyst (*continued*)
  corpus luteum, 265, 373, 375*f*
    ruptured hemorrhagic, 400*f*
  diagnostic aspiration of, 271
  follicle, 265
  germinal inclusion, 265
  physiologic, 265
  theca-lutein, 265
Cystic teratomas, 268
Cystitis, 161
  hemorrhagic, 309–310
Cystourethrography, 358
Cytomegalovirus, 228

Dactinomycin, complications from, 311
Decidua capsularis, 369
Decidua parietalis, 369
Deep venous thrombosis (DVT), diagnosis of, 180
Dehiscence, 283–285, 284*f*
Delivery in emergency department, 139
  delivery of placenta, 144–145
    episiotomy and repair in, 146–147*f*, 148–149*f*, 150
    oxytocin agents in, 145–146
  spontaneous vaginal delivery, 140*f*
    breech delivery, 152, 153*f*
    clamping of cord, 144
    delivery of head, 140*f*
      clearing the nasopharynx, 141, 142*f*
      nuchal cord, 141, 143*f*
      Ritgen maneuver, 140, 141*f*
    delivery of shoulders, 141, 143–144*f*
    lacerations of birth canal, 152–154
    shoulder dystocia
      documentation of, 152
      management of, 151*f*, 151–152
Demerol, in sedating children, 325
Depoprovera, for anovulation, 260
Dermatitis, seborrheic, 234–235
Dermatologic lesions, presenting as vaginal bleeding in children, 331
Dexon, 329
Diabetic ketoacidosis, 14
  diagnosis of, 14–15*t*
  emergency treatment of, 15–16
  hospital management of, 16
  pathophysiology of, 14
Diarrhea, in thyroid storm, 11
Diazepam, for eclampsia, 19

Diazoxide, for preeclampsia, 100
Dicloxacillin
  for mastitis, 160
  for postpartum infection, 159
Dilation and curettage (D&C), 259–260, 261
Diphtheroides, in prepubertal child, 316
Discriminatory hCG zone, 49, 52
DNA fingerprint analysis, 346
DNA probe technologies, 341
DNA virus, 228
Dobutamine, during cardiopulmonary resuscitation, 82*t*
Dopamine
  for cardiopulmonary resuscitation, 82*t*
  for pelvic inflammatory disease, 215
  for septic shock, 114–115
Dorsolithotomy position, genital examination of child in, 321*f*, 323
Double decidual sac sign, 369–370, 371*f*
Doxorubicin, complications from, 311
Drug therapy, during pregnancy. *See also specific drugs*
  analgesics in, 193
  antiasthmatics in, 191
  antibiotics in, 188–190
  anticoagulants in, 190–191
  anticonvulsants in, 192–193
  FDA pregnancy categories, 186, 187–188*t*
  gastrointestinal agents in, 194
  pediculoides in, 193
  principles of teratogenesis, 185–186
  scabicide in, 193
Duncan mechanism, 144
Dysfunctional uterine bleeding (DUB), 252
Dyspnea of pregnancy, 7
Dystocia, shoulder, 150–152

Eclampsia, 16–17
  as cause of postpartum seizures, 166–167
  management of seizures in, 18–19
Ectopic pregnancy, 268–269, 389–390*f*
  ambulatory evaluation and management of, 47–48
    culdocentesis, 50–52
    history, 48
    physical examination, 48

pregnancy tests, 48–49
ultrasonography, 49
cause and risk factors in, 42–43, 44t
clinical presentation in, 44–45
definition of, 41
diagnosis of, 45–47, 46t, 268–269, 278, 380, 383f, 384–385, 384–391f, 391
evaluation of, 203
and hemoperitoneum, 391f
incidence of, 41–42
management of, 53, 54f, 55f
sites of, 42f
suction curettage in, 52–53
Electrical injury, during pregnancy, 73–74
Electrolyte replacement, for diabetic ketoacidosis, 15
Embolism, air, 356
Embolus, pulmonary, 165–166, 301–302
evaluation and management of, 166
Embryo, visualization of cardiac activity in, 369, 371, 372f
Embryonal cell carcinomas, 266
Embryonic bradycardia, 379–380
Emergency care, psychosocial and development issues in, for children, 336–337
Emergency department. *See also* Delivery in emergency department
equipment needs in, 203–207
Endocarditis, 217–218
Endocervical curettage, 268
Endodermal sinus tumors, 266
Endometrial cancer, 257–258
Endometriosis, pain in, 279
Endometriotic cysts, 268
Endometritis, 156
as consequence of chorioamnionitis, 105
differential diagnosis of, 157
evaluation and management of, 157–159
imaging in diagnosis of, 395
and wound infections, 156–161
Endometrium, ablation of, 261–262
Endomyometritis, 156, 294
Endoparametritis, 156
Enemas
barium, 360
gastrografin, 360

Enteritis, regional, 238
Enterobacter
as cause of postpartum infection, 156
in urinary tract infection, 161
Enterococci, as cause of postpartum infection, 156
Enterocutaneous fistulas, 297
Epilepsy, effect of pregnancy on, 17
Epinephrine
for asthma, 9
for cardiopulmonary resuscitation, 82t
Episiotomy, 146
infection of, 159
repair of, 147, 148–149f, 150
timing of repair, 144f, 146–147f
Eppendorfer-type biopsy forceps, 268
Epstein-Barr virus, 228
Ergonovine, in achieving hemostasis, 146
Erythromycin
for chancroid, 230
during pregnancy, 189
Escherichia coli
in chorioamnionitis, 104
in pelvic inflammatory disease, 212
in postpartum infection, 156
in pyelonephritis, 108
in urinary tract infection, 161
Essential menorrhagia, 256–257
Estrogen, for anovulatory bleeding, 259
Etoposide, complications from, 311
Eversion, vaginal, 287–288
Evisceration, vaginal, 286

Fallopian tube
masses in, 265
torsion of, 275
False-negative pregnancy test, in ectopic pregnancy, 46
Fascitis, necrotizing, 289–291f
Fellatio, injuries caused in, 343–344f
Fellatio syndrome, 355–356
Fetal death, maternal death as cause of, 57
Fetal effects
of anticonvulsant medications, 17–18
of maternal cardiac arrest, 79–80
of maternal pyelonephritis, 109
of radiographic procedures, 67, 68t
Fetal evaluation
in chorioamnionitis, 105
in trauma, 66

416 ♦ INDEX

Fetal exposure
  as determinant of teratogenesis, 186
  timing of, 186
Fetal gestational age, calculation of, 172
Fetal hydantoin syndrome, 17–18
Fetal malformation, 133
Fetal maturity, as factor in preeclampsia, 98
Fetal monitoring
  in acute seizures, 20
  in diabetic ketoacidosis, 16
Fetal morbidity and mortality, 57
  in appendicitis, 28
  in penetrating abdominal trauma, 71
Fetal warfarin syndrome, 190–191
Fetomaternal hemorrhage, 63–64, 70
Fetus
  hypoxic injury to, 80
  radiation exposure to, 4–5
Fibroadenomas, 269
Fibroids, 255–256
Fistulas
  formation of, 308
  rectovaginal, 361
  ureterovaginal, 298, 361
  urologic, 309
  vesicovaginal, 298, 361
Fitz-Hugh-Curtis syndrome, 226
Flouro-uracil, complications from, 311
Follicle cyst, 265
Foreign bodies
  inadvertent residual, 302
  retained, 359
  vaginal, 246–247
Forensic medicine, for sexual assault, 341
Fractures, bilateral ischiopubic rami, 361
Frog-leg position, genital examination of child in, 321f, 347

Gallbladder disease, treatment of, 29
Gardnerella vaginalis, as cause of postpartum infection, 156
Gastrografin enemas, 360
Gastrointestinal agents, during pregnancy, 194
Gastrointestinal disease, production of pelvic mass by, 267–268
Gastrointestinal fistulas, 297–298
Gastrointestinal system, anatomic and physiologic changes associated with pregnancy in, 59, 60f

Genital condyloma, 333f
Genital examination, in children, 320–321f
Genital human papilloma, 331, 332f
Genital trauma, in children, 327–329f, 328f
Genital warts, 349
Genitourinary injuries resulting in postoperative emergencies, 298–300
Gen-probe, 345–346
Gentamicin
  for pelvic mass, 271
  for postpartum infection, 158–159
Germ cell tumors, 266
Germinal inclusion cyst, 265
Gestational trophoblastic disease, 269
  vaginal bleeding caused by, 306–307
Glucocorticoid
  for asthma, 9
  for thyroid storm, 13
GnRH agonist therapy, 255–256
Gonadal stromal tumors, 266
Gonococcemia, 216
Gonorrhea. *See Neisseria gonorrhea*
Granuloma inguinale (Donovanosis), 240–242
Graves' ophthalmopathy, 11
Group B streptococci, in chorioamnionitis, 104–105
Gunshot wounds
  diagnostic approach to, 178
  to pregnant abdomen, 71
Gynandroblastoma, 269

Haemophilus ducreyi, as cause of chancroid, 230
Haemophilus influenzae, in pelvic inflammatory disease, 212
Haemophilus vaginalis, 243
Head, delivery of, in spontaneous vaginal delivery, 140f, 140–141f, 142f, 143f
Head injuries, management of, 72–73
Heart rate, acceleration of maternal, in pregnancy, 58
Hegar's sign, in diagnosing ectopic pregnancy, 48
HELLP syndrome, as sign of preeclampsia, 96

Hematology, anatomic and physiologic changes associated with pregnancy in, 61
Hematomas
    detection of subchorionic, 132
    retroperitoneal, 360
    vulvar, 361–362f
Hematometra, acute, 198
Hematuria, in children, 330–331
Hemoconcentration, 290
Hemoperitoneum
    diagnosis of, 178
    ectogenic fluid in, 385, 391f, 393f
Hemorrhage
    evaluation and management of, 162–163
    fetomaternal, 63–64, 70
    intra-abdominal, 70–71
    postpartum, 145, 161–162
Hemorrhagic cystitis, 309–310
Heparin therapy
    for deep venous thrombosis, 165
    during pregnancy, 190–191
    for pulmonary embolus, 5–6, 166, 301–302
Hepatitis, risks of acquiring, 350
Hepatomegaly, in thyroid storm, 11
Hernia
    external, 296
    incisional, 286–287
Herpes, primary, 118
    diagnosis of, 119
    management of, 120t, 120–121
    outcome and sequelae in, 120
    pathophysiology in, 119
Herpes simplex virus (HSV) infection, 228–230, 238
    risks of acquiring, 350
HPV, risks of acquiring, 350
Huffman adolescent speculum, 324, 334
Human immunodeficiency virus (HIV). *See also* Acquired immune deficiency syndrome (AIDS)
    risks of acquiring, 350
Human menopausal gonadotropin (Pergonal), for ovulation induction, 279–280
Hydatidiform mole, 133
Hydralazine, for preeclampsia, 100
Hydrocortisone, for asthma, 9
Hydronephrosis, 398
Hydrops tubae profluens, 265
Hydrosalpinx, 395

Hymenal tearing, management of, 356
Hypercalcemia, in thyroid storm, 12
Hypercoagulability, 300
Hyperdefecation, in thyroid storm, 11
Hyperglycemia, in thyroid storm, 12
Hypertension
    as complications of preeclampsia, 100
    persistence of, 101
    as sign of preeclampsia, 96
Hyperthyroidism, thyroid storm in, 10
Hypoplastic vulvar dystrophy, 237
Hypotension, as complication in pulmonary emboli, 4
Hypothyroidism, 253
Hypoxic injury, to fetus, 80
Hysterectomy, 256. *See also* Abdominal hysterectomy; Vaginal hysterectomy
Hysterosalpingography, 395
Hysteroscopy, 261

Iatrogenic gynecologic trauma, 362
Idiopathic seizure disorders, 16
Idiopathic thrombocytopenic purpura, 255
I-fibrinogen, contraindication during pregnancy, 180
Ifosfamide, complications from, 311
Ileus, postoperative, 295–296
Imaging
    in diagnosis of
        appendicitis, 398, 401f
        endometritis, 395
        ovarian torsion, 398, 399f
        renal pathology, 398, 400, 401–403f
        ruptured ovarian cyst, 398, 400f
        salpingitis, 395, 396f
        tubo-ovarian abscess, 395, 396f, 397f
    modalities, 171–172f, 173f, 174t, 175f
    of acute abdomen, 179
    of bleeding during late pregnancy, 175–177f, 176f
    in maternal trauma, 178–179
    of thromboembolic complications, 180–182
    of pregnant patient, 367
        normal early intrauterine, 367, 369, 371–373
Impedance plethysmography, in diagnosis of deep venous thrombosis, 165

Incest, 346
Incisional hernia, 286–287
Infections
  chorioamnionitis, 103–104
    diagnosis of, 104
    management of, 105–107, 106t
    outcome and sequelae in, 105
    pathophysiology in, 104–105
  following illegal abortions, 199–200
  herpes simplex virus, 228–230
  postabortion, 199
  as postpartum emergency, 155–157
  primary herpes, 118
    diagnosis of, 119
    management of, 120t, 120–121
    outcome and sequelae in, 120
    pathophysiology in, 119
  primary varicella, 116
    diagnosis of, 116
    management of, 117–118
    outcome and sequelae in, 117
    pathophysiology in, 116–117
  pyelonephritis, 107
    diagnosis of, 107t, 107–108
    management of, 110–111
    outcome and sequelae in, 108–110, 109f
    pathophysiology in, 108
  septic shock, 111
    diagnosis of, 111–112
    management of, 113–115, 114t
    outcome and sequelae in, 113
    pathophysiology in, 112–113
Infertility, menotropin therapy for, 275
Infusion pyelography, in diagnosing urinary tract injury, 178
Insulin therapy, for diabetic ketoacidosis, 15
Interstitial pregnancy, imaging in diagnosing, 385, 394f, 395
Intestinal obstruction, 31–32
  management of, 32
  symptoms of, 32
Intra-abdominal hemorrhage, 70–71
Intra-abdominal soft-tissue injuries, 360
Intra-amniotic infection. *See* Chorioamnionitis
Intradecidual sac, imaging of, 367, 369, 370f
Intrapartum infection. *See* Chorioamnionitis

Intrauterine device (IUD), 43
  in preventing pregnancy following sexual abuse, 350–351
  and risk of pelvic inflammatory disease, 211–212
Intrauterine pregnancy, 278
Intravenous pyelography (IVP), in diagnosing pelvic masses, 269
Inversion, of uterus, 145
Ischemia, as cause of abdominal pain, 26
Isoimmunization, risk of, among women with antepartum bleeding, 129
Isotope scanning, in diagnosis of deep venous thrombosis, 165

Jarisch-Herxheimer reaction, 227
Jaundice
  in syphilis, 224
  in thyroid storm, 11

Kaposi's sarcoma, 219
Klebsiella, in urinary tract infection, 161
Klebsiella pneumoniae, in pyelonephritis, 108
Kleihauer-Betke test, 63–64, 70
Knee-chest position, in genital examination of child, 322f, 326, 347

Laboratory studies
  in diagnosing vaginal bleeding, 306
  in evaluating trauma, 66–67
Lactobacillus, in prepubertal child, 316
Laparoscopic bowel injury, 298
Laparoscopy
  in diagnosing pelvic masses, 270–271
  in intraperitoneal injury, 360
  in management of ovarian torsion, 279
Laparotomy
  in intraperitoneal injury, 360
  in managing pelvic mass, 272
Laparotomy tape, in diagnosing foreign bodies, 302
Large intestine, obstruction of, 297, 307–308
Levonorgestrel, for anovulation, 260
Lichen planus, 236–237
Lichen sclerosus, 237–238, 331, 332f
Lichen simplex chronicus, 236

Lidocaine, during cardiopulmonary resuscitation, 82t
Lindane, during pregnancy, 193
Listeria monocytogenes chorioamnionitis, 104
Liver failure, 312
Lymphadenectomy, pelvic, 266
Lymphocysts, 268
Lymphogranuloma venereum, 239, 240f

Magnesium sulfate
  for eclampsia, 19
  for postpartum seizures, 166–167
  for preeclampsia, 98, 100
Magnetic resonance imaging (MRI)
  in evaluating
    pelvic masses, 270
    urinary tract injury, 178
Malignancy. *See* Cancer
Mastitis, 159–160f
  evaluation and management of, 160
McRobert's maneuver, in management of shoulder dystocia, 151f
Meclizine, during pregnancy, 194
Medical history
  in abdominal pain, 35–36
  in ectopic pregnancy, 48
  in sexual assault, 342
Meigs' syndrome, 267
Menorrhagia
  definition of, 251
  essential, 256–257
  etiology of, 260t
  initial treatment for, 259–262t
Menotropin therapy, for infertility, 275
Menstrual dysfunction, and pelvic masses, 267–268
Menstruation
  irregular, 333–335
  normal, 251–252
Metaproterenol, during pregnancy, 191
Methergine, for postpartum hemorrhage, 205
Methotrexate, complications from, 311
Methylergonovine, in achieving hemostasis, 146
Methylergonovine maleate, for postpartum hemorrhage, 162
Methylprednisolone, for asthma, 9
Metritis, 156
Metronidazole
  for anaerobic bacteria, 310
  for bacterial vaginosis, 243
  for pelvic mass, 271
  for postpartum infection, 158–159
  during pregnancy, 190
  for trichomoniasis, 244–245
Military antishock trousers (MAST), during pregnancy, 65
Miller-Abbott tube, 296
Minority women, incidence of ectopic pregnancy in, 42
Mobiluncus vaginitis, 245–246, 247
Mortality, trauma as cause of maternal, 57
Mycoplasma, in pelvic inflammatory disease, 212
Mycoplasma hominis, as cause of postpartum infection, 156
Myomas, 263–264
  degeneration of, 278–279
  of uterus, 256, 268, 269
Myonecrosis, uterine, 292

Nalidixic acid, during pregnancy, 190
Naloxone, for septic shock, 115
Nasopharynx, clearing of, in spontaneous vaginal delivery, 141
Necrosis, subcutaneous, 290
Necrotizing fasciitis, 289–291f
Neisseria gonorrhea, 216–218, 349–350t
  in child, 316, 318, 327
    treatment of, 350t
  cultures for, 336, 344, 345–346, 348–349
  in pelvic inflammatory disease, 212
  in postpartum infections, 158
  and presence of foreign object, 247
  prevention of, 349–350t
  screening for, in adolescents, 335–336
  in sexual assault, 341
  treatment of, in children, 350t
Neonatal resuscitation, equipment needs for, 204–205
Nitrofurantoin, during pregnancy, 190
Nitroimidazoles, for trichomoniasis, 244–245
Nitroprusside, for preeclampsia, 100–101
Nonsexually related trauma, 360–362f
Norethindrone acetate, for anovulation, 260
Norplant, for anovulation, 260
Nuchal cord, 141, 143f

Obstruction
    intestinal, 31–32
    of large intestine, 297, 307–308
    of small bowel, 296, 307
    ureteral, 309
Oncologic emergencies, 305
    bowel emergencies, 307
        colostomy, 308
        complications of radiated, 308
        fistula formation, 308
        obstruction, 307–308
    complications of chemotherapy, 311
    complications of total parenteral nutrition, 311
    organ failure, 312
    postoperative complications, 310–311
    urologic
        fistulas, 309
        hemorrhagic cystitis, 309–310
        ureteral obstruction, 309
        urinary conduit complications, 310
    vaginal bleeding, 306–307
Open-chest cardiac massage, in cardiopulmonary resuscitation, 81
Oral contraceptives (OCP), in treating anovulation, 259–260
Oral-genital sex, complications of, 355–356f
Organ failure, 312
Osteomyelitis, 224, 361
Ovarian cancer, 33–34
    and small-bowel obstruction, 307
Ovarian cyst
    bleeding, 268–269
    rupture of, 47
        imaging of, 398, 400f
Ovarian hyperstimulation syndrome (OHSS), 275, 279–280
Ovarian masses, 265–266
Ovary, torsion of. See Torsion of ovary
Ovral, in preventing pregnancy following sexual abuse, 350–351
Oxygen therapy
    for asthma, 8
    for maternal and fetal trauma, 69–70
    for septic shock, 115
    for thyroid storm, 12
Oxytocin
    in achieving hemostasis, 146
    in delivery of placenta, 145–146
    for postpartum hemorrhage, 162

Paclitaxel (Taxol), complications from, 311
Pancreatitis, 30–31
    etiologic factors of, 30
    management of, 30
    severity of, 30–31
Papillary serous tumors, 269
Pap smear, 257
Paracentesis, needle placement during, 178
Parenteral therapy, for pyelonephritis, 110–111
Pederson-type speculum, 324
Pediatric speculum, in unanesthetized child, 322
Pediatric vulvar injuries, management of, 328
Pediculoides, during pregnancy, 193
Pelvic cellulitis and abscess, 292–293
Pelvic examination
    for adolescent and child, 318, 321f, 322f, 323–324f, 323f, 346–349, 347f
    in diagnosis of foreign body, 246
Pelvic fractures, 360
Pelvic inflammatory disease (PID), 211–216
    clinical presentation of, 211–212
    costs associated with, 211
    diagnosis of, 212–213f, 214f
        imaging in, 391, 395
    increase in incidence of, 43
    pain in, 278
    sites of disseminated, 217f
    treatment of, 214–215t
Pelvic lymphadenectomy, 266
Pelvic mass
    adnexal structure of, 263
    ascites with, 267
    common etiologies of, 263
    differential diagnosis of, 263–266, 264t, 267t
        aspiration of cysts in, 271
        history of, 266–268
        imaging in, 269–270
        initial evaluation of, 266
        laboratory studies in, 269
        laparoscopy in, 270–271
        physical examination in, 268
        special studies in, 268–269
    etiology of, 272
    management of, 271–272
    nongynecologic causes of, 266

Pelvic pain, in adolescent, 335–336
Penicillin
  for mastitis, 160
  for pelvic mass, 271
Peptic ulcer disease, 31
  diagnosis of, 31
  management of, 31
  symptoms of, 31
Peptococcus
  in pelvic inflammatory disease, 212
  in postpartum infection, 156
Peptococcus species, with symptoms of chorioamnionitis, 104
Peptostreptoccus
  in pelvic inflammatory disease, 212
  in postpartum infection, 156
Perfusion scanning, in diagnosing pulmonary embolus, 301
Perimenopausal woman, uterine masses in, 264
Perimortem cesarean section. See Cesarean delivery
Peritoneal irritation, 27–28
Peritoneal lavage, in evaluating, 68
Peritonitis, 26
  from inadvertent residual foreign bodies, 302
  in sexually related trauma, 360
Periurethral injuries, bleeding from, 328
Pfannenstiel incision, 358–359
Pharmacologic agents, for asthma, 9–10
Phenergan, in sedating children, 325
Phenobarbital
  during pregnancy, 192
  for seizures, 18
Phenylephrine neosynephrine hydrochloride, for postoperative complications, 310–311
Phenytoin
  during pregnancy, 192
  for seizures, 18
Phlebitis, 165
Physical examination. See also Genital examination; Pelvic examination
  in diagnosing abdominal pain, 35–36
  in sexual abuse
    of adult, 342–346, 343f, 344f, 345f
    of child, 346–349, 347f
Physiologic cysts, 265
Pitocin, after placental delivery, 204–205
Pityriasis rosea, 236

Placenta, delivery of, 144–145
Placental abruption
  maternal death from, 62–63
  as result of seizures, 20
Placenta previa
  ultrasound in diagnosis of, 134–137, 135f
  vaginal bleeding in, 175–176
Platelet disorder, 255
Pneumocystis carinii pneumonia, 219–220
Pneumoperitoneum, 356
Polycystic ovarian syndrome, 252–253
  evaluation for, 259
Polymicrobial pelvic inflammatory disease, 212
Postabortion infection, 199
Postabortion intrauterine bleeding, 198
Postmenopausal bleeding, in pelvic mass, 268
Postmortem cesarean section. See Cesarean delivery
Postoperative emergencies, 283
  gastrointestinal emergencies
    fistulas, 297–298
    ileus, 295–296
    laparoscopic bowel injury, 298
    obstruction of large intestine, 297
    small bowel obstruction, 296
  genitourinary injuries resulting in, 298–300
    urinary retention, 300
  infectious complications
    clostridial infections, 291–292f
    necrotizing fasciitis, 289–291f
    pelvic cellulitis and abscess, 292–293
    superficial wound infections, 288–289f
  mechanical wound complications
    dehiscence, 283–285, 284f
    incisional hernia, 286–287
    suture sinuses, 286
    vaginal evisceration, 286
  pulmonary embolus, 301–302
    inadvertent residual foreign bodies, 302
  septic pelvic thrombophlebitis, 293–295
  vaginal eversion, 287–288
  venous thrombosis, 300–301
Postoperative ileus, 295–296
Postoperative small bowel obstruction, 296

Postpartum emergencies, 155, 156f
  hemorrhage as, 145, 161–162
    evaluation and management of, 162–163, 205
  infection as, 155–157
    endometritis and wound infections, 156–161
  psychological reactions as, 167
  seizures as, 166–167
  thrombosis as, 163–166, 164f
Precipitous delivery, equipment needs for, 204–205
Preeclampsia, 16
  conditions associated with, 93
  criteria for severe, 94t
  diagnosis of, 93, 94–96, 97f
  incidence of, 93
  intrapartum management of, 98, 100–101
  pathophysiology of, 94
  postpartum management of, 101
  prepartum management of, 97–98, 99–100f
  prevention of, 101
Pregnancy. *See also* Ectopic pregnancy
  cervical, 254f, 391
  changes associated with, 58, 61t
    in cardiovascular system, 58–59
    in gastrointestinal system, 59, 60f
    in hematology, 61
    in reproductive system, 60–61
    in respiratory system, 59
    in urinary system, 59–60
  complications of first-trimester, 203–204
  cornual, 385, 394f, 395
  diagnosis of
    in adolescent, 335
    in management of pelvic masses, 271
  effect of, on epilepsy, 17
  imaging of, 367
    abnormal early intrauterine pregnancy, 373, 375, 376f, 377f, 378f, 378–380, 379f, 380f, 381f, 382f
    ectopic pregnancy, 380, 383f, 384–385, 384–391f, 391
    normal early intrauterine pregnancy, 367, 369, 371–373
  prevention of, following sexual assault, 350–351
  vaginal bleeding in, 253–255, 254f
Pregnancy tests, in diagnosing ectopic pregnancy, 48–49
Prehospital management, of trauma, 65–66
Premarin 25 mg IV, for pubertal bleeding, 335
Premature uterine contractions, in pyelonephritis, 110
Prepubertal child, rectal examination in, 322
Preterm labor, as sequel of maternal trauma, 63
Proctitis, 359
Proctoscopy, in examination for sexual abuse, 345, 359
Propranolol, 13
Propylthiouracil (PTU), for thyroid storm, 13
Prostaglandins, for postpartum hemorrhage, 205
Proteinuria, as sign of preeclampsia, 96
Proteus, in urinary tract infection, 161
Proteus mirabilis
  in postpartum infection, 156
  in pyelonephritis, 108
Prothrombin deficiency, 255
Pruritus, 236
Pseudogestational sac, 384, 385f, 386f
Pseudomonas, in urinary tract infection, 161
Pseudomonas aeruginosa, 294
Psoriasis, 235–236
Psychological support and counseling, following sexual abuse, 351
Pubertal bleeding, gynecologic emergencies in adolescent years, 333–335
Puberty, onset of, 317
Pubic hair development, Tanner staging for, 320f
Puerperal fever
  risk factors for, 155–156
  source of, 155
Pulmonary embolism, 301–302
  diagnosis of, 4–5, 180–181
  patient presentation in, 3–4
  therapy for, 5–6
Pulmonary metastasis, 312
Pulsus paradoxus, in asthma patient, 8
Pyelonephritis, 294
  acute, 32
  diagnosis of, 107–108, 107t
  fetal effects of maternal, 109

management of, 110–111
outcome and sequelae in, 108–110, 109f
pathophysiology in, 108
recurrent, 161
symptoms of, 32–33
ultrasound examination in acute, 400, 404f
Pyonephrosis, 403f
Pyosalpinx, 395, 396f
Pyuria, in appendicitis, 28

Quinolones, during pregnancy, 190

Radiated bowel, complications of, 308
Radiation exposure, to fetus, 4–5
Radiographic studies, 365
   in diagnosing abdominal pain, 37
   estimated fetal radiation exposure from, 175t
   procedures in evaluating trauma, 67, 68t
   technology in diagnosing obstetric emergencies, 172, 174
Rape. See Sexual assault
Rape crisis centers, 339
Rape kits, 329, 341
Rape trauma syndrome, 351
Rectal examination, in prepubertal child, 322
Rectosigmoid colon perforations, 360
Rectovaginal fistulas, 298, 361
Recurrent herpes zoster. See Varicella, primary
Regional enteritis, 238
Renal calculi, diagnosis of, 278–279
Renal function, changes in, during pregnancy, 26
Renal pathology, imaging in diagnosis of, 398, 400, 401–403f
Reproductive system, anatomic and physiologic changes associated with pregnancy in, 60–61
Respiratory system
   anatomic and physiologic changes associated with pregnancy in, 59
   anatomic and physiologic considerations in mother and fetus in, 79

Respiratory tract, effect of pregnancy on, 26
Retained products of conception from an incomplete abortion, 380, 380f, 381f
Retrograde pyelography, in diagnosing pelvic masses, 269
Retroperitoneal hematoma, 360
Rh sensitization, 129
   of mother, 63
   occurrence of, after abortion, 131
Ritgen maneuver, 140, 141f

Sacral colpopexy, 287–288
Salpingitis
   Chlamydia trachomatis as agent in acute, 43
   differentiating between ectopic pregnancy and, 46–47
   imaging in diagnosis of, 395, 396f
Saponification, 290
Sarcomatous degeneration, in uterine myomas, 264
Scabicide, during pregnancy, 193
Schultze mechanism, 144
Sclerocystic ovaries, 265
Seborrheic dermatitis, 234–235
Secondary syphilis, 238
Sedation, in children, 324–325t
Seizure disorders, 16–17
   effect of anticonvulsant medications on fetus, 17–18
   effect of pregnancy on epilepsy, 17
   management of patient with acute seizure, 18–20
Separation anxiety, 336
Sepsis
   maternal death due to, 130
   in pregnancy, 35
Septic arthritis, 216–217
Septic pelvic thrombophlebitis, 293–294
Septic shock, 294–295
   diagnosis of, 111–112
   management of, 113–115, 114t
   outcome and sequelae in, 113
   pathophysiology in, 112–113
Sexual abuse
   as cause of abnormal vaginal bleeding, 258
   chronic or recurrent, 346–347f
   signs of, 327

Sexual assault
  equipment needs for, 205–206
  examinations for, 340
Sexual assault victim, 339–340
  forensic medicine, 341
  multidisciplinary approach in, 339
  obtaining medical history, 342
  physical examination
    of adult, 342–346, 343f, 344f, 345f
    of child, 346–349, 347f
  prevention of pregnancy, 350–351
  prevention of venereal disease, 349–350t
  psychological support and counseling, 351
  treatment of, 349
  triage, 340–341
Sexually related trauma, 355–360, 356f, 357f, 358f, 359f
Sexually transmitted diseases
  acquired immune deficiency syndrome (AIDS), 218–222f, 220f
  chancroid, 230
  gonorrhea, 216–218
  herpes simplex virus infections, 228–230
  increase in incidence of, 43
  pelvic inflammatory disease, 211–216
    clinical presentation of, 211–212
    costs associated with, 211
    diagnosis of, 212–213f, 214f
    sites of disseminated, 217f
    treatment of, 214–215t
  screening for, 335–336
  syphilis, 223f, 223–227, 224f
Shingles. See Varicella, primary
Shock, during pregnancy, 35
Shoulder dystocia, 150
  documentation of, 152
  management of, 151f, 151–152
Shoulders, delivery of, in spontaneous vaginal delivery, 141, 143–144f
Sigmoidoscopy, in examination for sexual abuse, 345
Small bowel obstruction, 307
  postoperative, 296
Smead-Jones technique, 284
Sodium bicarbonate, during cardiopulmonary resuscitation, 82t
Somatization, 351
Sonography
  of ovarian torsion, 398
  of salpingitis, 395

Speculum examination, in diagnosing vaginal bleeding, 306
Spleen, rupture of, 178
Stab wound, to abdomen, 72
Staphylococcus aureus
  contamination of wound, 288–289f
  in postpartum infection, 156, 158, 159
  in septic shock, 115, 294
  in thrombophlebitis, 164
Staphyloccus epidermidis, in prepubertal child, 316
Status asthmaticus
  in asthma, 10
  avoidance of, 191
Status epilepticus, management of, during pregnancy, 192–193
Strawberry cervix, 244, 245f
Streptococci, as cause of postpartum infection, 156
Subchorionic hematoma, detection of, 132
Subchorionic hemorrhage, detection of, 373, 374f
Subcutaneous necrosis, 290
Subgluteal abscess formation, 157–158f
Suction curettage
  in diagnosis of ectopic pregnancy, 52–53
  equipment needed for, 204
Sulfonamides, during pregnancy, 189
Superficial thrombophlebitis, 300
Suprapubic pressure, in management of shoulder dystocia, 151
Surgical intervention, in treating pulmonary emboli, 6
Surgical needles, as inadvertent residual foreign body, 302
Surgical sponge, in diagnosing foreign bodies, 302
Suture sinuses, 286
Syphilis, 223–227, 223f, 224f
  secondary, 238
  therapy for, 226–227

TAC, topical, for local anesthesia, 328–329
Tachycardia
  presence of, in asthma patient, 8
  in thyroid storm, 10–11
Tampons, 360
Tampon test, 298

Tanner staging
  for breast development, 319f
  for pubic hair development, 320f
Teratogenesis, principles of, 185–186
Teratomas, cystic, 268
Terbutaline, during pregnancy, 191
Tetanus prophylaxis, 70
Tetracycline, during pregnancy, 189
Thalidomide tragedy, 186
Theca-lutein cyst, 265
Theophylline, during pregnancy, 191
Thermal burns, during pregnancy, 73
Thoracic injuries, management of, 72
Thoracotomy, in cardiopulmonary resuscitation, 81
Thorazine, in sedating children, 325
Thrombocytopenia, as warning sign for preeclampsia, 95–96
Thromboembolic complication, imaging modalities in diagnosing, 180–182, 181f
Thrombophlebitis
  septic pelvic, 293–294
  superficial, 163–164f, 300
Thrombosis, 163–166, 164f
  venous, 164, 300–301
    evaluation and management of, 165
Thyroid storm, 10
  common physical findings in, 12t
  diagnostic criteria of, 10–11
  differential diagnosis of, 11–12t
  events precipitating, 11t
  laboratory evaluation of, 12
  management of, 12–14, 13t
Ticarcillin-clavulanate, for anaerobic bacteria, 310
Tococardiography, in evaluating maternal trauma, 69
Toluidine blue staining, in examination for sexual assault, 344–345
Torsion of adnexa, 275
Torsion of ovary, 275
  causes of, 275, 276f
  clinical features of, 277–278
  differential diagnosis of, 278–279
  etiology of, 276–277t
  imaging in diagnosis of, 398, 399f
  special considerations in, 279–280
  treatment of, 279
Total parenteral nutrition (TPN), complications of, 311
Toxoplasmosis, diagnosis of, 221–222

Transvaginal sonography, in diagnosing pelvic masses, 269–270
Trauma
  anatomic and physiologic changes associated with pregnancy, 58, 61t
    cardiovascular system, 58–59
    gastrointestinal system, 59, 60f
    hematology, 61
    reproductive system, 60–61
    respiratory system, 59
    urinary system, 59–60
  blunt abdominal, 70–71
  burns during pregnancy
    electrical injury, 73–74
    perimortem cesarean section, 74
    thermal, 73
  as cause of maternal mortality, 57
  evaluation of mother and fetus, 66
  head injuries, 72–73
  imaging modalities in diagnosing, 178–179
  management of maternal and fetal, 69–70
  nonsexually related, 360–362f
  patterns of fetal and maternal injury, 62
    following blunt abdominal trauma, 62–64f, 65f
  penetrating abdominal, 71–72
  peritoneal lavage in evaluating, 68
  prehospital management, 65–66
  radiographic procedures in evaluating, 67, 68t
  routine laboratory studies in evaluating, 66–67
  sexually related, 355–360, 356f, 357f, 358f, 359f
  thoracic injuries, 72
  tococardiography in evaluating maternal, 69
  ultrasonography in evaluating, 68
Treponema pallidum, 223–227
Triage, for sexual assault, 340–341
Trichomonas vaginalis, 244
  as indication of sexual abuse, 349
  during pregnancy, 190
  treatment of, 190
Trichomoniasis, 244–245
Trimethadione, during pregnancy, 192
Trimethobenzamide, during pregnancy, 194

Trimethoprim, during pregnancy, 189–190
Triploidy, 133
Tubal sterilization, pregnancies following, 43
Tuberculosis, in AIDS patients, 220
Tubo-ovarian abscess
 imaging in diagnosis of, 395, 396f, 397f
 rupture of, 214
Tumor markers, 266, 269
Tumors. *See* Cancer

Ulcerative disease of vulva, 238–242
Ultrasound
 in evaluating
  abdominal pain, 37
  abortion, 131–132
  deep venous thrombosis, 165
  ectopic pregnancy, 49
  endometritis, 395
  failed pregnancy, 373, 375, 376f, 377f, 378f, 378–380, 379f, 380f, 381f, 382f
  maternal trauma, 68
  obstetric emergencies, 171
  pelvic inflammatory disease, 391, 395
  pelvic masses, 269–270
  pregnant patient, 367
  pyelonephritis, 400, 404f
  threatened abortion, 128–129
  thrombophlebitis, 164
  tubo-ovarian abscess, 395
 to rule out placenta previa, 134–135
 transabdominal scanning, 365, 366f
 transvaginal scanning, 365, 367, 368f
Umbilical cord, clamping of, 144
Unilateral adnexectomy, 279
Ureaplasma urealyticum, as cause of postpartum infection, 156
Ureteral obstruction, 309
Ureterovaginal fistulas, 298, 361
Urethral avulsions, 361
Urethral prolapse, 330f, 330–331
Urinary calculi, treatment of, 33
Urinary conduit complication, 310
Urinary retention, 300
Urinary system
 anatomic and physiologic changes associated with pregnancy in, 59–60
 disorders of, 32–33
 infections in
  postpartum emergency, 161
  ureteral obstruction, 309
Urologic emergencies
 fistulas, 309
 hemorrhagic cystitis, 309–310
 ureteral obstruction, 309
 urinary conduit complications, 310
Urosepsis, 294, 309
Uterine bleeding, association of abnormal, with pelvic mass, 267–268
Uterine endometrial sampling, 259
Uterine malignancy, 264–265
Uterine mass, benign, 263–264
Uterine myonecrosis, 292
Uterine rupture, 63
Uterus
 avulsion of, 360
 developmental abnormalities of, 265
 inversion of, 145
 myomas of, 256, 268, 269

Vaginal atrophy, 357
Vaginal bleeding, 306–307
 abnormal, 258
 after 20 weeks in pregnancy, 134–137
 in AIDS female, 221
 in bowel emergencies, 307
 in children, 325–331, 326t, 328f, 329f, 330f, 332f, 333f
 in ectopic pregnancy, 44
 in first 20 weeks of pregnancy, 127–133. *See also* Abortion
 laboratory test for, 132
 during late pregnancy, 175–177f, 176f
  imaging modalities in diagnosing, 175f, 175–177f
 in pregnancy, 253–255, 254f
 ultrasound diagnosis of, 136–137
 urologic causes of, in children, 330f, 330–331
Vaginal cuff cellulitis, 310
Vaginal delivery spontaneous
 clamping of cord, 144
 delivery of head, 140f
  clearing nasopharynx, 141, 142f
  nuchal cord, 141, 143f
  Ritgen maneuver, 140, 141f
 delivery of shoulders, 141, 143–144f

Vaginal disease
  bacterial vaginosis, 242–243
  candidiasis, 243–244
  foreign bodies in, 246–247
  mobiluncus vaginitis, 245–246
  trichomoniasis, 244–245
Vaginal eversion, 287–288
Vaginal evisceration, 286
Vaginal foreign bodies, 246–247
Vaginal hysterectomy, complications following, 286
Vaginal infections, 133
Vaginal lacerations, management of, 357
Vaginal penetration, physical findings suggestive of, 344–345
Vaginal prolapse, 287–288
Vaginal sponges, in diagnosing foreign bodies, 302
Vaginal vault, spontaneous rupture of, 357
Vaginal voiding, 330
Vaginitis, 325–327, 326t
  mobiluncus, 245–246
Vaginosis, bacterial, 242–243, 247
Valproate, for seizures, 18
Vancomycin, during pregnancy, 190
Varicella, primary
  diagnosis of, 116
  management of, 117–118
  outcome and sequelae in, 117
  pathophysiology in, 116–117
Varicella zoster, 228
Vascular injury, 300
Vasculitis, 239
Venereal disease, prevention of, 349–350t
Venography in diagnosis of
  deep venous thrombosis, 165
  thrombophlebitis, 164
Venous thrombosis, 300–301
Ventilation scan, 180
Versed, in sedating children, 325
Vesicovaginal fistulas, 298, 361
Vicryl, 329
Vinblastine, complications from, 311
Viral hepatitis, 226
Virchow's triad of stasis, 300
von Willebrand's disease, 255, 334, 335
Vulvar dermatoses
  lichen planus, 236–237
  lichen sclerosus, 237–238
  lichen simplex chronicus, 236
  pityriasis rosea, 236
  psoriasis, 235–236
  seborrheic dermatitis, 234–235
  secondary syphilis, 238
  ulcerative disease of vulva, 238–242
    diagnostic identification of, 242t
Vulvar disease, 233
  Bartholin gland cysts and abscesses, 233–234, 235f
  vulvar dermatoses
    lichen planus, 236–237
    lichen sclerosus, 237–238
    lichen simplex chronicus, 236
    pityriasis rosea, 236
    psoriasis, 235–236
    seborrheic dermatitis, 234–235
    secondary syphilis, 238
    ulcerative disease of vulva, 238–242
      diagnostic identification of, 242t
Vulvar hematomas, 361–362f
Vulvar injuries, 361
Vulvar ulcerative disease, diagnostic identification of, 242t
Vulvovaginitis, obtaining cultures in, 326–327

Warfarin, during pregnancy, 190–191
Warm shock, 111, 214–215
Water skiing injury, 360
Wilms' tumor, 330
Woods corkscrew maneuver, in management of shoulder dystocia, 151
Woods light, 342–343, 344
Wound complications
  dehiscence in, 283–285, 284f
  eversion in, 287–288
  evisceration in, 286
  incisional hernia in, 286–287
  suture sinuses in, 286
Wound infections, 291–292f
  superficial, 288–289f

Yolk sac
  imaging of, 369, 371, 372f
    in diagnosing abnormal pregnancy, 375, 377f, 378, 378f

Zavanelli maneuver, in management of shoulder dystocia, 151–152